Treatment of
partially edentulous patients

Treatment of partially edentulous patients

LOUIS J. BOUCHER, Ph.D., D.D.S., F.A.C.P., F.A.D.P.

Associate Dean, Professor and Director of Prosthodontics,
School of Dental Medicine, State University of New York
at Stony Brook, Stony Brook, New York; on attending staff of Long Island
Jewish-Hillside Medical Center, New York, and
University Hospital, Health Sciences Center, State University of New York
at Stony Brook, Stony Brook, New York; Consultant to the Veterans
Administration, United States Air Force, United States Army,
Surgeon General of the United States Air Force, HEW Public Health
Service Bureau of Health Resources Development; Consultant to the
Commission on Accreditation and Chairman of the Prosthodontic
Advisory Committee to the Commission on Accreditation of the
American Dental Association; Associate Editor and Section Editor of
the Journal of Prosthetic Dentistry; Diplomate of the American Board
of Prosthodontics; formerly Director of Maxillofacial Prosthetics,
Director of the Graduate Program in Dentistry, and Director of Postgraduate
Education, Marquette University School of Dentistry, Milwaukee, Wisconsin;
Director of Graduate Studies and Research, University of Kentucky College of
Dentistry, Lexington, Kentucky; Associate Dean, Medical College of Georgia School of
Dentistry, Augusta, Georgia; Dean and Director of Graduate Prosthodontics,
Fairleigh Dickinson University School of Dentistry, Hackensack, New Jersey;
Associate Dean and Acting Chairman of Prosthodontics, College of
Medicine and Dentistry of New Jersey, New Jersey Dental School, Newark, New Jersey

ROBERT P. RENNER, D.D.S.

Associate Professor of Prosthodontics and Director of Removable Prosthodontics,
Department of Restorative Dentistry, School of Dental Medicine,
State University of New York at Stony Brook, Stony Brook, New York;
Consultant to the Veterans Administration and University Hospital,
Stony Brook, New York; formerly Adjunct Assistant Professor of Dentistry,
Division of Prosthodontics, School of Dental and Oral Surgery,
Columbia University, New York, New York, and Staff Prosthodontist,
Northport Veterans Hospital, Northport, New York

With **651** *illustrations*

The C. V. Mosby Company

ST. LOUIS · TORONTO · LONDON   1982

A TRADITION OF PUBLISHING EXCELLENCE

Editor: Darlene Warfel
Assistant editor: Margaret Heppermann
Manuscript editor: Alan Sorkowitz
Book design: Susan Trail
Production: Carolyn Biby, Kathleen Teal

The C.V. Mosby Company
11830 Westline Industrial Drive, St. Louis, Missouri 63141

Library of Congress Cataloging in Publication Data

Main entry under title:

Treatment of partially edentulous patients.

    Bibliography: p.
    Includes index.
    1. Partial dentures, Removable. I. Boucher,
Louis J., 1922-   . II. Renner, Robert P.,
1943-   . [DNLM: 1. Denture, Partial, Removable.
2. Jaw, Edentulous, Partially—Therapy. WU 515
T784]
RK665.T73   617.6'92   81-19016
ISBN 0-8016-0821-X   AACR2

C/CB/B 9 8 7 6 5 4 3 2 1   02/C/265

Contributors

DEWEY H. BELL, Jr., D.D.S., F.A.C.D.

Professor and Chairman, Department of Removable Prosthodontics, Virginia Commonwealth University, Medical College of Virginia School of Dentistry, Richmond, Virginia; Consultant to Walter Reed Army Medical Center; Chairman of the Board of Directors, Education and Research Foundation of Prosthodontics; formerly Consultant in Prosthodontics to the United States Army, Veterans Administration, United States Navy, National Institutes of Health, and Commission on Accreditation of the American Dental Association

LOUIS J. BOUCHER, Ph.D., D.D.S., F.A.C.P., F.A.D.P.

Associate Dean, Professor and Director of Prosthodontics, School of Dental Medicine, State University of New York at Stony Brook, Stony Brook, New York; on attending staff of Long Island Jewish-Hillside Medical Center, New York, and University Hospital, Health Sciences Center, State University of New York at Stony Brook, Stony Brook, New York; Consultant to the Veterans Administration, United States Air Force, United States Army, Surgeon General of the United States Air Force, HEW Public Health Service Bureau of Health Resources Development; Consultant to the Commission on Accreditation and Chairman of the Prosthodontic Advisory Committee to the Commission on Accreditation of the American Dental Association; Associate Editor and Section Editor of the Journal of Prosthetic Dentistry; Diplomate of the American Board of Prosthodontics; formerly Director of Maxillofacial Prosthetics, Director of the Graduate Program in Dentistry, and Director of Postgraduate Education, Marquette University School of Dentistry, Milwaukee, Wisconsin; Director of Graduate Studies and Research, University of Kentucky College of Dentistry, Lexington, Kentucky; Associate Dean, Medical College of Georgia School of Dentistry, Augusta, Georgia; Dean and Director of Graduate Prosthodontics, Fairleigh Dickinson University School of Dentistry, Hackensack, New Jersey; Associate Dean and Acting Chairman of Prosthodontics, College of Medicine and Dentistry of New Jersey, New Jersey Dental School, Newark, New Jersey

ROBERT J. CHAPMAN, D.M.D.

Associate Clinical Professor and Head, Section of Removable Partial Dentures, Tufts University School of Dental Medicine, Boston, Massachusetts

EARL E. FELDMANN, D.D.S., F.A.C.D., F.I.C.D., F.A.C.P.

Professor and Chairman, Department of Prosthodontics, Dental School, The University of Texas Health Science Center at San Antonio, San Antonio, Texas

ARTHUR MICHAEL LaVERE, D.D.S., F.A.C.D., F.I.C.D., F.A.C.P.

Professor and Chairman, Department of Removable Prosthodontics, University of the Pacific School of Dentistry, San Francisco, California; Consultant to the Veterans Administration; Diplomate of the American Board of Prosthodontics

JOHN J. LUCCA, D.D.S., F.A.C.D., F.I.C.D., F.A.C.P.

Professor and Director, Division of Prosthodontics, Columbia University School of Dental and Oral Surgery, New York, New York; on attending staff of Presbyterian Hospital; Consultant to Westchester County Medical Center, Veterans Administration, and United States Public Health Service; Diplomate of the American Board of Prosthodontics

GLEN P. McGIVNEY, D.D.S., F.A.D.P.

Professor and Chairman, Removable Prosthodontics, Marquette University School of Dentistry; Attending Dentist, Milwaukee County General Hospital, Milwaukee, Wisconsin; Consultant to the Veterans Administration and the Council on Dental Education and member of the Advisory Committee Commission on Dental Accreditation of the American Dental Association; Diplomate of the American Board of Prosthodontics; formerly Assistant Professor and Acting Chairman, Removable Prosthodontics, Northwestern University Dental School

A.T. MORSTAD, D.D.S., M.S., F.I.C.D.

Professor and Chairman, Department of Removable Prosthodontics, University of Minnesota School of Dentistry; on attending staff of University Hospital, University of Minnesota, Hennepin County Medical Center, Minneapolis, Minnesota; Consultant to the Veterans Administration; formerly at School of Dentistry, University of Iowa, Iowa City, Iowa

ROBERT P. RENNER, D.D.S.

Associate Professor of Prosthodontics and Director of Removable Prosthodontics, Department of Restorative Dentistry, School of Dental Medicine, State University of New York at Stony Brook, Stony Brook, New York; Consultant to the Veterans Administration and University Hospital, Stony Brook, New York; formerly Adjunct Assistant Professor of Dentistry, Division of Prosthodontics, School of Dental and Oral Surgery, Columbia University, New York, New York, and Staff Prosthodontist, Northport Veterans Hospital, Northport, New York

HENRY C. RIVETTI, D.D.S., F.A.C.D.

Professor and Chairman, Department of Prosthodontics, Fairleigh Dickinson University School of Dentistry, Hackensack, New Jersey; Visiting Professor, College of Medicine and Dentistry of New Jersey, Newark, New Jersey; Consultant in Prosthodontics to the Veterans Administration

NICHOLAS ANTHONY VERO, D.D.S.

Assistant Clinical Professor and Director of Removable Prosthodontics Preclinical Program, Division of Prosthodontics, School of Dental and Oral Surgery, Columbia University, New York, New York

KENNETH E. WICAL, D.D.S., M.S.D.

Professor and Chairman, Department of Removable Prosthodontics, School of Dentistry, Loma Linda University, Loma Linda, California; Consultant to the Veterans Administration; formerly Director of Monument Valley Extension Clinical Program, Monument Valley, Utah

A.A. YURKSTAS, D.M.D., F.A.D.P., F.I.C.D., F.A.C.D.

Professor and Chairman, Department of Complete Dentures, Tufts University School of Dental Medicine, Boston, Massachusetts; Consultant to the Veterans Administration

Preface

The examination, diagnosis, treatment planning, and clinical procedures related to patients requiring treatment with removable partial dentures constitute the most important aspects of this text. In contrast to other textbooks of removable partial denture prosthodontics currently in print, which are concerned primarily with dental laboratory procedures, this textbook deals primarily with patient-related procedures. It will serve as a source of current authoritative information and explain basic prosthodontic concepts and principles for the clinical management of the patient who requires treatment with a removable partial denture.

A concerted effort has been made to keep this text as short and concise yet as comprehensive as possible. An extensive bibliography is included for those students and dental practitioners who desire additional information or original sources.

Dental laboratory procedures, although important to the success of any removable partial denture, are deemphasized, since several excellent, profusely illustrated dental laboratory manuals and texts on this subject are currently available to the dental student and practitioner. Similarly, space in this text is not devoted to cleft palate and maxillofacial prostheses, intracoronally retained (precision) removable partial dentures, correction of interceptive occlusal contacts, or the overdenture concept.

Although dental plaque control and periodontal health are two of the most important factors in the long-term success of a removable partial denture, neither dental plaque control techniques nor periodontal therapy is emphasized in this text. There are several reasons for this. First, it is assumed that a removable partial denture will be used only in a patient for whom optimal dental plaque control can be practiced. Second, numerous sources are available in the current dental literature that deal with periodontal therapy and dental plaque control. The ultimate objective of successfully treating a patient with a removable partial denture is to prevent the further destruction of the remaining oral structures and tissues. This text provides the dental student and practitioner with the necessary clinical information to obtain this objective.

Appreciation is extended to all those people who helped make this book possible. We extend our thanks to our outstanding and dedicated contributors and colleagues; to Eugene McDermott, Senior Medical Photographer, who provided the excellent quality of prints; to John B. Jones, Jr., Graphic Illustrator; to Kris Vandenberg, Cathy Retzger, Rosanne Randazzo, and Vivian Cavaluzzi, our secretaries, who typed and retyped the manuscript; and to our patients, dental assistants, and dental laboratory technicians. To our wives, Mel and Fran, who provided patience and understanding, our very special thanks.

Louis J. Boucher
Robert P. Renner

Contents

4 Examination, diagnosis, and treatment planning, 89

5 Mouth preparations for removable partial dentures, 128

6 Impressions: trial fitting of the framework, 161

Treatment of
partially edentulous patients

1 Introduction

REASONS FOR LOSS OF NATURAL DENTITION

Perhaps the most fundamental question to raise in a textbook about removable partial dentures (RPDs) is "What is the need for this type of restorative service?" Regrettably, the answer that dentists and dental educators come to is that the need is great. Surveys conducted in the United States with regard to oral health status of adult patients indicate that: (1) of the total civilian population in the United States in 1975, an estimated 21% wear some type of prosthodontic restoration; (2) as age increases, RPDs and complete dentures are still very prevalent, with some 50% of the population over 60 years of age being treated with an RPD or complete denture; (3) the number of denture wearers per family is affected by both the family income and the level of education of the head of the family unit. As income or level of education rises, the percentage of denture wearers in that family unit decreases; and (4) there is a slightly higher percent of women who wear an RPD or complete denture than men in the general population (ADA, 1976).

The reasons for tooth loss among large segments of the population are many and varied but can be classified conveniently into two broad categories: (1) the public's attitude toward oral health and (2) the availability of treatment and reasonableness of dental costs for the preservation of the patient's natural teeth. Even in the younger adult age groups, who have benefited from fluoridation, increased dental health advertising, and wide availability of dental care facilities, still only 30% to 40% seek treatment only when they are troubled by their dentition. It is not surprising, therefore, for the dentist to find that this type of patient prefers to have a painful posterior tooth extracted rather than restored.

In the United States, the availability of dental treatment designed to preserve the dentition is related to ready access to dental treatment, dentist-patient ratios, government assistance in the delivery system, and the provision of funds for the practice of preventive dentistry. Coupled with these factors is the inability of the patient to afford the cost of treatment rendered by the dentist.

There is a great need to change the attitude of the public toward dental health care. Much of the responsibility lies with parents, who influence a child with regard to the regularity of dental care and attitudes toward dentistry. Unfortunately a poor dental attitude and irregular dental care will be perpetuated for years to come by parents who have a low dental IQ and are partially or completely edentulous. Regretfully, we can predict with a great degree of certainty that providing patients with RPDs will be a common restorative service well into the forseeable future.

PATTERN OF TOOTH LOSS

The loss of a patient's natural dentition usually follows a characteristic, predictable pattern. Generally, the maxillary teeth are lost before the mandibular teeth. According to Brewer (1980), an all too typical restorative sequence for an "average" patient is: (1) loss of the maxillary posterior teeth and their replacement with a maxillary RPD; (2) loss of the remaining maxillary anterior teeth and some mandibular posterior teeth and restoration with a complete denture; (3) loss of the remaining mandibular posterior teeth and their replacement with a mandibular RPD; and finally (4) loss of the mandibular anterior teeth and treatment of the patient with complete dentures.

PARTIAL VERSUS COMPLETE EDENTULISM

There is a higher percentage of people today who are completely edentulous compared with those who are partially edentulous (ADA, 1976). This phenomenon is a paradox because of improved restorative materials, techniques, and instrumentation (improved amalgam and composite materials, pin-retained amalgams, overdentures, better methods of plaque control, fluoridation, etc.). All of these factors can help patients maintain their teeth and avoid the sequela of complete edentulism. Therefore, it behooves the dentist to treat patients with the type of fixed or removable partial dentures that will best preserve their remaining teeth for the longest period of time.

THE PARTIALLY EDENTULOUS STATE

The loss of teeth most often results from the patient's failure to maintain adequate oral hygiene and plaque-control measures. This is often coupled with the loss of an adequate periodontium, which is necessary to retain the teeth. This situation may be exacerbated by destructive parafunctional habits.

Normal occlusal function is usually intermittent and fleeting and is mainly directed in a vertical direction through the long axes of the teeth. Parafunction (bruxism, clenching, and grinding), however, is frequently horizontal in direction and may be excessively prolonged. It occurs diurnally and nocturnally. In parafunc-

tion there is an abnormal increase in the magnitude, frequency, and duration of the occlusal force. The bruxing movement is often concentrated close to the tips of the occluding teeth. This creates a concentration of forces that tends to abnormally displace the tooth in its alveolus. This force is of a greater magnitude than a force that is normally directed through the long axis of the tooth. Such forces may be beyond the adaptive responses of the tooth, especially if it is an abutment tooth for an RPD.

When part of the natural dentition is lost, the integrity of the masticatory system is altered (Fig. 1-1). Also altered is the individual's ability to respond and adapt to a reduced dentition and a depleted periodontal support for that dentition. More important, this partially edentulous state must have a sufficient adaptive capacity to withstand occlusal forces without causing further breakdown in the system. This reserve capacity is especially important when the dentist intervenes with a prosthodontic restoration of the masticatory system. The long-term success of the dentist's restorative efforts can be predicted on the basis of the total residual area of support for the prosthesis. This support is derived from the periodontal ligament, which must adequately support the load transmitted from the now-restored dentition to

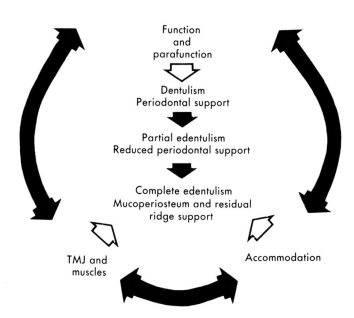

Fig. 1-1. Integrity of masticatory system is altered when part or all of natural dentition is lost.

the remaining dentition and portions of the residual ridge and hard palate. It is unclear at what point a partially edentulous dentition, prosthodontically restored with a fixed or removable partial denture, fails to adapt to the dictates of the required support (periodontal ligament, residual ridge, and hard palate).

SEQUELAE OF PARTIAL EDENTULISM

Partial or complete loss of the natural dentition is, in all practicality, the result of disease of the calcified tooth surfaces (dental caries) or disease of the supporting tissues (periodontal disease). Both disease processes are usually chronic and attack individuals during different times of their lives. Attack by dental caries usually occurs early in a person's life, whereas periodontal disease ensues in middle or later life. Both disease processes and their effects on the individual's face become increasingly noticeable as he or she looses natural teeth and progresses from the partially to the completely edentulous state.

When individuals lose some of their teeth, the remaining teeth and the periodontium, muscles, ligaments and temporomandibular joints may also be affected. This in turn may create functional problems. The consequences of partial loss of the natural dentition are numerous and varied. Most clinicians are in general agreement as to the consequences of loss of the natural dentition. These are: (1) esthetic alterations; (2) decrease in masticatory efficiency; (3) tipping, migration, and rotation of the remaining dentition; (4) extrusion of teeth; (5) loss of support for the teeth; (6) deviation of the mandible; (7) tooth depression and attrition; (8) loss of occlusal vertical dimension and shortening of the morphologic face height; (9) temporomandibular joint dysfunction; and (10) loss of alveolar bone and reduction of the residual ridges (Zarb, 1979).

Although the loss of the natural dentition may bring patient complaints about loss of masticatory function or speech problems, these are almost always secondary to esthetic alterations (poor cosmetics).

The loss of natural teeth may alter the patient's occlusion in several ways. It may affect the remaining teeth by causing their tipping, migration, rotation, extrusion, depression, or attrition. Tooth loss may also cause a deviation of the mandible. Some of the above factors, especially tipping and migration of teeth, may result in reduced periodontal support for those teeth. This can result in loss of alveolar bone. Some of the sequelae could create a loss of vertical dimension of occlusion, a collapsed morphologic face height and temporomandibular joint problems. Most can cause a loss of masticating efficiency. These conditions adversely affect the individual's comfort, health, and well-being.

THE REMOVABLE PARTIAL DENTURE

An RPD (Fig. 1-2), as its name implies, is a prosthodontic restoration that supplies teeth and associated structures to a partially edentulous arch and that can be removed and inserted by the patient. In general, an RPD is made from a combination of several common dental materials. The basic substructure or framework of an RPD is fabricated from one of several commercially available dental alloys, such as gold, aluminum, or the more popular chromium-cobalt alloys. To this underlying RPD framework are attached the supplied replacement teeth, usually fabricated from dental porcelain, acrylic resin, or combinations of acrylic resin and a dental gold alloy. The replacement denture teeth are retained either chemically or mechanically to the RPD framework by means of acrylic resin or dental cement.

In general, there are two broad types of RPDs, their classification being based on their type of fixation to the natural dentition. An RPD can be retained (or fixed) to the remaining dentition either by extracoronal or intracoronal means. In clinical practice, most RPDs constructed today are retained by extracoronal means. That is to say, retention is achieved by the RPD's retaining units.' engaging certain portions of the natural teeth on their external contours. Intracoronal retention (Fig. 1-3) of an RPD is achieved by having at least one part of the retentive unit placed within the confines of a restored natural tooth. Inherent in the use of intracoronal retention is the need to use cast restorations on the natural teeth that are used to retain the RPD. RPDs can be further classified according to the type of support they derive from the remaining dentition and associated soft tissues (mucoperiosteum and residual

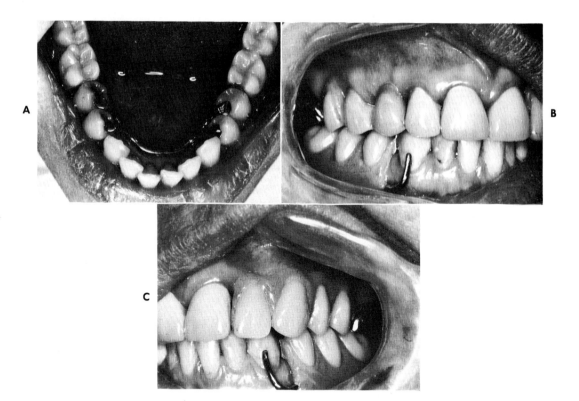

Fig. 1-2. **A,** An RPD is a restoration that supplies teeth and associated structures to a partially edentulous arch; it can be removed and inserted by patient at will (occlusal view, Kennedy Class I RPD). **B,** Right lateral view of maxillary RPD and mandibular Kennedy Class I RPD in centric occlusion. Fixed partial denture connects maxillary right first premolar to left central incisor. **C,** Left lateral view of maxillary RPD and mandibular Kennedy Class I RPD in centric occlusion. Maxillary RPD replaces maxillary left lateral incisor through left second premolar and is retained in part by precision attachments in fixed partial denture.

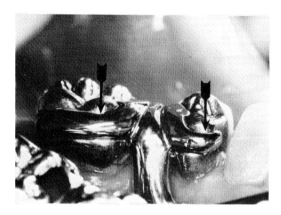

Fig. 1-3. Reciprocal arms *(arrows)* of this embrasure clasp are placed within confines of mandibular molar gold crown and first premolar porcelain-fused-to-metal crown (lingual view).

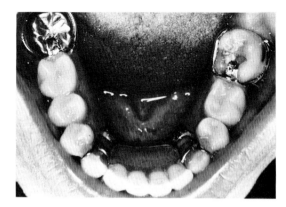

Fig. 1-4. Tooth-borne RPD (Kennedy Class III, modification I) retained by mandibular molars and canines bilaterally (occlusal view).

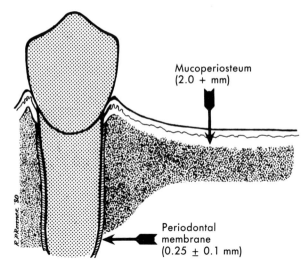

Fig. 1-5. Essential displacement differentials between periodontal ligament of natural tooth and mucoperiosteum covering residual ridge.

ridge). Many RPDs derive all of their support from the remaining natural teeth and are referred to as tooth-borne (supported) RPDs; others derive their support from both the teeth and associated residual ridge tissues and are termed tooth-tissue–borne (supported) RPDs (or distal-extension RPD). Between these two extremes of support are a range of RPDs that derive a varying amount of support from both the natural dentition and associated residual tissues.

DISSIMILARITIES IN TOOTH-BORNE AND TOOTH-TISSUE–BORNE REMOVABLE PARTIAL DENTURES

The essential dissimilarities of the tooth-borne RPD (Fig. 1-4) and the distal-extension base (tooth-tissue–borne) RPD (Fig. 1-2) must be recognized by the dentist. In the tooth-borne prosthesis, occlusal stresses (functional or parafunctional) are transmitted to the bone physiologically by way of the periodontal ligament. Because all of the edentulous spaces are bound by natural teeth, this type of prosthesis functions in a manner similar to a fixed partial denture. This relatively unyielding type of support allows the dentist to choose components of the RPD based on convenience and their ability to provide rigidity and stability to each remaining tooth.

In contrast, the distal-extension base RPD must depend on two completely different types of tissue for its support. The teeth represent a relatively immobile support, whereas the tissues of the edentulous ridge have variable degrees of displaceability (Fig. 1-5). The problem of designing an RPD that will protect both tissue types from eventual destruction constantly plagues the dentist. This problem is less severe in the maxillary arch, because, in general, the residual ridges are larger and broader than those in the mandibular arch. This provides for a greater area of potential denture base coverage and thus a greater degree of tissue support. In addition, the maxillary hard palate affords an additional area of support. By close adherence to sound basic prosthodontic principles and concepts, the dentist can generally provide a satisfactory RPD for the maxillary arch.

A mandibular RPD, however, presents problems that are quite different and unique. Any yielding of the mucosa that permits displacement of the denture base may result in tilting or torquing stresses' being transferred to the abutment teeth. In their normal position and natural environment, teeth and their periodontium are designed to resist vertical stress but they respond poorly to lateral and torquing types of occlusal stress. The residual ridge in the edentulous area changes in form by varying degrees as it responds to many stimuli. Pressure or compressive stresses transmitted through the RPD are some of the external stimuli. When the remaining soft tissues, teeth, and the residual ridge are stressed beyond their physiologic tolerance, the resulting changes can include mucosal irritation, tooth mobility and increased bone resorption (residual ridge reduction).

Many methods have been proposed for preserving the supporting tissues, the abutment teeth, and the residual ridge while permitting them to function satisfactorily for an extended period of time. Primarily, these approaches attempt to control the tipping and torquing stress to which the teeth and tissues are subjected.

THE FIXED PARTIAL DENTURE

The decision to treat the patient with a fixed (Fig. 1-6) or removable partial denture prosthesis is dependent in large measure on the quality of the abutment teeth. The preliminary selection of the abutment teeth is based on the following factors: location of the teeth in the dental arch; amount of bony support; condition of the mucoperiosteum; shape and length of the roots; condition and form of the crowns; position of the abutment teeth in relation to other teeth, as influenced by extrusion, migration, or tipping; and vitality of the teeth. Also involved in the dentist's decision are the patient's plaque-control ability, age, and periodontal and systemic health, as well as cost factors.

Inherent in the dentist's decision-making process when a patient is treated with a fixed partial denture is the intraoral environment in which the restoration is to be placed. Any fixed partial denture must be placed in a biologic environment that is clinically healthy. The fixed partial denture restoration that is placed must be correctly designed so that the restored function of the masticatory system does not exceed the adaptive capacity of the patient. It is also the dentist's responsibility to see to it that the patient can maintain the health and integrity of the supporting tissues around the fixed partial denture and the remaining dentition in the oral cavity. Although not stressed, this general philosophy is implied when a dentist treats a patient with any type of RPD or fixed partial–removable partial denture combination.

FIXED PARTIAL–REMOVABLE PARTIAL DENTURE COMBINATIONS
(see Fig. 1-2, *B* and *C*)

The dentist will encounter in many clinical situations the need to treat a patient with both a fixed and a removable partial denture restoration simultaneously. In a given partially edentulous arch with missing teeth in both anterior and posterior arch segments, it is often advisable to restore the anterior edentulous areas with a fixed partial denture and the posterior arch segments with an RPD. This is done for several reasons: (1) to prevent rotation of the RPD around a fulcrum associated with the

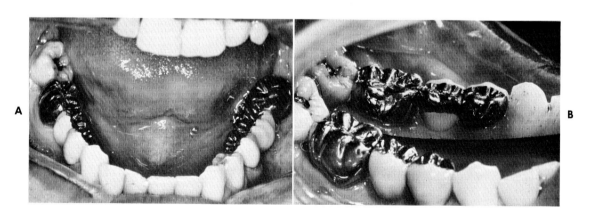

A   B

Fig. 1-6. A, Dentist's decision to treat patient with fixed partial denture or RPD is dependent in large measure on quality of abutment teeth and their supporting structures. In this instance, patient was treated with bilateral mandibular fixed partial dentures (occlusal view). **B,** Lingual view of mandibular right fixed partial denture described in **A.**

most distal abutment teeth; (2) to permit the development of better esthetics anteriorly; (3) to allow the patient to remove the distal-extension RPD for tissue rest without sacrificing esthetics; and (4) to allow any necessary alterations to the RPD to be made without the patient's being embarrassed socially.

There are other clinical situations that indicate the use of a fixed-removable partial denture combination or just a fixed partial denture. These include: (1) patients in whom it is necessary to prevent an isolated terminal abutment situation (such as a lone-standing second premolar with an adjacent anterior edentulous area and natural anterior teeth); (2) patients requiring anterior guidance to coordinate mandibular movements and the development of a satisfactory posterior occlusal scheme, since this guidance can best be produced by the use of an anterior fixed partial denture rather than an RPD; (3) patients in whom splinting is needed to provide adjacent teeth and cross-arch stability for the natural teeth and the RPD; (4) patients in whom RPD retainers, whether extracoronal or intracoronal, are placed into cast restorations for biomechanical or esthetic reasons; and (5) situations in which a patient has a unilateral edentulous area bounded by teeth that are adequate abutment teeth for a fixed partial denture.

OBJECTIVES OF A SOUND REMOVABLE PARTIAL DENTURE SERVICE

The ultimate success of any RPD depends on a mutual understanding and shared responsibility between the dentist, the dental laboratory technician, and the patient. The dentist's obligation begins with the diagnosis necessary to identify the anatomic, physiologic, and psychologic conditions that are unique and individual to that patient. This is accomplished through an organized, detailed, and thorough medical and dental examination. The dentist must establish goals and institute a treatment plan that will be prudent and realistic for each individual patient. The goals should:

1. Preserve the teeth and tissues that will *enhance* the RPD design and promote oral health
2. Improve masticatory function
3. Distribute the occlusal load equitably

4. Improve esthetics
5. Improve phonetics
6. Provide restorations that are comfortable to the patient
7. Improve the health and general well-being of the patient

A SYSTEMATIC APPROACH TO DIAGNOSIS

A reduction in the function of the masticatory system is generally attributed to tooth loss, periodontal disease, dental caries, tooth wear, malarticulation of the teeth, or trauma. With the exception of trauma, the dentist's obligation is to intercept these processes and prevent them from running their full course. Our purpose as dentists is to assist the patient to attain and maintain the best physiologic oral health possible. Too often, however, the concept of preventive dentistry is thought of solely in terms of preventing dental caries and eliminating adverse periodontal conditions. This, of course, must be of primary consideration in all treatment procedures. However, notwithstanding the importance of these services, the patient who requires a distal-extension base RPD presents a far more complex situation than can be treated with this generally accepted philosophy. The partially edentulous patient requires the widest application of preventive procedures (Fig 1-7), which includes procedures to combat:

1. Tooth loss
2. Periodontal disease
3. Dental caries
4. Residual ridge reduction
5. Dental arch collapse
6. Occlusal plane distortion
7. Loss of occlusal harmony
8. Temporomandibular joint dysfunction

Since a high percentage of patients who are partially edentulous require RPDs the most reasonable course of action is to plan dental treatment from the perspective of how the design of the prosthesis can best preserve and maintain the residual oral tissues or significantly enhance their longevity.

The dentist must organize his or her thoughts and methods before treating a patient with an RPD. To accomplish any procedure, the dentist must have a logical goal, must plan a systematic approach to achieving the most

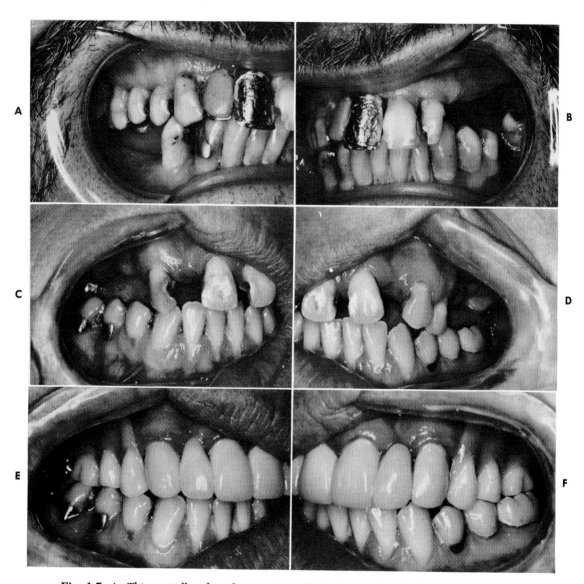

Fig. 1-7. A, This partially edentulous patient will challenge dentist's diagnostic and treatment planning ability and application of preventive procedures to utmost degree (right lateral view). **B,** Left lateral view of patient shown in **A. C,** This partially edentulous patient presents serious challenge to provide functional restoration that will preserve remaining intraoral tissues (right lateral view). Note rampant dental caries, severe periodontal destruction, and residual ridge reduction in maxillary edentulous areas. **D,** Left lateral view of patient shown in **C. E,** Restoration of this patient's dentition (**C** and **D**) to optimum level involved treating patient with combination maxillary fixed and removable partial denture after periodontal therapy, dental caries control, preventive procedures, home care instruction, and treatment of abused tissues of edentulous areas (right lateral view). **F,** Left lateral view of patient shown in **E.**

satisfactory RPD design for the dental conditions individual to that patient, and must develop, in sequence, the methods and means of achieving that design.

In developing a treatment plan and the approach to achieving it, the dentist must not lose sight of reality. To justify any treatment plan, two questions should be answered:

1. Is it necessary to replace lost teeth and associated tissues with an RPD?
2. Are these procedures and the potential prognosis realistic and prudent for this patient?

The degree of successful treatment depends on the physiologic, anatomic, and psychologic conditions of the patient and the attitude and ability of the dentist. Within these limits, the dentist's obligation is to attain and maintain the best physiologic health possible for the patient. Because of the potential for failure that can result from inadequate diagnosis and treatment planning, the first phase in treating a patient with an RPD is to establish *a systematic approach to diagnosis*. Three basic types of considerations—physiologic, anatomic, and psychologic—are necessary in accomplishing routine diagnostic procedures related to RPD service.

Physiologic considerations

The dentist's objective in regard to physiologic considerations is to thoroughly examine and evaluate the patient and to weigh the findings in relation to their potential for satisfying the requirements of a biologically acceptable RPD. Diagnostic factors of particular interest are:

1. The general and oral health of the patient
2. The patient's known diseases and disorders
3. Diseases and disorders of which the patient is unaware, detected during examination
4. The patient's basic physiologic functioning and coordination, as evaluated by the dentist

The accumulation of the necessary diagnostic factors is not satisfied only by a simple clinical or radiographic examination. Accurate diagnosis for patient treatment with RPDs should also include a:

1. Dental history
2. Medical history
3. Clinical examination (both visual and digital)
4. Roentgenographic examination
5. Mounted diagnostic cast examination, including analysis of horizontal and vertical jaw relationships (clinical vs. mounted diagnostic casts) and survey analysis (surveying of the diagnostic casts)

Anatomic considerations

The second and most important physical consideration is a thorough evaluation of the clinical entities that will influence the design of the RPD. This evaluation should assess:

1. The need to restore maxillomandibular relationships
2. The need to restore function
3. The availability of structures to oppose the vertical and lateral components of occlusal force
4. The condition of those oral structures capable of providing support and stability
5. The availability and location of retentive areas
6. The need for mouth preparation to accommodate the basic principles of design and for the correct placement of the component parts of the RPD

Psychologic considerations

Basically, there are three categories to be evaluated under psychologic considerations: patient attitude, patient education, and patient motivation.

It is the dentist's responsibility to inform the patient of the extent of his or her dental problems and to outline a treatment plan to correct them. In so doing, the dentist must make the patient aware of the limitations and longevity of the prosthesis and thoroughly inform the patient of his or her responsibility for the continuing care of the teeth and the RPD. This will ensure a successful prognosis and longevity of the treatment. The dentist must continually reinforce instruction in the importance of dental plaque removal, oral hygiene maintenance, and the necessity of prosthodontic recall. It is simply not enough for the patient to have a need for an RPD. The patient must also want the prosthesis and be willing to assume his or her share of the responsibility for its success.

REASONS FOR FAILURE OF A REMOVABLE PARTIAL DENTURE

When an RPD no longer continues to function as designed by the dentist or as anticipated by the patient, it is generally considered to be in one of varying stages of failure. Most often, these failures are the direct result of an omission or deficiency in its design or of the alteration of the supporting tissues during or after fabrication of the prosthesis. The causes of failure can be categorized under inadequate diagnosis and treatment planning, inadequate mouth preparation, or communication failures.

Inadequate diagnosis and treatment planning

Unfortunately, too many removable partial dentures are designed without the use of a dental surveyor (Fig. 1-8). Without question,

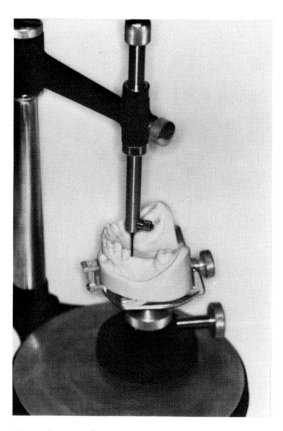

Fig. 1-8. Dental surveyor is an essential instrument for dentist to use to ensure adequate diagnosis and design analysis for an RPD.

the dental surveyor is an essential instrument that aids the dentist in making an accurate diagnosis. Surveying identifies those areas of the mouth that need to be modified to accommodate the design of a prosthesis that will promote and maintain oral health.

Inadequate treatment planning is most often identified as the cause of failure when the need for a specific mouth preparation was not recognized or not accomplished by the dentist or when components of the RPD were errantly selected or improperly applied to its design. An additional area reflecting inadequate diagnosis and treatment planning is the dentist's failure to identify irritated or distorted tissue in the edentulous areas.

Inadequate mouth preparation

The second category of failure results when the dentist does not provide for adequate tooth support by the proper positioning and contouring of the clasp (direct retainer) or for proper tissue support by tissue conditioning methods and corrected impressions. Also included in this category is the failure of the dentist to create occlusal harmony of the remaining natural dentition before mouth preparation for the RPD.

Communication failures

The third category of failure involves communication between the dentist and the patient and between the dentist and the dental laboratory technician. If the dentist fails to educate and motivate the patient regarding the limitations of the prosthesis and the patient's responsibility for plaque control and maintenance of the oral tissues and prosthesis, the potential for failure increases considerably. The dentist must also provide the dental laboratory technician with the necessary information on the dental laboratory prescription (work authorization) to fabricate the RPD framework. The dentist must provide the dental laboratory technician with dental stone casts that are accurate reproductions of the existing intraoral anatomy. Also, the dental laboratory technician must follow these instructions precisely to ensure compliance with the indicated design.

Singularly or in combination, these categories constitute the most common causes of failure in treating patients with RPDs.

THE FUTURE OF THE REMOVABLE PARTIAL DENTURE SERVICE

The dental profession has still not developed a universal cure for dental disease, either for dental caries or periodontal disease. The profession has come a long way in developing therapeutic methods, agents, and devices to reduce the prevalance of these disease states. But in spite of these advances in dental science there are and will still be a large number of partially edentulous patients well into the twenty-first century. The demand for RPD service will in all likelihood increase both as life expectancy increases and as a greater number of individuals become not completely but only partially edentulous. It will be dentistry's obligation to continue to educate and train sufficient numbers of competent clinical practitioners who will be able to successfully treat these large numbers of partially edentulous patients. The future clinician must be educated to make a rational choice when restoring a partially edentulous dentition. It is a choice between treating the patient and risking the production of iatrogenic disease or not treating the patient and perhaps risking far more damaging sequelae to the remaining dentition. The thrust of dental education still must be twofold: to educate dentists so that they can make rational clinical judgments on when and how to treat a partially edentulous patient and to educate patients to maintain their oral tissues in as good a state of health as practical so that they do not become completely edentulous.

2 Classification of partially edentulous arches and components of a removable partial denture

CLASSIFICATION OF PARTIALLY EDENTULOUS ARCHES

The fact that a definite need exists for an acceptable classification of partially edentulous arches is evidenced by the number of classifications that have been proposed in the dental literature over the years. A universally accepted classification would not only make it easier for dentists to communicate among themselves in describing the multitude of combinations that may exist in partially edentulous arches, but it would also help them visualize the teeth that are to be replaced with a removable partial denture (RPD). Some of the best known classifications that have been proposed are those of Cummer, Kennedy, Bailyn, Neurohr, Mauk, Godfrey, Beckett, Friedman, Skinner, Austin and Lidge, Applegate (a modification of Kennedy's), and Swenson. Unfortunately, none of these has been universally accepted by the dental profession.

Miller (1970), in a survey of American dental schools in 1967, found that the classification that was most often taught was that of Kennedy. Clinical experience has shown that the Kennedy classification is simple, logical, and workable. In view of its simplicity and its wide acceptance, the Kennedy classification is the one described and used in this textbook. Many dentists, however, place too much importance on the relationship between the classification of partially edentulous arches and the application of an RPD design. This is one reason that RPDs fail, because the classification does not indicate the amount and type of support for the RPD.

Kennedy classification

Kennedy (1928) divided all partially edentulous arches into four classes according to their frequency of occurrence, Class I being the most common type of partially edentulous arch and Class IV the least common.

Class I: A partially edentulous arch in which there are bilateral edentulous areas located posterior to the remaining natural teeth (Fig. 2-1)

Class II: A partially edentulous arch in which a unilateral edentulous area is located posterior to the remaining natural teeth (Fig. 2-2)

Class III: A partially edentulous arch in which there is a unilateral edentulous area with natural teeth remaining both anterior and posterior to it (Fig. 2-3)

Class IV: A partially edentulous arch in which a single edentulous area, located anterior to the remaining natural teeth, crosses the midline (Fig. 2-4)

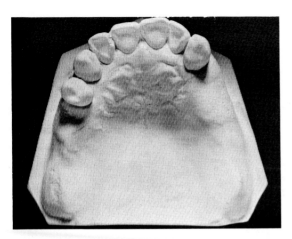

Fig. 2-1. Kennedy Class I partially edentulous arch.

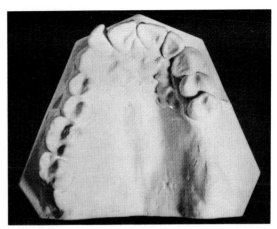

Fig. 2-2. Kennedy Class II partially edentulous arch.

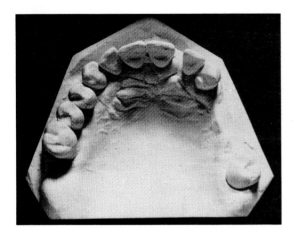

Fig. 2-3. Kennedy Class III partially edentulous arch. Maxillary right second molar is not to be replaced because opposing mandibular right second molar is missing and is not to be restored.

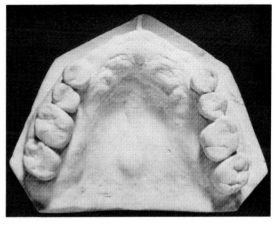

Fig. 2-4. Kennedy Class IV partially edentulous arch.

Applegate's rules governing the application of the Kennedy classification

Applegate (1954) found that some uncertainty often arose in the use of the Kennedy classification, and as a result he devised the following eight rules for the purpose of clarification.

Rule 1: Classification should follow mouth preparation, since further extractions would alter it.

Rule 2: If the third molar is missing, that edentulous area is not considered in making the classification, since third molars are not to be replaced.

Rule 3: Third molars, if present and to be used as abutments, are considered in the classification.

Rule 4: Missing second molars are sometimes not replaced. When the occluding second molar is also missing and is not to be restored, this edentulous area is not considered in the classification.

Rule 5: When there are additional edentulous areas in the same dental arch, the most posterior area (excepting third molars) governs the classification.

Rule 6: Edentulous areas in addition to those that determine the primary classification are indicated as modifications of that class and are designated by their number (Fig. 2-5).

Rule 7: The extent of the modification area has no bearing: it is the number of such areas that is the determining factor.

Rule 8: Only Classes I, II, and III can have modifications, since any additional edentulous areas must lie posterior to the "single, bilateral edentulous area" of the Class IV type and would determine the classification.

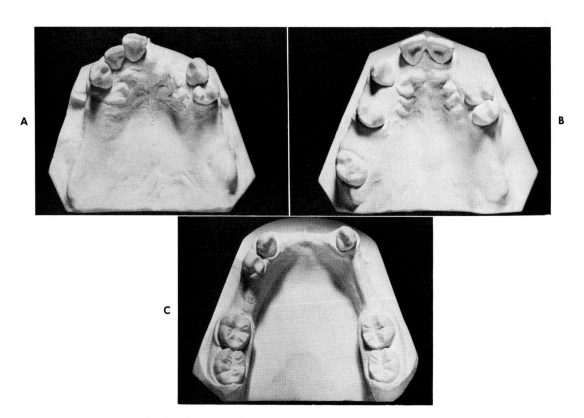

Fig. 2-5. Kennedy classification with examples of modification spaces. **A,** Class I, modification 1. **B,** Class II, modification 4. **C,** Class III, modification 2. There is no modification space for Class IV, because any additional edentulous areas must be posterior to "single, bilateral edentulous area" of Class IV and these would determine classification.

COMPONENTS OF A REMOVABLE PARTIAL DENTURE

The common types of clasp assemblies and components of an RPD are identified in this chapter. In Chapter 3, they are explained in detail.

The typical RPD (Fig. 2-6) usually consists of:

1. Major connector
2. Minor connectors
3. Rests
4. Direct retainers
5. Indirect retainer(s)
6. Denture base(s)

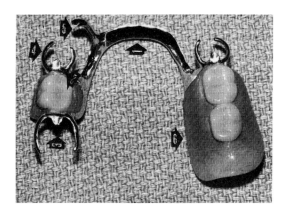

Fig. 2-6. Mandibular RPD with its components identified. *1*, Lingual bar major connector; *2*, minor connector; *3*, occlusal rest; *4*, direct retainer; *5*, indirect retainer; *6*, denture base.

Major connectors

A major connector is that part of the RPD which connects the components on one side of the arch to the components on the opposite side of the arch. It is that portion of the RPD to which all other components are attached.

Maxillary major connectors

Maxillary major connectors are classified into five basic types:

1. Single palatal strap or bar (Figs. 2-7 and 2-8)
2. U-shaped palatal connector (Fig. 2-9)
3. Anteroposterior palatal bar (Figs. 2-10 and 2-11)
4. Posterior palatal strap (Fig. 2-12)
5. Complete palatal plate (Figs. 2-13, 2-14, and 2-15)

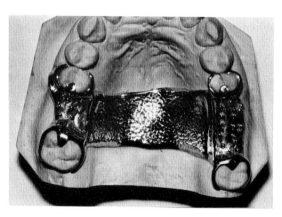

Fig. 2-7. Single palatal strap major connector. It should be made flat yet wide and thick enough so that it is rigid.

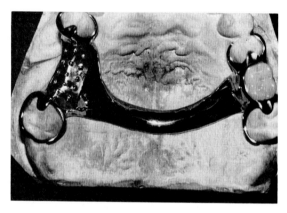

Fig. 2-8. Narrow single palatal bar major connector. This type of connector is usually contraindicated because added thickness and bulk required to make it rigid often proves annoying to patient.

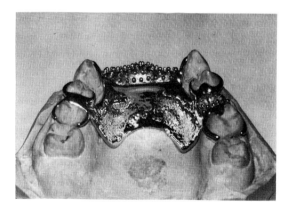

Fig. 2-9. U-shaped palatal major connector. Because of the many limitations of this type of connector, it should be used only when it is not possible to use another type of major connector.

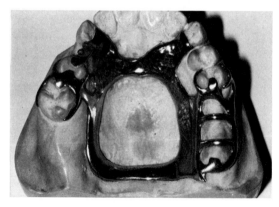

Fig. 2-10. Anteroposterior palatal bar. It is indicated where remaining natural teeth have good periodontal support and large amount of palatal support is not required.

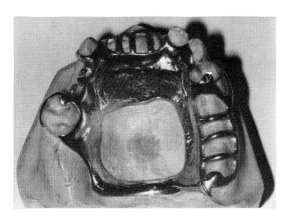

Fig. 2-11. Closed horseshoe palatal bar. This maxillary major connector is a modification of anteroposterior palatal bar and can be used where both anterior and posterior teeth are missing.

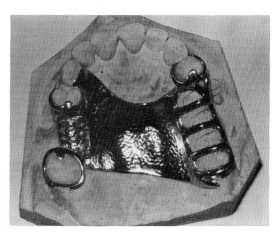

Fig. 2-12. Posterior palatal strap major connector. Because of its many advantages and its versatility of design, this major connector should be used extensively in RPD construction.

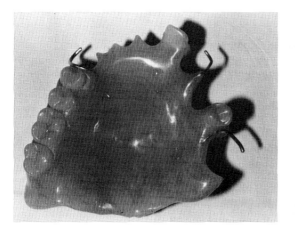

Fig. 2-13. Complete acrylic resin palate (Every denture). This connector is used when economic or other factors prevent use of cast framework or when patient is treated with transitional RPD.

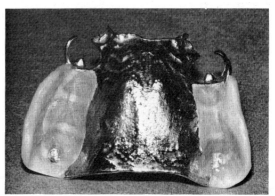

Fig. 2-14. All cast complete palate. This major connector can be made thinner than a complete acrylic resin palate and as a result is usually more comfortable to wear. Added weight of metal may contraindicate its use for some patients.

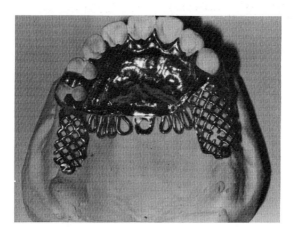

Fig. 2-15. Cast framework for combination cast and acrylic resin complete palate. This major connector combines strength, support, and comfort of metal in anterior part of palate with lightness of acrylic resin in posterior part of palate.

Mandibular major connectors

There are four types of mandibular major connectors in common use today:

1. Lingual bar (Fig. 2-16)
2. Linguoplate (Figs. 2-17 and 2-18)
3. Continuous bar (or Kennedy bar) (Fig. 2-19)
4. Sublingual bar (Fig. 2-20)

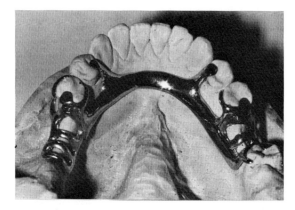

Fig. 2-16. Lingual bar major connector is simplest type of mandibular major connector and constitutes basic design for the other types of mandibular major connectors. It should be considered the mandibular major connector of choice where floor of mouth and structures that support RPD are considered favorable.

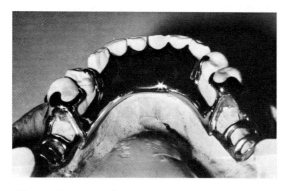

Fig. 2-17. Linguoplate major connector is structurally similar to lingual bar except that thin metal plate is added to bar superiorly, which covers (plates) lingual surfaces of anterior teeth.

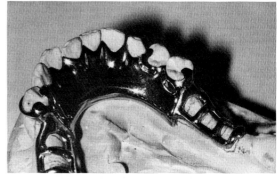

Fig. 2-18. Plating is not only confined to anterior teeth, but also may be extended onto posterior teeth. Indications for its use are similar to those of the linguoplate.

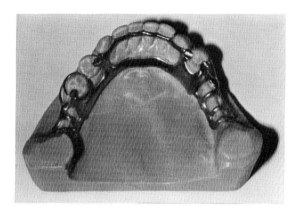

Fig. 2-19. Kennedy, or continuous, bar major connector is structurally similar to lingual bar. It is indicated when large interproximal spaces exist between mandibular anterior teeth that would make a linguoplate esthetically unacceptable.

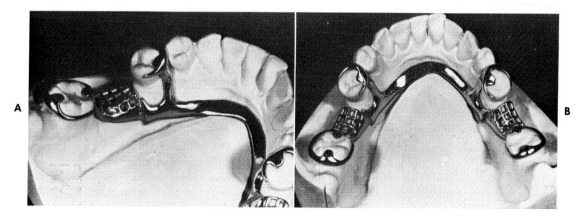

Fig. 2-20. A, Sublingual bar (mediolateral view). **B,** Sublingual bar (occlusal view). (Courtesy Dr. J.D. Walter, Guys Hospital, London, U.K.)

Minor connectors

A minor connector is the connecting link between the major connector or base of an RPD and other units of the prosthesis, such as clasps, indirect retainers, and occlusal rests (Fig. 2-21). The minor connectors most commonly used to connect the denture base to the major connector are of three types:

1. Open latticework (Fig. 2-22)
2. Mesh (Fig. 2-23)
3. Metal base (Fig. 2-24)

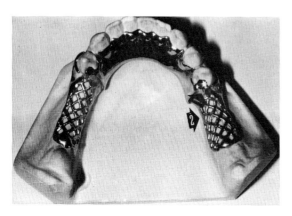

Fig. 2-21. Two different types of minor connectors. *1,* Minor connectors that attach direct retainer to major connector; *2,* minor connectors that attach denture base to major connector.

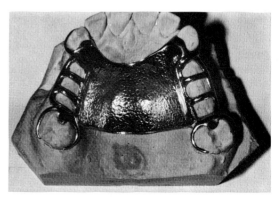

Fig. 2-22. Open latticework type of minor connector. Metal retention loops should be made large and should extend to buccal side of crest of residual ridge. This connector produces greatest amount of retention for acrylic resin.

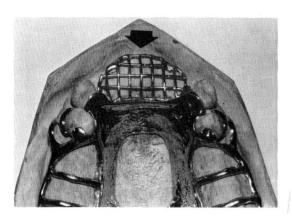

Fig. 2-23. Mesh type of minor connector. Because metal loops of mesh are smaller in diameter than metal loops of open latticework, mesh type of connector is indicated where acrylic resin must be made very thin but must be reinforced with metal to provide sufficient strength to withstand functional forces exerted on RPD.

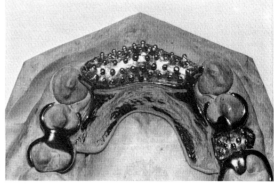

Fig. 2-24. Metal base minor connectors should be used extensively on well-healed residual ridges that have abutments located on both sides of edentulous spaces. They should not be placed on distal-extension edentulous spaces or where future relining of denture base is anticipated.

Rests

A rest is a rigid extension of an RPD that contacts a remaining tooth or teeth to dissipate vertical or horizontal forces. Rests are the supporting elements of an RPD that prevent the vertical displacement of the denture in a gingival direction. The various types of rests in common use are:

1. Occlusal rest (Fig. 2-25)
2. Onlay rest (Fig. 2-26)
3. Lingual rest (Fig. 2-27)
4. Cingulum rest (Fig. 2-28)
5. Incisal rest (Figs. 2-29 and 2-30)
6. Internal rest (Fig. 2-31)

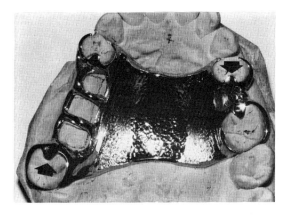

Fig. 2-25. Occlusal rests are rigid extensions of RPD framework that contact occlusal surface of posterior teeth. They provide support for RPD and prevent vertical displacement of prosthesis in gingival direction.

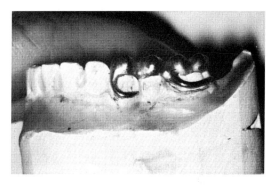

Fig. 2-26. Onlay rests are placed on posterior teeth to create more favorable occlusal plane. Onlay rest is used most frequently to restore occlusion and provide vertical support on tooth that has been tipped or rotated below plane of occlusion.

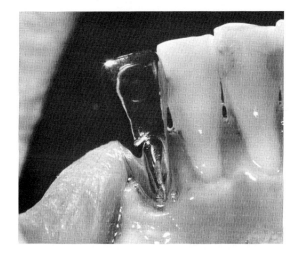

Fig. 2-27. Lingual rest has been placed in this cast restoration on mandibular lateral incisor. In most instances where mandibular incisors must be used to provide support for RPD, multiple rests placed on cingulum of crowns on several incisors are preferable to a rest on a single incisor.

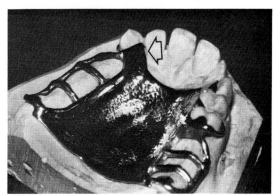

Fig. 2-28. Cingulum rest on maxillary canine. Morphologic features of maxillary canines will usually permit adequate rest preparation for lingual rest to be prepared in enamel of these teeth.

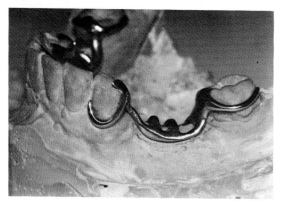

Fig. 2-29. When used in conjunction with circumferential clasps, incisal rests are usually placed on distoincisal angle of abutment teeth.

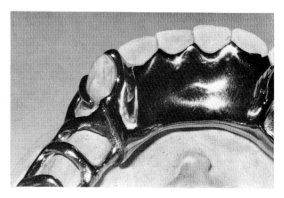

Fig. 2-30. When used in conjunction with a bar clasp, incisal rests are usually positioned on mesioncisal angle of abutment tooth to ensure 180-degree encirclement of clasp on abutment tooth.

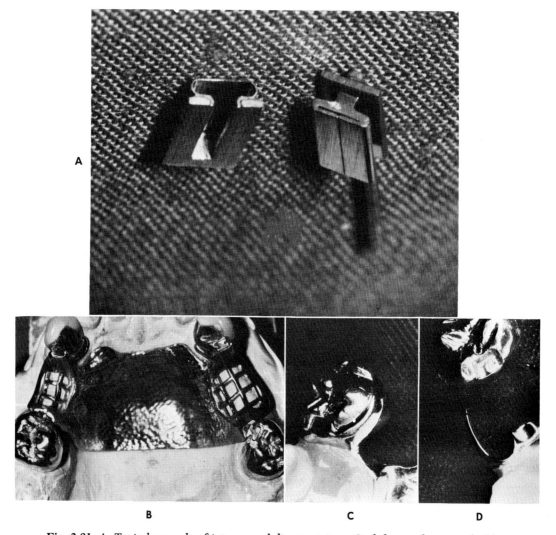

Fig. 2-31. A, Typical example of intracoronal direct retainer. On left, metal receptacle (slot, female portion) is positioned in abutment tooth. On right, closely fitting part (flange, male portion) is located on RPD. **B,** Cast framework of RPD showing intracoronal direct retainers in position on abutment teeth. **C,** Semiprecision internal rest filled with RPD framework. **D,** Occlusal view of rest without RPD in situ.

Extracoronal direct retainers (clasps)

Clasps are those parts of an RPD that act as direct retainers, stabilizers, or both for the denture by partially encircling or contacting the abutment teeth.

Basic requirements of a clasp

A properly designed clasp should provide:

1. Support (Fig. 2-32)
2. Stabilization (Fig. 2-33)
3. Reciprocation (Fig. 2-34)
4. Encirclement (Fig. 2-35)
5. Passivity
6. Retention (Fig. 2-36)

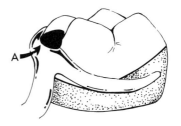

Fig. 2-32. Support. *A*, Occlusal rest provides support through long axis of tooth and prevents clasp from being displaced in gingival direction.

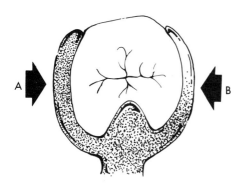

Fig. 2-33. Stabilization. All rigid parts of clasp contribute to this property and resist displacement of clasp in horizontal direction. Stippled portion of clasp indicates those parts of clasp that contribute to stabilization. *A*, Reciprocal clasp arm; *B*, retentive clasp arm.

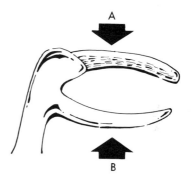

Fig. 2-34. Reciprocation. *A*, Reciprocal clasp arm; *B*, retentive clasp arm. Force exerted on abutment tooth by retentive clasp arm must be opposed by reciprocal clasp arm or some other rigid component of RPD, such as minor connector or linguoplate. Reciprocal component should be located on tooth opposite retentive clasp arm and should always contact tooth before retentive clasp arm when clasp is being seated on tooth.

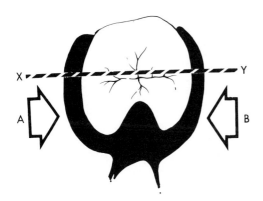

Fig. 2-35. Encirclement. *A*, Reciprocal clasp arm; *B*, retentive clasp arm. Clasp must engage minimum of 180 degrees of circumference of abutment tooth to prevent tooth from moving out of contact with clasp. Line *XY* represents more than 180 degrees of circumference of abutment tooth from origin of clasp.

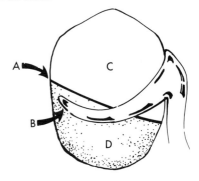

Fig. 2-36. Retention. *A*, Height of contour (survey line); *B*, retentive clasp arm; *C*, suprabulge area; *D*, infrabulge area. For a clasp to be retentive, its arm must flex (distort) as it passes over height of contour of tooth and engage undercut in infrabulge area of tooth.

Common types of clasps used in clinical removable partial denture prosthodontics

Circumferential type

1. Cast circumferential clasp (Akers, or Class I, clasp) (Figs. 2-37 through 2-41)
2. Ring clasp (see Figs. 3-49 and 3-50)
3. Back-action clasp (see Fig. 3-51)
4. Embrasure clasp (Fig. 2-42)
5. Half-and-half clasp (see Fig. 3-53)
6. Mesiodistal clasp (see Fig. 3-54)
7. Rest–proximal plate–Akers retentive arm (RPA) clasp (see Fig. 3-55)
8. Circumferential C clasp (hairpin clasp) (Fig. 2-43)

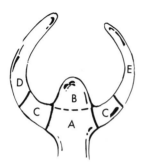

Fig. 2-37. Components of circumferential clasp. *A,* Body of clasp; *B,* occlusal rest; *C,* shoulders of clasp; *D,* reciprocal clasp arm; *E,* retentive clasp arm.

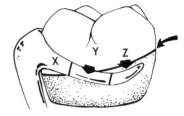

Fig. 2-38. Parts of retentive circumferential clasp arm. *X,* Proximal third, or shoulder, which must be rigid and located above survey line; *Y,* middle third, which is slightly flexible and transverses survey line; *Z,* terminal third, which must be flexible and engage retentive undercut on tooth below height of contour *(arrow).*

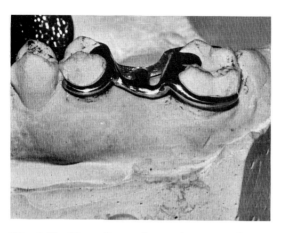

Fig. 2-39. Circumferential cast clasp is used most frequently on teeth adjacent to modification space where usable undercut on abutment tooth is located on side of tooth away from edentulous area.

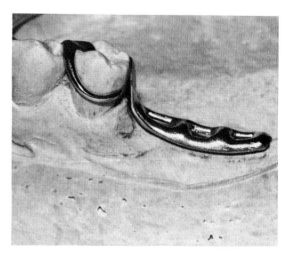

Fig. 2-40. Cast circumferential clasp arm can be used to engage distobuccal undercut on abutment tooth adjacent to distal-extension edentulous space when large buccal tissue undercut contraindicates use of bar clasp.

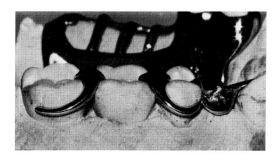

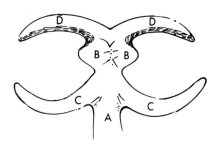

Fig. 2-41. Cast circumferential clasp being used in quadrant where no edentulous space exists. Clasps that pass over occlusal embrasure are subject to fracture unless sufficient clearance between opposing teeth and rests is obtained during mouth preparation so that clasp can be made thick enough to provide for adequate strength.

Fig. 2-42. Embrasure clasp is essentially two cast circumferential clasps joined together. *A,* Body of clasp; *B,* occlusal rests; *C,* reciprocal clasp arms; *D,* retentive clasp arms.

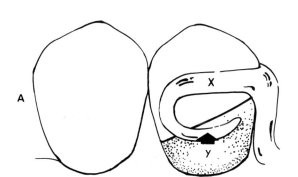

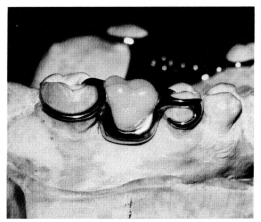

Fig. 2-43. A, Retentive arm of C clasp turns back upon itself to make C-shaped loop so that it can engage proximal undercut on side of tooth where clasp originates. Upper half of clasp arm *(X)* should not taper and should be rigid. Lower half *(Y)* should have uniform taper to make it flexible so that it can engage usable undercut on tooth. **B,** C clasp is used most often on abutment tooth adjacent to tube-type denture tooth or metal pontic or where soft tissue undercuts prevent use of bar clasp.

Bar type
  1. T-bar clasp (Fig. 2-44)
  2. Modified T-bar clasp (Fig. 2-45)
  3. I-bar clasp (Fig. 2-46)
  4. RPI-bar clasp (Fig. 2-47)
  5. RII-bar clasp (Fig. 2-48)

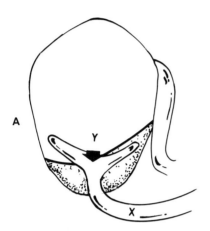
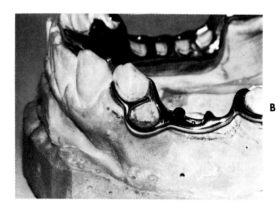

Fig. 2-44. **A,** T-bar clasp derives its name from the fact that its form resembles letter T. Approach arm *(X)* should have uniform taper and contact retentive terminus at approximately a right angle. Retentive terminus *(Y)* should taper toward its end, and tip should be rounded and point occlusally. One half of retentive terminal should engage retentive undercut and other half should be located above survey line. **B,** T-bar clasp on mandibular first premolar. This type of clasp is indicated when usable undercut on abutment tooth is located on side of tooth adjacent to edentulous space.

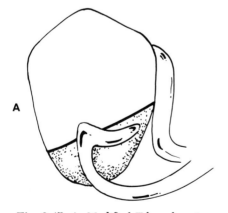
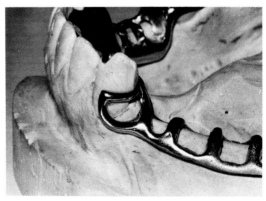

Fig. 2-45. **A,** Modified T-bar clasp is essentially T-bar clasp with that half of retentive terminal which lies above survey line removed. It is often used instead of T-bar clasp because it is more acceptable esthetically. **B,** Modified T-bar on mandibular canine. Like T-bar clasp, its use is contraindicated where approach arm must cross soft tissue undercut or where survey line is located high on abutment tooth.

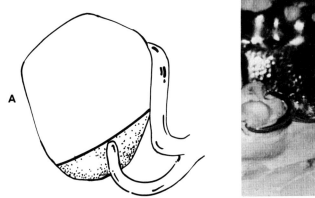
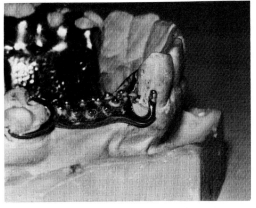

Fig. 2-46. A, I-bar clasp derives its name from the fact that its shape resembles letter I. Minimum amount of contact this type of clasp makes with tooth not only makes it more acceptable esthetically than most other clasp designs, but also reduces chance of dental caries' occurring beneath clasp. **B,** I-bar clasp on mandibular canine. Care must be used in design of this type of clasp to ensure that clasp provides for more than 180-degree encirclement of abutment tooth.

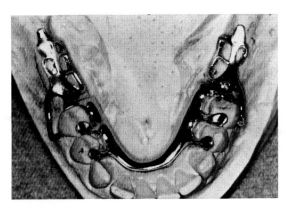
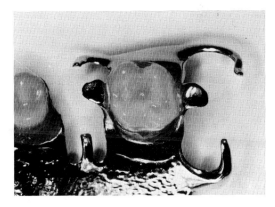

Fig. 2-47. RPI clasp. This distal-extension RPD is retained by two RPI clasps on mandibular second premolars with two indirect retainers on first premolars (occlusal view).

Fig. 2-48. RII clasp. Occlusal view of two RII clasps on this maxillary tooth-borne RPD.

Combination type
1. Wrought wire clasp (Fig. 2-49)
2. Combination bar and cast circumferential clasp (see Fig. 3-61)
3. Vertical reciprocal–horizontal retentive clasp (Fig. 2-50)

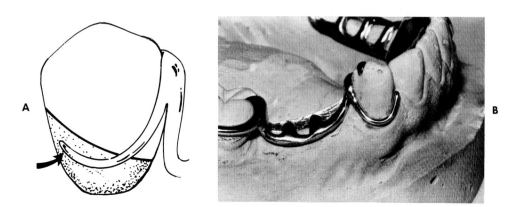

Fig. 2-49. A, Wrought wire clasp arm. Retentive clasp arm of combination clasp is made of 18-gauge round platinum-gold-palladium (PGP) wrought wire rather than cast metal. Being round in form, it has ability to flex in all spatial planes. Because this characteristic permits wrought wire clasp to dissipate torsional forces exerted on abutment tooth, this clasp is usually considered clasp of choice when retentive undercut on abutment tooth adjacent to distal-extension base is located on side of tooth away from denture base. **B,** Because wrought metal has greater strength than cast metal, wrought wire clasp arm can be made smaller in diameter and more resilient than cast retentive arm. These two features make it more acceptable esthetically than cast clasp arm because wrought wire clasp arm is smaller in size, can be located closer to gingival margin of tooth, and has less tooth contact.

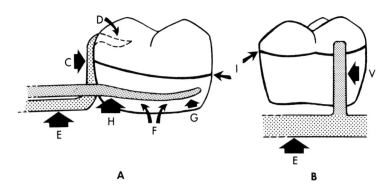

Fig. 2-50. Vertical reciprocal–horizontal retentive clasp. **A,** Survey line, *I;* major connector, *E;* minor connector, *C;* occlusal rest, *D;* retentive area, *F;* retentive area, *G;* retentive clasp, *H.* **B,** Survey line, *I;* major connector, *B;* reciprocal arm, *V.*

Indirect retainers

Indirect retainers help control the masticatory or seating forces that are applied to an RPD. The axis of rotation around which the RPD rotates is called the fulcrum line (Fig. 2-51). Indirect retainers (Fig. 2-52) located on the opposite side of the fulcrum line from the denture base of a distal-extension RPD are used to help control dislodging or unseating forces, such as gravity, the pull of sticky foods, or forces created by muscle action that act on the RPD.

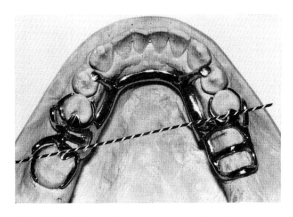

Fig. 2-51. Fulcrum line is imaginary line that passes through most distal rest seat on most posterior abutment tooth on each side of dental arch; RPD can rotate around this line. To be most effective, indirect retainer should be located on opposite side of fulcrum line from distal-extension base and should be positioned at right angles to and as far from fulcrum line as possible.

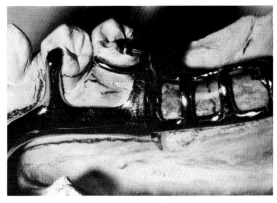

Fig. 2-52. Indirect retainer located in mesial fossa of mandibular first premolar. Mesial fossa of lower first premolar makes ideal location for indirect retainer, because there is usually no opposing maxillary cusp that occludes into this fossa.

Denture base (Figs. 2-53 through 2-57)

A denture base is that part of the RPD which rests on the oral mucosa and to which the teeth are attached.

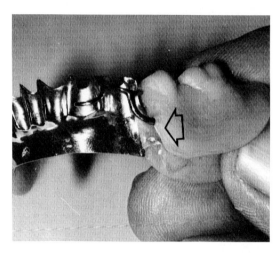

Fig. 2-53. Anterior border of buccal denture flange should be thinned and tapered toward soft tissues to make junction between denture base and soft tissues as imperceptible as possible.

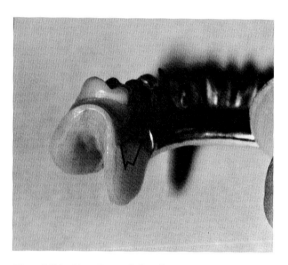

Fig. 2-54. Distolingual border of distal-extension partial denture should be beveled so that it makes smooth junction with soft tissues and is as inconspicuous as possible to tongue.

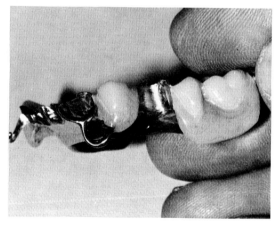

Fig. 2-55. Denture bases that cover modification spaces should not provide for maximum tissue coverage of edentulous space but should be designed so that they prevent food from accumulating beneath denture, enhance esthetics, and restore only natural soft tissue contours that were lost following extraction of teeth. Borders should be tapered toward tissue to make them as thin and indistinct as possible.

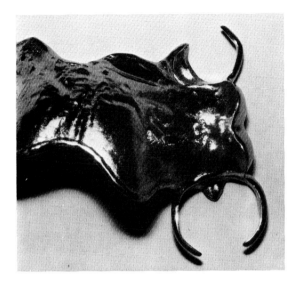

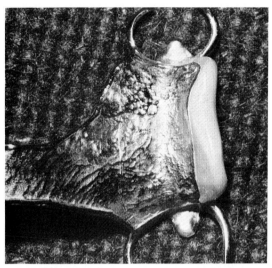

Fig. 2-56. All cast metal base tends to promote better tissue response than acrylic resin because it is easier to keep clean, has a higher thermal conductivity, and can be cast more accurately to a master cast than acrylic resin can be processed to one. Because it is very difficult to reline or rebase, all cast metal base should not be used for distal-extension RPDs in patients who have had extractions within 2 to 3 years. Its use should be limited to modification spaces where edentulous ridges are well healed.

Fig. 2-57. Combination cast metal and acrylic resin denture base. Because metal portion of this denture base covers large amount of residual ridge and tends to create favorable tissue response, this type of denture base is excellent choice for modification spaces where edentulous ridges are well healed. Inasmuch as this type of denture base is difficult if not impossible to reline or rebase, it should be used with discretion as denture base for distal-extension RPD.

3 Survey and design analysis

ANALYSIS OF STRESS AND FUNCTION
Forces acting on the distal-extension removable partial denture

A systematic approach to designing a clasp (extracoronal) type of removable partial denture (RPD) should be based on a thorough understanding of the various forces that will act on the RPD. After the dentist completely analyzes the direction and potential magnitude of these forces, he or she can select the components of the RPD and position them to counteract, control, or minimize these stresses. The dentist designs and positions the components to ensure that the health of the remaining teeth and their supporting structures will be preserved as well as to satisfy the other objectives of an RPD service.

In general, three possible movements may occur singly or in combination in a distal-extension RPD:

1. Rotation of the prosthesis around a fulcrum line passing through the two principal occlusal rests of the direct retainer or through the points where the minor connectors adjacent to the edentulous areas break contact with the tooth surface (Fig. 3-1).

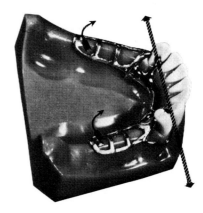

Fig. 3-1. Forces acting on distal-extension base RPD. Rotation occurs around fulcrum line *(long arrow)*. See Table 3-1.

TABLE 3-1
Forces around the fulcrum line

Force activated by	Resultant force	Counteracted by
Sticky foods	Vertical lift	Retention
Tongue and muscle forces	Vertical lift	Adequate denture base coverage
Gravity (maxillary)	Vertical lift	Indirect retainers
		Denture tooth placement
		Gravity (mandibular)
Occlusal load	Movement toward the residual ridge	Occlusal, cingulum, and incisal rests
		Adequate denture base coverage
		Choice of connector

2. Rotation of the prosthesis around the longitudinal axis formed along the crest of the residual ridge (Fig. 3-2).
3. Rotation of the prosthesis around an imaginary perpendicular axis located near the center of the dental arch (Fig. 3-3).

Unfortunately, these rotational movements are not activated singularly, nor do they occur individually during function. In reality, the dynamics of these basic movements are not completely understood. One can surmise, however, that the forces resulting from these

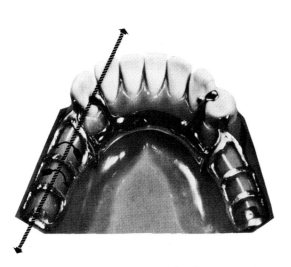

Fig. 3-2. Forces acting on distal-extension base RPD. Rotation occurs around longitudinal axis formed by crest of residual ridge. See Table 3-2.

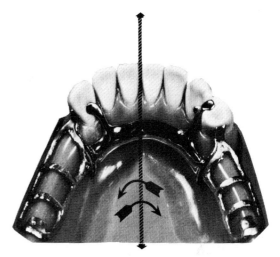

Fig. 3-3. Forces acting on distal-extension base RPD. Rotation occurs around imaginary perpendicular axis near center of dental arch. See Table 3-3.

TABLE 3-2
Forces around the longitudinal axis

Force activated by	Resultant force	Counteracted by
Occlusal force on one side of the arch causes lifting forces on the contralateral side of the arch	Twisting, tilting	Rigid connectors Direct retainer design Denture base coverage Denture tooth placement Contour of the denture base

TABLE 3-3
Forces around the perpendicular axis

Force activated by	Resultant force	Counteracted by

Masticatory stress	Twisting and spreading of the RPD	Adequate bracing:
		  Rigid connectors
		  Connector choice
		Denture base coverage
		Occlusal balance
		Contour of the denture base

movements can induce stress to the supporting edentulous tissues and abutment teeth, not only in varying degrees of magnitude but also in directions varying from vertical or horizontal to combinations of torquing movements. Primarily, the forces acting on an RPD are activated by occlusal loading during mastication or from patient habits (Fig. 3-1) or muscle influences, primarily from the tongue, on the borders of the prosthesis (Fig. 3-2). Other minor activating factors could include the effect of sticky foods on the prosthesis and gravity in the case of the maxillary distal-extension base RPD.

The first consideration in a systematic approach to RPD design is for the dentist to apply the information gained from a systematic approach to diagnosis. The dentist must identify those clinical entities within the oral cavity that can withstand the stress generated by occlusal loading and the movements of the distal-extension base RPD. In particular, the dentist must know which teeth remain, the relationship of the remaining teeth to the edentulous areas, and the relationship of the remaining teeth to each other, in both their proximity and occlusion.

Each of these diagnostic entities must be interpreted in relationship to:

1. The periodontal health of the teeth and the health of the edentulous tissues (Table 3-4)
2. The morphologic features of the crowns and roots of the teeth (Figs. 3-4 and 3-5)
3. The crown-to-root ratio
4. The integrity of the dental arch
5. The previous response of the teeth and the tissue to stress
6. The age of the patient
7. The application of common sense and the exercise of prudent judgment

TABLE 3-4
Evaluation of periodontal health

Entity evaluated	Criterion used
Oral health	Age of the patient
Soft tissue	Previous response of the tissue to stress
Bone	Common sense
Tooth mobility	Common sense

Methods of reducing stress to abutment teeth and supporting tissues

A second consideration in a systematic approach to RPD design is how the existing clinical entities might be altered by selective *mouth preparation* to make them more capable of *withstanding* stresses. Methods of reducing stress (Kratochvil, 1971) are as follows:

1. *Decreasing the mobility of the abutment teeth by:*
   a. Performing an occlusal equilibration
   b. Splinting the teeth either by cast restorations or by the prosthesis itself
   c. Preparing and positioning guiding planes properly
   d. Designing and positioning rests properly
2. *Improving the supportive ability of the edentulous area by:*
   a. Performing impression-making procedures properly
   b. Maximizing the coverage of the residual ridges
   c. Relining or rebasing the prosthesis in a timely fashion
3. *Reducing the amount of force applied to the abutment teeth and residual ridges by:*
   a. Reducing the number of posterior artificial teeth
   b. Reducing the buccolingual width of the artificial teeth
   c. Maintaining the sharpness of the cusps
   d. Providing adequate sluiceways after occlusal corrections
4. *Creating a favorable distribution of the load between the abutment teeth and the ridges by:*
   a. Providing a physiologic development of the edentulous denture base area
   b. Providing extensive stress distribution through use of a rigid RPD design
   c. Selecting a type of clasp assembly that provides direct retention
   d. Using a stress-breaking prosthesis

A SYSTEMATIC APPROACH TO DESIGN
Establishing support

The decision about the type of support for the RPD, whether it be tooth support or tooth-and-tissue support, must be made based on the

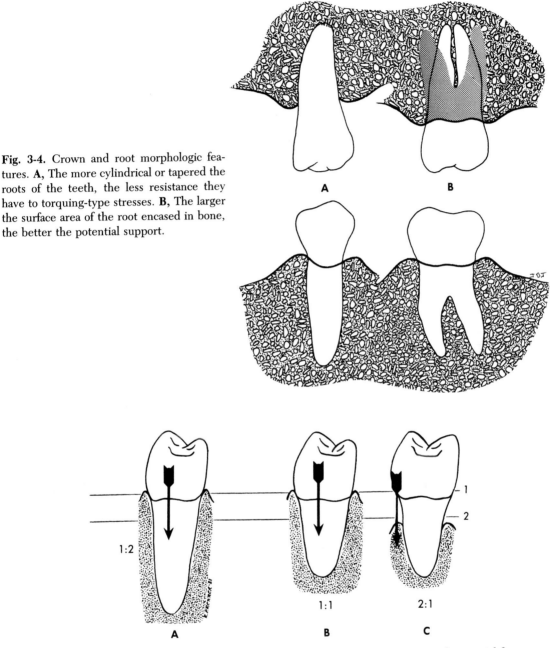

Fig. 3-4. Crown and root morphologic features. **A,** The more cylindrical or tapered the roots of the teeth, the less resistance they have to torquing-type stresses. **B,** The larger the surface area of the root encased in bone, the better the potential support.

Fig. 3-5. Crown-to-root ratio. **A,** Crown-to-root ratio of *1:2* demonstrates good potential for support and stability. Crown's size and its alignment directly over circumference of root will provide for proper axial loading of tooth and for proper rest contour and placement. **B,** Crown-to-root ratio of *1:1* indicates only fair potential for support and stability. Alignment and size of crown in relation to circumference of root will present some problems for proper axial loading of abutment tooth without tooth modification. **C,** Crown-to-root ratio of *2:1* indicates poor potential for support and stability. Alignment and size of crown in relation to circumference of root will present serious problems for proper axial loading even with tooth modification. NOTE: When alveolar bone resorbs from line *1* to line *2*, crown-to-root ratio is increased.

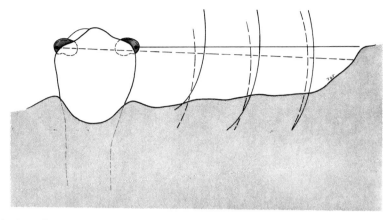

Fig. 3-6. Arc of rotation around principal rest increases the closer rest is positioned to edentulous area.

diagnostic data collected. Once the dentist decides on the type and amount of support for the prosthesis, the components of the RPD that are to provide this support can be *located* and *designed* on the diagnostic casts.

Tooth support

In an entirely tooth-supported RPD, *rests* should be located in such a manner that any load applied to the prosthesis is directed along the long axes of the abutment teeth so that movement of the prosthesis in an apical direction can be effectively resisted (see Fig. 1-4). At the same time, direct retainers and minor connectors must be designed so that the least possible lateral or torquing stress will be transmitted to the abutment tooth. The best rest location in a tooth-supported prosthesis is on the occlusal, cingulum, or incisal surfaces of the abutment teeth directly adjacent to the edentulous areas. To ensure sufficient bulk for adequate strength, each rest should be visualized and prepared on mounted diagnostic casts before mouth preparation is done. Tooth enamel, cast restorations, and well-condensed, highly polished amalgam alloy are suitable materials in which to place RPD rest seats. In a toothborne prosthesis, the amount of the framework latticework in the edentulous area should be kept to a minimum. The design requires only that it be strong enough to prevent fracture under occlusal loading.

In a prosthesis that is designed to be tooth-tissue—supported, the rest preparations must still be designed and located so that the occlusal load is directed through the long axes of the

abutment teeth and so that the least possible lateral or torquing stress is transmitted to the abutment teeth. This is an important guideline in designing a distal-extension base RPD, because the rests can and do act as points of rotation of the prosthesis. The closer the rest is to the edentulous area, the greater is the arc of rotation around the rest (Fig. 3-6). In clinical practice, this rotation is controlled by the location of the rest and the amount of contact of the minor connectors to the tooth surfaces adjacent to the distal-extension base area (Fig. 3-7). Whenever possible, rests should be placed in a position where they will act in concert with the minor connectors to reduce or flatten the arc of rotation. Rests placed on the abutment tooth surfaces adjacent to the distal-extension base may cause distal movement of the abutment tooth if the supporting minor connectors are not properly positioned to contact the prepared tooth surfaces (guiding planes) and adequate tissue support for the prosthesis is not established (Kratochvil, 1963). This distal tooth movement may cause loss of dental arch continuity (dental arch collapse), with resultant food entrapment and periodontal disorders (Figs. 3-8 and 3-9).

In a distal-extension RPD, it is often advisable to place the rest on the mesial aspect of the primary abutment tooth (Kratochvil, 1963, 1971; Krol, 1973a). This, in conjunction with a properly designed minor connector located adjacent to the edentulous area, will flatten the arc of rotation. The resultant force on the prosthesis will tend to move the tooth mesially and be reciprocated by the dental arch (Fig. 3-10).

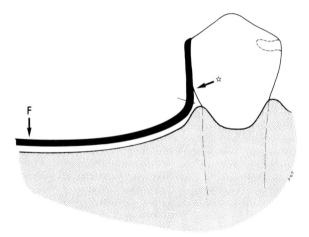

Fig. 3-7. Point of rotation *(star)* for an occluding force is located where minor connector breaks contact with tooth surface. Stresses from these forces are transferred horizontally throughout adjacent teeth. *F*, Occluding force.

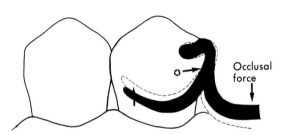

Fig. 3-8. Rests placed adjacent to edentulous area when supporting minor connectors do not contact prepared tooth surfaces (guiding planes). Point of rotation *(star)* resulting from occlusal forces will be at primary rest. Action of clasp assembly will cause posterior movement of abutment tooth and result in food impaction between premolars.

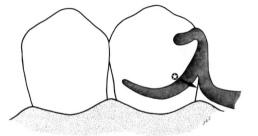

Fig. 3-9. Rest placed adjacent to edentulous area when supporting minor connector will contact prepared tooth surface (guiding plane) from marginal ridge to junction of middle and gingival thirds of crown. Point of rotation *(star)* resulting from occlusal forces will be transferred horizontally to adjacent teeth.

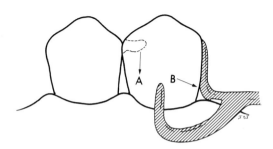

Fig. 3-10. *A*, Rest located on mesial aspect of primary abutment tooth is designed to direct forces of occlusion toward long axis of tooth. *B*, Proximal plate minor connector is designed to contact prepared tooth surface (guiding plane) adjacent to edentulous area from marginal ridge to junction of middle and gingival thirds of crown. Point of rotation resulting from occlusal forces will be transferred horizontally *(arrow)* to adjacent teeth.

Theoretically, this should allow for greater support from the edentulous tissues, reduce the stress to the periodontium of the abutment teeth, and aid in better control of the lateral and torquing stresses resulting from occlusal loading and muscle pull.

If it is necessary to place the rest on a tooth surface adjacent to the edentulous area, it should be designed to control the direction and the distribution of the forces from occlusal loading and from the movements of the distal-extension base without damaging the abutment tooth (Fig. 3-8). To do this, the residual tissues covered by a distal-extension denture base must be capable of providing the necessary support to help oppose vertical, lateral, and torquing forces of occlusion and movement of the prosthesis resulting from muscle pull.

Once tooth support units have been identified and the location of the rest preparations established, the dentist should draw them on the diagnostic cast and note their preparation and outline in the treatment plan record. Rest preparation should follow the basic design principles as previously outlined.

TYPES OF RESTS. The various types of rests used in dental practice can be classified as (1) occlusal, (2) onlay, (3) lingual, (4) incisal, or (5) internal rests.

OCCLUSAL RESTS. Occlusal rests are rigid extensions of the RPD framework that contact a prepared receptacle in the occlusal surface of the posterior teeth (see Fig. 2-25).

An occlusal rest should be roughly triangular (or spoon-shaped), with its apex nearest the center of the tooth. It should be approximately as long as it is wide. The buccolingual width of an occlusal rest should be approximately the same size as half the distance between the buccal and lingual cusp tips of the posterior tooth in which it is placed. When viewed laterally, an occlusal rest should be spoon-shaped and incline slightly toward the center of the abutment tooth. The angle formed by the proximal and occlusal portion of the rest in contact with the marginal ridge of the tooth enamel should be rounded rather than sharp and should be less than 90 degrees. An occlusal rest should be at least 1 mm thick at its thinnest portion to ensure adequate strength to resist fracture. The critical area of occlusal rest fracture is the marginal ridge area. Rests should not interfere with normal occlusal contacts, that is, they

should not alter the occlusal vertical dimension. The occlusal surface of the rest should be concave rather than convex so that its shape follows the normal occlusal surface contour of the abutment tooth. The occlusal rest should fit the rest preparation accurately, and the margins should be finished so that they resemble the margins of a well-fabricated inlay. The relation of the occlusal rest to the abutment tooth should simulate a shallow ball and socket so as to provide only occlusal support for the RPD, while not transmitting horizontal forces to the abutment tooth. Components of the RPD other than the occlusal rest must be used to resist these potential destructive forces, especially on distal-extension RPDs.

ONLAY RESTS. An onlay rest is a rest that covers most or all of the occlusal surface of the abutment tooth (see Fig. 2-26). Onlay rests are most often used to restore the plane of occlusion and the occlusal morphologic features of the tooth and to provide vertical support for teeth that have rotated or been tipped below the existing plane of occlusion. They can be used on multiple teeth to provide a more favorable occlusal plane. Because of the high incidence of dental caries found beneath onlay rests, it is essential that patients who are treated with an RPD with onlay rests practice meticulous oral hygiene. In addition, as an adjunct to dental caries control, the occlusal surface of the teeth beneath these rests should be brushed daily with a 0.4% stannous fluoride gel; any deep fissures or grooves should be restored or have occlusal sealants placed.

LINGUAL RESTS. Where clinically possible, it is preferable to use occlusal rests on posterior teeth to provide vertical support for an RPD rather than to use rests on anterior teeth. In many partially edentulous situations, however, this is not always possible, and the canines or other anterior teeth must be used as an abutment for direct retainers (clasps), indirect retainers, or auxiliary rests. Because of the greater amount of periodontal supporting apparatus, canines should be used as abutments for an RPD instead of incisors whenever possible. In instances where the incisors must be used to support an RPD, multiple rests (see discussion of the mesiodistal clasp assembly) placed on several incisors are preferable to one rest on a single incisor. Rest seats can sometimes be prepared in the lingual enamel surface of the incisors; however, in most instances the lingual morphologic features and enamel surface thickness of these teeth will not permit this. Conservative restorations (silver amalgam alloy or gold inlay) with definite rest seats prepared in them should be used when the lingual anatomy is not favorable in order to ensure that the forces exerted on the teeth by the prosthesis are directed through the long axes (see Fig. 2-27).

The most common type of lingual rest used on anterior teeth is the cingulum rest (see Fig. 2-28). Cingulum rests may be used on any anterior tooth, but they find their greatest use on maxillary canines. Morphologically, maxillary canines usually have a gradual lingual surface incline and a prominent cingulum. These morphologic characteristics usually permit adequate tooth preparation in enamel for a lingual rest. Mandibular canines, on the other hand, usually do not have a prominent cingulum, and the lingual surface incline is more vertical than on the maxillary canines. Their anatomic form therefore does not permit an adequate rest seat preparation to be made in the enamel of these teeth. As a result, cast restorations with included cingulum rest preparations are usually indicated if cingulum rests are to be placed on mandibular canines (see Fig. 2-28).

INCISAL RESTS. Although incisal rests can be used on any anterior tooth, they are most commonly used on mandibular anterior teeth and on mandibular canines in particular. Incisal rests are usually employed on sound abutment teeth when both a lingual enamel rest seat preparation and the construction of a cast restoration with a prepared lingual rest are contraindicated. Incisal rests should be positioned on either the mesial or distal incisal angle of the abutment teeth in a rest seat prepared in the enamel. Incisal rests can be used as an auxiliary rest, indirect retainer, or a component of a direct retainer. When used as a part of a circumferential clasp, they are usually placed on the distal incisal angle of the abutment tooth (see Fig. 2-29). When an incisal rest is used in conjunction with a bar-type clasp assembly (rest, proximal plate, I bar [RPI] clasp assembly), it should be positioned on the mesial incisal angle of the abutment tooth (see Fig. 2-30). The margins of these rests should always be finished intraorally to make them as inconspicuous and comfortable as possible for the patient.

When the option of selecting either a lingual or an incisal rest for an abutment tooth is available, the lingual rest is usually considered the rest of choice for several reasons. A lingual rest is located in the gingival third rather than on the incisal edge of the abutment tooth. This places the rest closer to the center of rotation on the tooth and can reduce the effect of horizontal or rotational forces that are transmitted to the tooth by the prosthesis. Lingual rests are also more esthetic and less subject to distortion or breakage, because they are of greater bulk than are incisal rests.

INTERNAL RESTS (see Fig. 2-31, *C* and *D*). An internal rest (either a semiprecision or a precision rest) consists of a male portion (soldered to or cast as part of an RPD) that fits into a female receptacle of a cast restoration placed on the abutment tooth (Becker and associates, 1978; Blatterfein, 1969; Cecconi and associates, 1975; Cohn, 1956; Gilson and associates, 1965; Grosser, 1953; Harris, 1955; Knowles, 1963; Koper, 1973; Leff, 1952; McLeod, 1978; Prieskel, 1971, 1979; Zinner, 1979). These rests, because of their boxlike form, transmit both the vertical and lateral forces exerted on the RPD to the abutment teeth. The precision fit of these rests in their recesses in the abutment teeth in general contraindicates their use on distal-extension RPDs because of the torquing effect created on the abutment teeth by this type of prosthesis when it moves in function. The use of internal rests should therefore be limited to tooth-borne RPDs or to clinical situations where esthetics is a primary consideration. Additionally, adequate tissue support for the RPD permits the use of internal rests (as in a maxillary distal-extension RPD, where the horizontal part of the palate will assist in the support).

Tissue support

It is essential that a thorough evaluation of the proposed abutment teeth and the residual ridge be made based on the relative ability of each to provide support for the prosthesis and resist stress. In the final design, each tissue should receive an equitable share of the load so that the total dental health of the patient is maintained for an optimal period of time. Since a distal-extension base RPD derives a great deal of its support from the residual ridge, it is essential that the distal-extension base should

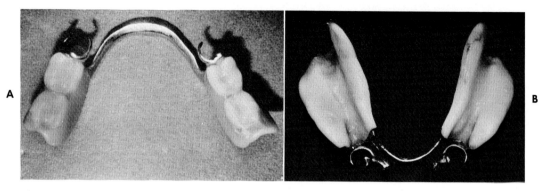

Fig. 3-11. A, Minimal tissue coverage by distal-extension RPD. **B,** Maximal tissue support is obtained by covering greatest surface area of edentulous ridge possible without impinging on movable tissue. Denture teeth should not be placed on steep incline anterior to retromolar pad.

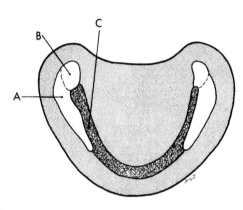

Fig. 3-12. Primary support areas of mandible. *A,* Buccal shelf area; *B,* retromolar pad (depending on tissue consistency); *C,* slopes of residual ridge (secondary support).

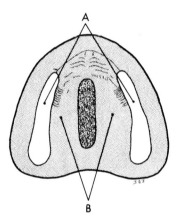

Fig. 3-13. Primary support areas of the maxilla. *A,* Posterior residual ridge area; *B,* horizontal part of palate.

cover the greatest surface area without impinging on movable tissues (Fig. 3-11) (Applegate, 1955, 1960b; Hindels, 1952; Holmes, 1970; Leupold and Kratochvil, 1965). Maximum tissue support can be obtained only by using broad, accurate-fitting denture bases (Cecconi and associates, 1971c).

Considerations in evaluating the potential of tissue support for RPDs are discussed in the following.

LENGTH AND CONTOUR OF THE RESIDUAL RIDGE. In distal-extension RPDs, the length of the edentulous area exerts a definite influence on the available support. The denture base area in close approximation to the abutment teeth is primarily supported by the abutment teeth. Proceeding away from the abutment teeth, support for the distal-extension base is primarily derived from the underlying tissue. The support areas for an RPD in the *mandible* (Fig. 3-12) are:

1. Buccal shelf area (primary support)
2. Retromolar pad area (primary or secondary support, depending on tissue consistency)
3. Slopes of the residual ridge (secondary support)

The support areas for an RPD in the *maxilla* (Fig. 3-13) are:

1. Slopes of the residual ridge (secondary support)
2. Horizontal portion of the hard palate (primary support)

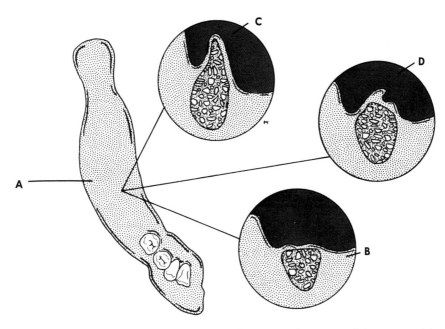

Fig. 3-14. A, The longer the edentulous area, the greater the potential for increased lever action on abutment teeth. **B,** Flat ridge: good support, poor stability. **C,** Sharp spiny ridge: poor support, poor to fair stability. **D,** Redundant tissue on ridge: poor support, poor stability.

3. Crest of the posterior residual ridge (primary support)

CONTOUR OF THE EDENTULOUS BASE AREA. The contour of the edentulous base area exerts an influence on tissue support equal to that of its length and breadth. The ideal residual ridge contour is one that has a broad, smooth, rounded ridge crest with nearly vertical buccal and lingual slopes. Residual ridge crests that are parallel to the opposing residual ridges or the occlusal plane provide the most advantageous position for distribution of stress. Residual ridges that are flat may offer secondary support but will provide little, if any, lateral stability. Residual ridges that are sharp and spiny provide the poorest anatomy for both the support and stability of a prosthesis (Fig. 3-14).

QUALITY OF THE SUPPORTING BONE AND OVERLYING MUCOSA. The quality of the underlying residual ridge provides a definite influencing factor on the support that can be derived from the distal-extension base. Absence of cortical bone in specific areas usually indicates a poor response of the residual bone to stress. A radiographic evaluation of the bone can provide the dentist with an index of how the bone is currently reacting to the forces of occlusion and the movements of an existing distal-extension RPD and can provide an estimate of how the bone might perform as a supporting unit for a new prosthesis (Fig. 3-15).

Since a distal-extension RPD must derive part of its support from the residual ridge, the mucosal covering of the residual ridge plays an important role in the quality of that support. Some areas of the mucoperiosteum covering the residual ridge are firm with limited displaceability, whereas others are very displaceable (Fig. 3-14). The tissues covering the residual ridges should be recorded in their dynamic form; that is, both the functional form of the primary support areas and the anatomic form of the displaceable areas should be recorded in the impression (Fig. 3-16). This approach to making an impression of the residual tissues provides assurance that the primary stress-bearing areas of the residual ridge will provide their fair share of support for the distal-extension RPD.

FORCES ON SUPPORTING TISSUES. Distribution of occlusal loading to the available tissue support area is determined by the relation of

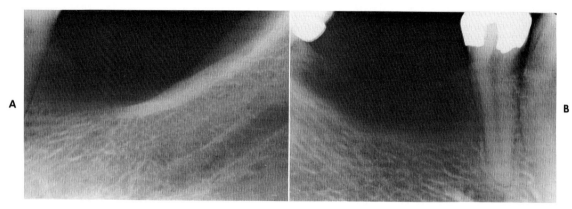

A   B

Fig. 3-15. A, Radiograph of distal-extension base area demonstrating absence of cortical bone. This area has been subjected to stress from RPD for 2 years. There has been a negative bone response. **B,** Radiograph of edentulous area demonstrating questionable continuity to cortical plate. Poor support can be anticipated from this type of bone.

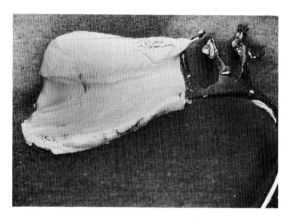

Fig. 3-16. Altered cast impression that has recorded edentulous tissues in their dynamic form. Buccal shelf area has been recorded in its functional state, and crest of residual ridge and other investing tissues have been recorded in their resting anatomic states.

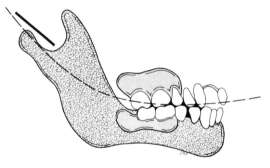

Fig. 3-17. RPD fabricated to improperly oriented occlusal plane. Forces of occlusion in denture base area will not be directed at right angles to primary support area (buccal shelf) of residual ridge.

the opposing residual ridges or teeth and by the forces transferred to the residual ridges by occlusion and rotational movements of the distal-extension RPD (see Figs. 3-1 through 3-3). Dental arch collapse, in the form of rotated or tilted teeth and an altered occlusal plane resulting from extruded teeth or residual ridges, can result in occlusal forces that cannot be controlled or directed to the long axes of the abutment teeth or support areas of the edentulous ridges (Fig. 3-17). Proper recontouring of the tissues or the restoration or extraction of the

teeth may be necessary to properly reorient the plane of occlusion or to correct the dental arch form and thus control the direction of the forces of occlusion. To satisfy the primary objective of preservation, it is necessary to control the direction of the occlusal forces so that they can be directed along the long axes of the primary abutment teeth and at right angles to the primary support areas.

PREVIOUS RESPONSE TO STRESS. An evaluation of the residual ridges to determine the amount of residual ridge reduction that has oc-

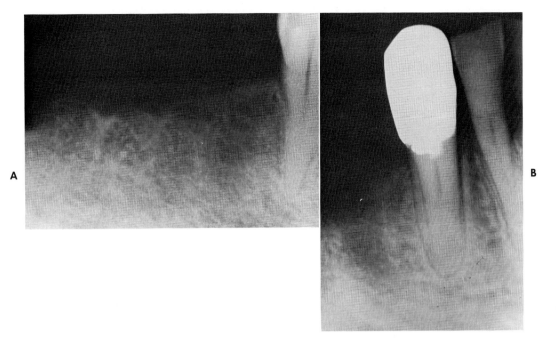

Fig. 3-18. Previous response to stress. **A,** Mandibular right first premolar supported a distal-extension base RPD for 8 years. RPD had circumferential clasps with distal rests. Note response of supporting bone in edentulous area. **B,** Mandibular left first premolar supported a distal-extension base RPD for 1½ years. RPD had I-bar type of clasp with distal proximal plate and mesial rest. Note poor response of supporting bone in edentulous area.

curred over time will give the dentist some indication of the resistance of bone to resorption after tooth loss (Fig. 3-18). Obviously, where the edentulous areas have been subject to additional stress from a previous RPD (prosthodontic load factors), their morphologic change will have an even greater predictive value. The evaluation should provide the dentist with an index of how the bone is currently reacting to stress and give an estimate of how the bone may perform as a supporting unit for a prosthesis.

Support of the prosthesis should be the primary consideration in designing a distal-extension RPD (Hindels, 1952; Holmes, 1970; Lammie and Osborne, 1954; Leupold and Kratochvil, 1965). In general, tooth support provides a greater potential for control of occlusal forces than does tissue support. This is demonstrated by the relatively high percentage of success of tooth-borne RPDs as opposed to distal-extension RPDs. The dentist can satisfy the objectives of an RPD service if he or she interprets from the diagnostic findings the means that are available to satisfactorily oppose and control the vertical, lateral, and torquing components of occlusal forces. Put succinctly, the dentist must diagnose what type of tooth and tissue support is available to oppose and control these forces.

Connecting support units

The next phase in a systematic approach to design is for the dentist to decide how the tooth and tissue support units should be connected. The connection of supporting units is facilitated by *major* and *minor* connectors. Their design and placement must comply with accepted prosthodontic standards and structural detail previously indicated.

Some dentists recommend that, when edentulous areas are connected, similar or like areas be connected rigidly and dissimilar or unlike edentulous areas be connected semirigidly (Blatterfein, 1969; Koper, 1973; McLeod, 1978; Zinner, 1979). These individuals feel that the connection of dissimilar edentulous support areas should be designed so that the connectors

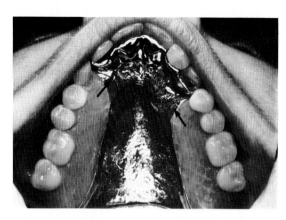

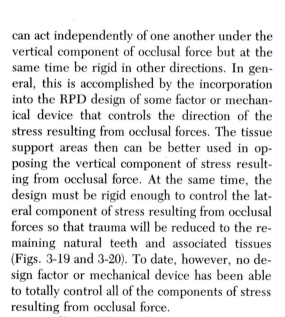

Fig. 3-19. Split maxillary palatal major connector *(arrow)* designed to control forces that result from occlusion. Theoretically, residual ridge areas will provide primary support to resist vertical stresses from occlusion.

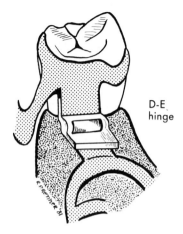

Fig. 3-20. Hinge-type mechanical device incorporated into prosthesis design to control vertical occlusal forces.

can act independently of one another under the vertical component of occlusal force but at the same time be rigid in other directions. In general, this is accomplished by the incorporation into the RPD design of some factor or mechanical device that controls the direction of the stress resulting from occlusal forces. The tissue support areas then can be better used in opposing the vertical component of stress resulting from occlusal force. At the same time, the design must be rigid enough to control the lateral component of stress resulting from occlusal forces so that trauma will be reduced to the remaining natural teeth and associated tissues (Figs. 3-19 and 3-20). To date, however, no design factor or mechanical device has been able to totally control all of the components of stress resulting from occlusal force.

Regardless of philosophies in connecting like or unlike edentulous areas, major and minor connectors should satisfy several specific basic requirements. They should be designed so that:

1. They are rigid and strong enough to withstand masticatory forces and patient handling.
2. They conform to and do not interfere with the normal anatomic structures of the mouth.
3. They avoid food entrapment.

4. They do not interfere with mastication or occlusion.

Major connectors

A major connector is that part of the RPD which connects the components of the prosthesis on one side of the dental arch to the components on the opposite side of the dental arch. It is that portion of the RPD to which all other components are attached.

It is essential that the major connector be made rigid so that the forces exerted on the RPD will be distributed more uniformly over the abutment teeth (direct and indirect abutments) and other natural teeth and soft tissues covered by the RPD. Major connectors that are flexible can cause damage to the periodontal supporting apparatus of the abutment teeth, injury to the soft tissues and the residual ridges covered by the RPD, and discomfort to the patient.

Clinical experience has shown that if the border of the major connector terminates or impinges on the free gingival margin, it will interfere with the blood supply to the gingival tissues, which can result in inflammatory changes of these tissues. To avoid these tissue changes, the superior border of a maxillary major connector should end at least 6 mm from the natural teeth and run parallel to the gingival mar-

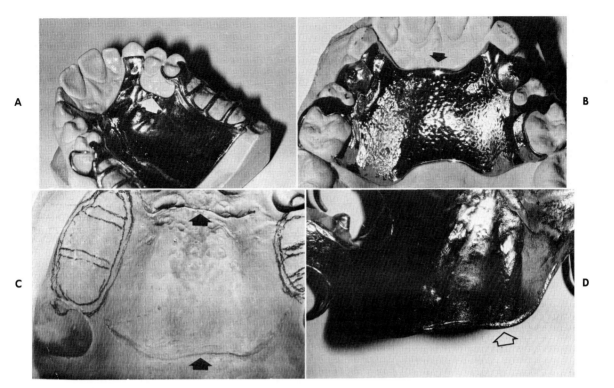

Fig. 3-21. Design considerations for maxillary major connectors. **A,** Borders should be placed a minimum of 6 mm away from free gingival margins. **B,** Both anterior and posterior connectors should cross midline at right angles. **C,** Internal edges of connectors' palatal borders should be placed at junction of vertical and horizontal surfaces of palate. (In flat, gently curved palate, this landmark must be approximated. These borders should be on same vertical level to prevent patient discomfort caused by tongue interferences.) **D,** Palatal strap should be a minimum of 8 mm in width. Thickness of metal should be uniform throughout the palate. Generally, no relief is required. Borders should be beaded to a depth of 0.5 mm. Metal should never be highly polished on tissue side. All borders of maxillary major connector should be tapered slightly toward tissue. Finished borders of metal should be smoothly curved and never irregular. If anterior bar is used, it should be flat or straplike and located so that anterior border follows existing valleys between crests of rugae. If posterior bar is used, it should be half-oval in shape and located as far posteriorly on hard palate as possible without infringement on movable tissues of soft palate.

gins of these teeth (Fig. 3-21, *A*). A clearance of at least 3 to 4 mm should always exist between the superior border of a mandibular lingual bar major connector and the free gingival margin of the mandibular teeth (Fig. 3-22, *A*).

In those mouths where it is not possible to provide adequate space between the mandibular major connector and the free gingival margin of the teeth, the major connector (lingual plate) can be extended onto the lingual surfaces of the teeth or a sublingual bar can be used. Whenever the lingual surfaces of the teeth are covered by the lingual plate major connector, inflammation of the underlying gingival tissue

may result from either the loss of the natural stimulation of these tissues normally provided through contact with food and muscle action or inadequate dental plaque removal and denture hygiene by the patient. The risk of dental caries' developing on the natural teeth is also increased if the patient does not effectively remove dental plaque when any major connector design is used. Stimulation of the gingival tissues through daily oral physiotherapy as well as meticulous dental plaque control of both the natural teeth and the RPD is essential if the health of the supporting tissues is to be preserved.

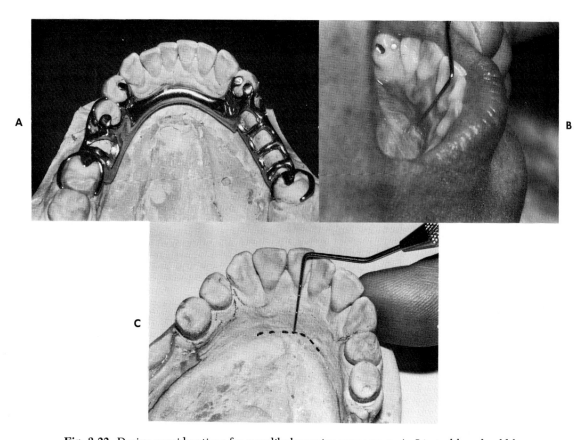

Fig. 3-22. Design considerations for mandibular major connectors. **A,** Lingual bar should be half-pear shaped and tapered superiorly, with inferior border rounded. Superior margin of lingual bar should be located 4 mm from free gingival margin and parallel to that margin. **B** and **C,** Inferior border should be located above moving tissues in floor of mouth. (If this cannot be done, because of height of mouth floor, linguoplate should be considered.) Relief wax (28 gauge) should be provided to avoid impingement of major connector into tissues if settling of base occurs. (Bar should never contact mucosa when it is in its terminal position.) For linguoplate, (see Figs. 2-17 and 2-18) entire lingual area should be surveyed, including areas between teeth, and all undercut areas blocked out. Upper border of plate should contact lingual surfaces of teeth tightly. Free gingival margin and inferior aspect of plate should be relieved slightly.

Sharp corners or angles on a major connector should be avoided because they tend to cause food entrapment. The border outline of the major connector should consist of smooth, gentle curves and should taper toward the tissues to make it as inconspicuous as possible to tactile sensation.

Major connectors, therefore, should be selected on the basis of their ability to provide support and rigidity to the RPD and their compatibility with anatomic structures of the maxilla and mandible.

DESIGN CONSIDERATIONS FOR MAXILLARY MAJOR CONNECTORS. Maxillary major connec-

tors should be designed with the comfort of the patient in mind. Connectors that are made thin, wide, and as uniform in thickness as possible without compromising rigidity are more comfortable than those that are made narrow and thick (Campbell, 1977; LaVere and Krol, 1973). DeVan (1952a) suggested that the importance of using the support potential of the hard palate whenever possible cannot be overemphasized. He recommended the use of broad, thin, ribbonlike connectors to take advantage of this additional support for the RPD. To use as much support from the hard palate as possible, the tissue side of the major connector should not be relieved (that is, it should be in intimate contact). Relief should be provided only in those areas where the major connector covers a palatal torus or a prominent median palatal suture. Free gingival margins and gingival crevices, however, should always be relieved when they are traversed by the major connector.

Coverage of the anterior area of the hard palate should be avoided whenever possible. This area plays a very important role in determining the patient's speech patterns, because the tip of the tongue, contacting the palatal rugae, anterior area of the palate, and teeth, acts as an articulator during speech production (Martone, 1957). However, when it is necessary to include this area on the RPD, it is better to cover it completely by plating the lingual surfaces of the anterior teeth with the major connector than it is to end its anterior border on the soft tissues just lingual to the maxillary anterior teeth. If it is necessary to partially cover the palatal rugae, the palatal major connector should follow the outline of the valleys and crests of the palatal rugae. The borders of the major connector should end level with the crest of the palatal rugae so that the junction between the major connector and the soft tissues is made as inconspicuous as possible to the patient's tongue (Fig. 3-21, *B* and *C*). If it is necessary to cross a ruga with the major connector, the ruga should be crossed abruptly.

A bead on the tissue surface of the major connector should be prepared along the peripheral outline of a maxillary major connector so that the major connector will slightly displace the underlying soft tissues to provide a tissue seal. This is accomplished by scoring the master cast, upon which the RPD is to be constructed, to a depth and width of approximately 0.5 to 1.0 mm along the border outline of the maxillary major connector. The beading should stop approximately 6 mm from the gingival margins of the teeth so as not to interfere with the blood supply to the gingival tissues. The compressibility of the palatal tissues covered by the major connector should be evaluated clinically and the depth of the bead determined according to tissue displaceability. The depth of the bead should be made slightly greater along the lateral slopes of the hard palate and slightly less along the horizontal portion of the hard

palate where it crosses the median palatal suture (Fig. 3-21, *C*).

Beading of a maxillary major connector accomplishes the following functions (Fig. 3-21, *C* and *D*):

1. It helps to prevent food debris from collecting beneath the major connector.
2. The additional thickness of metal along the bead permits the edges of the polished surface of the connector to be tapered so that a smooth junction with the soft tissues is created and yet the edges remain rounded rather sharp. The beaded edge of the major connector will usually adapt to the soft tissues after the RPD has been worn, which makes the junction between the major connector and the palatal tissues even less apparent to the patient.
3. The bead serves as a finishing line for the dental laboratory technician during the finishing and polishing of the metal framework.

Maxillary major connectors should not cover tissues that have undergone or will undergo residual ridge reduction and should never depend on the gingival tissues for their support. Fig. 3-21 presents the basic considerations of a maxillary major connector design.

Palatal straps, anteroposterior palatal straps (closed horseshoes), or complete palatal plates are the major connectors of choice for most maxillary RPD designs, since they provide excellent support and rigidity (LaVere, 1973). Because of their structure and contour, these types of major connectors are capable of distributing occlusal forces over a wide area. Increased retention may be achieved because of increased interfacial surface tension through intimate tissue contact between the major connector and the oral mucosa. Unfortunately, because of increased palatal coverage by the major connector, some patients may have minor speech interferences and may require varying lengths of time to adapt to the major connector. Anteroposterior palatal bars provide poor RPD support and are uncomfortable because they must be narrow and bulky if they are to be sufficiently rigid.

Rigidity of the major connector is necessary to effectively transfer the stress of mastication from one side of the dental arch to the other. Support is a necessary attribute of a major connector to prevent the RPD framework from

TABLE 3-5

Ability of major connectors to provide support and rigidity

Type of connector	Support	Rigidity
Palatal strap	Good to excellent	Good to excellent
Closed horseshoe (anteroposterior palatal strap)	Good	Excellent
Complete palate plate	Excellent	Excellent
Anteroposterior palatal bar	Poor	Good
Palatal bar	Poor	Poor
Horseshoe	Poor	Poor
Lingual bar	Poor	Good
Linguoplate	Poor	Good to excellent

moving in a tissueward direction. The ability of each of the various types of major connectors to provide support and rigidity is listed in Table 3-5.

Although the design of the maxillary major connector will vary according to the conditions found in the mouth, most maxillary major connectors can be classified into five basic types. Each is discussed below.

SINGLE PALATAL BAR OR STRAP. The single palatal bar (see Fig. 2-7) is indicated for Kennedy Class III RPDs, where only a few posterior teeth are missing and the periodontal support of the abument teeth is good. It is not indicated where both anterior and posterior teeth are missing or for distal-extension RPDs. The strap should be made flat yet wide (minimum of 8 mm) and thick enough so that it is rigid. Narrow palatal bars (see Fig. 2-8) must be made bulky to be rigid. As a result, the added bulk often proves to be annoying to the patient. The use of a narrow palatal bar is therefore contraindicated.

U-SHAPED, OR HORSESHOE-SHAPED, PALATAL MAJOR CONNECTOR. The U-shaped palatal major connector (see Fig. 2-9) may be indicated where anterior or both anterior and posterior teeth are missing and the RPD is supported posteriorly by natural teeth. It is also used when splinting of the anterior teeth is required, when a torus palatinus interferes with the placement of the major connector, and when the patient cannot tolerate complete palatal coverage or a posterior palatal bar. Because of the horseshoe shape of the major connector, it often lacks the necessary rigidity across the midline for adequate cross-arch stress distribu-

tion. Its use is therefore contraindicated for distal-extension RPDs unless some other type of major connector cannot be used. Because it covers the anterior portion of the palate, it often interferes with speech production and is often uncomfortable to the patient. If it is necessary to cover (plate) the lingual surfaces of the maxillary natural anterior teeth with this major connector, it may cause irritation of the gingival tissues covered by the prosthesis. Because of its many limitations, this type of major connector should be used only when it is not possible to use another type.

ANTEROPOSTERIOR PALATAL BAR. The anteroposterior palatal bar (see Fig. 2-10) may be indicated where the remaining maxillary natural teeth have adequate periodontal support and a large amount of palatal support is not required. It is also used when the patient objects to a large amount of palatal coverage or when a large torus palatinus exists. It is often used when replacement of the maxillary anterior teeth is required and when it is necessary to cover the entire palatal rugae area with the anterior bar. When it is used in this way, it is called a closed horseshoe palatal connector (see Fig. 2-11). Structurally it is a very rigid major connector and can be used on either distal-extension or long-span, tooth-supported RPDs. The anterior bar should be flat, and its borders should be coordinated with the valleys and peaks of the palatal rugae. The posterior bar, which is narrow, should be half oval to make it rigid. It should be located just anterior to the vibrating line. The large amount of border area of both of the palatal bars, the coverage of the anterior portion of the hard palate, and the increased thickness of the palatal bars contribute to patient discomfort when this type of major connector is used. It therefore has very limited applications.

POSTERIOR PALATAL STRAP. The posterior palatal strap (see Fig. 2-12) is a very versatile major connector because it can be used in a variety of RPD designs. In patients whose periodontal support of the teeth has been compromised, this major connector can be designed to cover a large area of the hard palate to help distribute the forces of occlusion over a broad area. Where periodontal support is good and the edentulous areas are small, it can be made narrower in width. This major connector can be used in either an all tooth-supported or a distal-extension RPD. Because of its large contact area with the hard palate, it derives excellent palatal support. Its wide area of tissue contact aids in the retention of the RPD through the forces of adhesion and cohesion. Because it is broad, it can be made thin and still maintain rigidity, which promotes patient comfort. This is an excellent major connector and should be used extensively in the design of RPDs. It should be kept in mind that major connectors should be selected on the basis of support and rigidity, not on which teeth are remaining.

COMPLETE PALATAL PLATE. The complete palatal plate (see Figs. 2-13 through 2-15) provides greater rigidity and support than any other maxillary major connector. It should be used in partially edentulous situations when: (1) the remaining natural teeth have lost extensive periodontal support; (2) the residual ridges have undergone severe resorption; (3) the anatomic form of the hard palate is flat; (4) there are long-span, bilateral, posterior edentulous areas; (5) a cleft palate patient is treated with an RPD; and (6) an RPD is considered a transitional prosthesis before a maxillary complete denture. The large amount of palatal coverage makes it less comfortable to wear than other types of major connectors (Campbell, 1977). Therefore, it should be used only in those patients who require maximum palatal support. Structurally this kind of connector can be designed as one of three types:

1. *Complete acrylic resin palate (the Every denture).* This type of major connector (see Fig. 2-13) is used when economic factors prevent the use of a cast framework or when the supporting structures of the remaining teeth require the use of a lightweight prosthesis.

2. *The complete cast palate.* This major connector (see Fig. 2-14) can be made very thin and is consequently the most comfortable to wear. The added weight of this major connector may contraindicate its use in some patients.

3. *Combination cast and acrylic resin complete palate.* This major connector (see Fig. 2-15) combines the advantages of the other two types by using the strength and comfort of the metal in the anterior portion of the hard palate and the lightness of the acrylic resin in the posterior area of the hard palate.

DESIGN CONSIDERATIONS FOR MANDIBULAR MAJOR CONNECTORS. The mandibular major connectors, like the maxillary major connectors, should be properly located in relation to gingival and movable tissues in the floor of the mouth. Major connectors should not cover tissues that have undergone or will undergo residual ridge resorption, and they should never depend on gingival tissues for their support.

There are four types of mandibular major connectors commonly used in dental practice today. Each is discussed below.

LINGUAL BAR. The lingual bar (see Fig. 2-16) is the simplest mandibular major connector to use. Because it has no tooth and soft tissue contact, the lingual bar reduces the patient's susceptibility to dental caries and gingival irritation from the food stagnation and dental plaque accumulation often associated with the wearing of an RPD. It should therefore be considered as the mandibular major connector of first choice except where there are definite contraindications for its use, such as a high floor of the mouth. It has its greatest use in Kennedy Class III RPDs and where the structures that support the RPD are considered favorable.

Structurally, the lingual bar constitutes the basic design for the other types of mandibular major connectors. It should be half-pear shaped in cross section, with the thicker inferior portion located as far below the free gingival margin of the lower anterior teeth as possible (at least 3 to 4 mm) without interfering with the normal functional activity of the tissues in the floor of the mouth. It should be at least 4 mm in superior-inferior width and thick enough to make it rigid. If the major connector is long or there are extensive edentulous areas, the lingual bar may require additional thickening to maintain its rigidity. The thinner superior border of the lingual bar should be located at least 3 to 4 mm below the lingual free gingival margins of the mandibular anterior teeth.

Because of the importance of locating the exact position for the placement of the inferior border of the lingual bar, a periodontal probe should be used to measure the distance between the lingual free gingival margin of the mandibular anterior teeth and the tissues in the floor of the mouth. Because the tissues in the floor of the mouth should be recorded at their functional level, the tip of the patient's tongue should be elevated so that it touches the roof of the palate when these measurements are being made (see Fig. 3-22). These measurements should then be recorded on the diagnostic or master cast to indicate where the inferior border of the lingual bar should be placed (see Fig. 3-22).

Adequate relief must be provided between the lingual bar and the lingual mucoperiosteum if injury to the underlying tissues during function is to be avoided (Fig. 3-23). The amount of relief required will vary with the inclination or degree of undercut of the soft tissues lingual to the mandibular anterior teeth. Mandibular major connectors used on distal-extension RPDs require more relief than those on tooth-borne RPDs because of the potential for rotation of the distal-extension section, causing injury to the mucoperiosteum. Mandibular tori, provided that surgical procedures are contraindicated and a major connector is to be placed over them, also require additional relief. In mouths in which the lingual mucoperiosteum is inclined vertically, minimal relief (32 gauge) of the lingual bar major connector is all that is necessary. More than the usual relief is required where the soft tissues slope lingually. Depending on the angle of the incline, 26- to 28-gauge wax relief is usually required to provide the necessary amount of tissue clearance. Where the lingual soft tissues are undercut, no relief is required except to block out the undercut area.

LINGUOPLATE. The linguoplate major connector has the same structural requirements as the lingual bar, except that a thin metal plate is added to the superior portion of the bar and covers the lingual surfaces of the mandibular anterior teeth (see Fig. 2-17).

The linguoplate should be used in preference to the lingual bar only when there is a

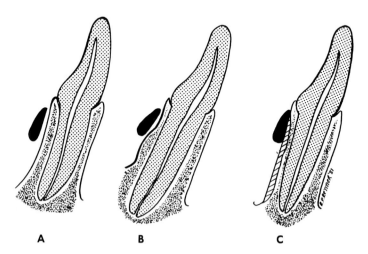

Fig. 3-23. Relief for mandibular major connectors. Generally, less relief is required for tooth-borne partial dentures. **A,** When lingual soft tissues slope toward floor of mouth, more than usual relief may be required. **B,** If lingual tori exist, there should be sufficient relief of major connector to avoid irritation of thin tissue that covers these tori. **C,** When lingual soft tissue is undercut, relief should be provided in undercut area only.

definite indication for its use. Some of these are:

1. When the floor of the mouth is shallow or gingival recession of the mandibular anterior teeth contraindicates the use of a lingual bar
2. When adequate rigidity cannot be obtained by the use of a lingual bar alone
3. When the mandibular posterior teeth have been lost and the major connector must be used to supply indirect retention on properly prepared anterior rest seats
4. When periodontally weakened mandibular anterior teeth require stabilization, that is, the linguoplate's use with the swing lock attachment (Antos and associates, 1978)
5. When extrusion of the mandibular anterior teeth must be prevented, in cases where rests are placed on the anterior teeth
6. When the future replacement of one or more mandibular anterior teeth is anticipated (Antos and associates, 1978)
7. When there is severe resorption of the residual ridges and a distal-extension RPD is to be constructed
8. When the prosthesis is to be constructed to circumvent covering mandibular tori
9. When the patient objects to a lingual bar

A linguoplate should be made as thin as possible, and it should duplicate the contours of the lingual surfaces of the mandibular anterior teeth and the interproximal embrasures. The superior border of the linguoplate should cover the cingula of the mandibular anterior teeth. The linguoplate should not be placed higher than the middle third of the teeth, except for the projections, which cover the interproximal spaces and extend up to the contact points of the teeth. It should have a scalloped appearance with sharp-pointed projections, and it should make intimate contact with the teeth. The linguoplate must be placed above the survey line on the teeth to avoid food entrapment. All areas below the survey line must be blocked out parallel to the path of insertion of the prosthesis, and the area of the free gingival margin must be relieved slightly (32-gauge wax) to avoid irritation. Proximal surfaces must also be blocked out to prevent wedging of the teeth. The linguoplate should be supported bi-

laterally, with either lingual or incisal rests on the canines or occlusal rests placed in the mesial fossae of the mandibular first premolars.

The linguoplate may be confined to the mandibular anterior teeth or it may also extend onto the posterior teeth (see Fig. 2-18). One reason to extend the linguoplate onto the lingual surfaces of the posterior teeth, in addition to the reasons for using a linguoplate on the mandibular anterior teeth, is to prevent food entrapment in the small spaces that sometimes exist between the lingual bar and other components of the RPD. The gingival tissues usually remain healthier if these spaces are covered with metal than if the small space is permitted to remain. Meticulous dental plaque control and adequate stimulation of the gingival tissues through daily oral physiotherapy procedures must be stressed during patient counseling if optimal health and preservation of the tissues covered by the linguoplate are to be achieved.

CONTINUOUS BAR (or Kennedy Bar). The continuous bar is another modification of the lingual bar major connector. However, instead of having a continuous plate cover the lingual surfaces of the mandibular anterior teeth, as does the linguoplate, it has a continuous bar that rests on the cingula of these teeth (see Fig. 2-19).

The continuous bar is used primarily in those mouths where periodontal disease has created large interproximal spaces between the mandibular anterior teeth with no mesial or distal contacts remaining and where the use of a linguoplate is indicated but would not be esthetically acceptable to the patient. Although this continuous bar is more rigid than a lingual bar, it is not as rigid as a linguoplate. Patients sometimes find not only that the space between the two bars tends to collect food, which causes gingival irritation, but also that the superior bar is often annoying to the tongue. For these reasons, a linguoplate is the preferred major connector, and the continuous bar should be used only when a linguoplate would not be esthetically acceptable.

SUBLINGUAL BAR. The sublingual bar (see Fig. 2-20) is an additional variation of the lingual bar major connector that is used fairly extensively in Europe, although its use in North America has been limited. The idea of placing a lingual bar at the floor of the mouth was first suggested to the dental profession by Tryde and Brantenberg in 1965. In essence the sublingual bar is structurally similar to a lingual bar, except that it is placed lower than a conventional lingual bar. The sublingual bar is placed in a functional, well-developed lingual sulcus impression, and it is designed to fill the entire registration of the lingual sulcus. These bars are well tolerated by patients, provided that the patient has a rounded lingual sulcus. When the lingual sulcus is flat, a sublingual bar cannot be used.

Minor connectors

Minor connectors are rigid structures or struts that arise from a major connector and join it with other parts of the RPD. They transfer vertical, horizontal, and torquing types of stresses between the abutment teeth and the supporting tissues of the edentulous area.

DESIGN CONSIDERATIONS. Like major connectors, minor connectors have basic design requirements (Figs. 3-24 through 3-30). Designs for minor connectors should ensure that there is 5 mm of space between adjacent vertical minor connectors to prevent food impaction. Minor connectors must contact the guiding plane surfaces of the teeth to facilitate a predictable path of placement for the components of the RPD and provide bracing, thus ensuring stability. Minor connectors should cross gingival tissues abruptly and join the major connector at rounded right angles. This allows them to cover as little of the gingival tissues as possible and to transmit the stresses of occlusion to the supporting rests.

Several design situations arise where it is impossible to space adjacent minor connectors the minimum of 5 mm apart and still comply with the other basic requirements of design. These situations generally occur in the maxillary or mandibular canine or premolar areas. Proper design in these cases can be achieved by covering (plating) the entire lingual surface of the tooth or teeth (see Fig. 2-18).

The minor connectors most commonly used to connect the denture base to the major connector are discussed below.

OPEN LATTICEWORK. Dunny and King (1975) found that the open latticework type of minor connector produced the greatest amount of retention for acrylic resin and that the larger the size of the openings, the greater the relative strength of the acrylic resin. When an open latticework is used to retain the acrylic resin denture base, the metal retention loops should extend to the buccal side of the crest of the residual ridge to provide maximal retention of the acrylic resin (see Fig. 2-22).

MESH. Mesh can be used interchangeably with an open latticework minor connector in

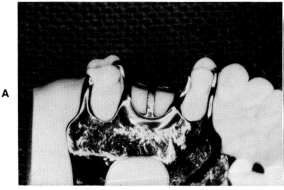 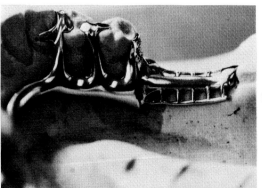

Fig. 3-24. Minor connector design considerations. Minor connectors should be rigid and strong enough to withstand masticatory stress and patient handling. **A,** They should be positioned in interproximal spaces to avoid tongue interference and should pass vertically from major connector to other components. They should be thickest toward lingual surface and taper toward contact area. (They should not be located on convex surfaces.) **B,** There should be a minimum of 5 mm of space between vertical minor connectors.

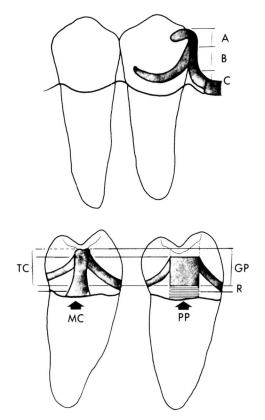

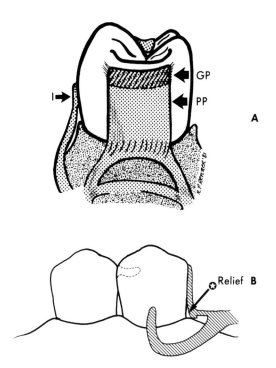

Fig. 3-25. Minor connectors that connect rests to major connectors and give rise to clasp arms should be tapered to tooth below origin of clasp. Minor connectors should contact guiding plane for a minimum of two thirds of crown's length, extending from rest to junction of middle and gingival thirds of crown. *A,* Occlusal third; *B,* middle third; *C,* gingival third; *TC,* tooth contact; *GP,* guiding plane; *R,* relief; *MC,* minor connector with clasp and rest; *PP,* proximal plate minor connector.

Fig. 3-26. A, Minor connectors that do not connect rests (proximal plates) should contact guiding plane surfaces of abutment teeth for a minimum of two thirds of crown's length, extending from below marginal ridge area to junction of middle and gingival thirds of crown. Superior edge of these proximal plates should not extend above occlusal surface of teeth. *GP,* Guiding plane; *PP,* proximal plate; *I,* I-bar retentive arm. **B,** An undercut should exist below guiding plane to prevent strangulation of free gingival tissues.

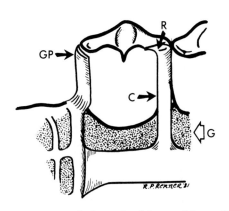

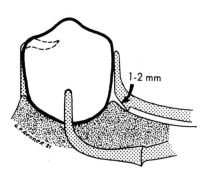

Fig. 3-27. Proximal plates should extend lingually far enough so that, together with minor connector that supports the rest, they will prevent lingual migration of tooth. This extension is generally located at junction of lingual and proximal surfaces of tooth. *GP,* Guiding plane; *G,* gingival tissue; *R,* rest; *C,* minor connector on lingual surface of the tooth.

Fig. 3-28. Minor connector including proximal plate should extend 1 to 2 mm onto mucosal surface next to abutment to facilitate proper placement of finishing line. Metal that extends onto residual ridge and serves as means of attachment for acrylic resin should be designed so that it will not interfere with tooth arrangement but will be strong enough to support and retain acrylic resin. Tissue stops used on extension base partial dentures are designed to hold free end of frame in position while acrylic resin is packed in flask.

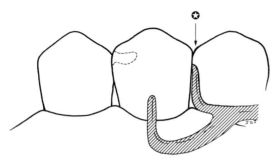

Fig. 3-29. When denture tooth is to be placed against minor connector, it should contact abutment tooth with only a thin layer of minor connector's metal intervening. Greatest bulk of metal should be located toward lingual aspect of abutment tooth.

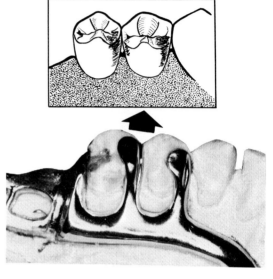

Fig. 3-30. When minor connectors contact tooth surfaces on either side of embrasure, they should be tapered to teeth and contact only prepared tooth surfaces. When 5 mm of horizontal clearance between minor connectors cannot be achieved, area should be plated.

any given clinical situation. However, with mesh, because of the small size of the openings between the metal, the strength of the attachment of the acrylic resin is reduced in comparison to that achieved with the open latticework type of minor connector. Therefore, the routine use of mesh is not recommended (see Fig. 2-23).

METAL BASE. Because of the large amount of metal contacting the residual ridge, metal base minor connectors are considered better able to promote tissue health and should be used extensively for residual ridge areas that are well healed and have abutment teeth on both sides of the edentulous space (see Fig. 2-24). Bead-type mechanical retention on the metal base minor connector provides better retention for the acrylic resin and interferes less with tooth arrangement than either "nailhead" or loop-type mechanical retention. Although bead-type mechanical retention provides less retention for the acrylic resin than either the open latticework or mesh, clinically it functions adequately. When a metal base minor connector is used over the residual ridge areas of an RPD, relining is difficult if not impossible. Therefore, a metal denture base is generally not used to cover distal-extension edentulous areas or tooth-supported edentulous areas where relining of the denture base in the future is anticipated.

FINISHING LINES. Finishing lines should be placed on the cast metal framework of all three types of minor connectors wherever the acrylic

resin joins the cast framework, both on the tissue surface (internal finishing line) as well as on the polished surface (external finishing line), specifically at the junction of the denture base and the major connector. The external finishing line on the polished surface of the framework (Fig. 3-31) should form an acute angle so that it creates a slight undercut in the metal. The internal finishing line on the tissue surface of the framework (Fig. 3-32) is formed by placing a layer of 24-gauge relief wax on the edentulous area of the master cast before making the refractory cast.

Using strain gauges to measure the stresses on the major connectors during function, Sekine and associates (1965) found that the greatest stress was concentrated at the junction of the mandibular lingual bar major connector and the denture base. Although the stresses on maxillary major connectors are somewhat varied in comparison to those on the mandibular, the same factors that cause stress to be concentrated at the junction of the major connector and the denture base in the mandible could cause stress to be concentrated on a similar area in the maxilla. Therefore, when finishing lines are placed on a framework, they should

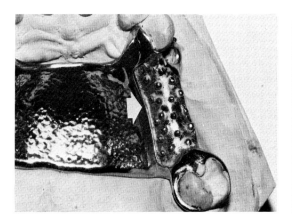

Fig. 3-31. Finishing line should be placed on metal framework wherever acrylic resin comes in contact with major connector. Finishing line on polished surface of RPD framework should form acute angle so that it creates slight undercut in metal.

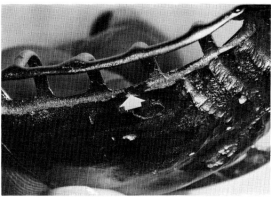

Fig. 3-32. Finishing line on tissue surface of RPD framework is formed by placing 24-gauge relief wax on saddle area of master cast before making refractory cast.

not be placed directly above one another but should be offset slightly so as not to jeopardize the strength or cause possible fracture of the cast framework in the area where the greatest amount of stress is concentrated. Finishing lines should provide a butt joint of sufficient bulk for the acrylic resin. Tissue-surface finishing lines should be located furthest away from the abutment tooth.

Providing retention

The next phase of the systematic approach to design is to decide how the RPD is to be retained. Retention is defined as resistance to dislodgement in an occlusal direction. This definition should be viewed in proper perspective. Retention must be provided so that the remaining teeth and their supporting structures are not subjected to excessive trauma from the prosthesis. To achieve this, it is essential not only to provide adequate support but also to ensure that the prosthesis is stable and will resist reasonable dislodging forces. There are two generally accepted means by which retention is achieved: *tissue seal* and *mechanical retention*. Tissue seal comes from the denture base, and its effectiveness is related to the amount of denture-bearing area covered by the denture base and the intimacy of the denture borders' contact with the underlying or adjacent tissues. Mechanical retention comes from direct retainers—clasp assemblies, attachments, or other

mechanical devices applied to the abutment teeth to hold an RPD in a predetermined position and to resist its movement away from the supporting tissues. Basically, there are two types of direct retainers: intracoronal and extracoronal.

Intracoronal direct retainers (precision or internal attachments)

An intracoronal direct retainer consists of a metal receptacle and a closely fitting male part that fits into the receptacle; the former is usually contained within the normal or expanded contours of an abutment tooth crown, and the latter is attached to the RPD framework (see Fig. 2-31). Retention of the RPD against dislodging forces is created through frictional resistance between the vertical walls of the receptacle and the closely fitting part on the prosthesis.

Intracoronal direct retainers have several advantages over extracoronal direct retainers. They are more esthetic because retention is obtained through frictional resistance and not by visible retentive arms located around the tooth contours. They provide for more effective cross-arch stabilization of the abutment teeth. They direct the vertical forces of occlusion more nearly through the long axes of the abutment teeth because their rest seats are located within the contours of the abutment teeth and closer to the horizontal axes of rotation.

However, intracoronal direct retainers also have several disadvantages and limitations that severely compromise their use clinically:

1. They require the placement of cast restorations on the abutment teeth, which limits their use for many patients. Because the retentive effectiveness of this type of retainer is directly proportional to its length, its use is contraindicated on short teeth.
2. They should not be placed on teeth with large pulps, because the amount of tooth structure required to be removed so that normal anatomic contours can be developed on the cast restoration in which the attachments are placed might result in pulp exposure.
3. They frequently tend to loosen during use, with a resultant loss of retention and increased torquing stress to the teeth.
4. The clinical and laboratory procedures required for their construction are complicated and complex.
5. They are expensive and difficult to repair, reline, or replace.

Intracoronal retainers are similiar in design to internal rests. Their use is therefore contraindicated on distal-extension RPDs unless an effective type of stress-breaking device is used between the denture base and the intracoronal retainer. A stress-breaking device is necessary in this clinical situation to relieve the abutment teeth of all or part of the torquing forces exerted on them by the movable distal-extension denture base.

Dental manufacturers of precious metals have made a most valuable contribution to dentistry by the development and manufacture of a wide variety of intracoronal retainers. They not only have developed the technology for these retainers, but also have provided excellent descriptive literature and technique manuals (see Fig. 2-31, *A* and *B*) that describe their use.

Extracoronal direct retainers (clasp assemblies)

A clasp assembly is that part of an RPD which acts as a retainer, stabilizer, or both for the prosthesis by partially encircling or contacting the abutment tooth. Most RPDs fabricated in clinical practice today derive their retention from the use of extracoronal rather than intra-

coronal retainers. In light of this fact, the term *direct retainer* hereinafter refers to extracoronal retainers (clasps) specifically.

This section identifies and discusses the various types of direct retainers and the situations that indicate their use, demonstrates their proper structural design, and explains why they might be selected for a particular situation. It is of paramount importance in this section on direct retainers to remember that we are referring to retention against reasonable dislodging forces.

Basically, there are three categories of extracoronal direct retainers: circumferential (suprabulge) clasps, bar (infrabulge) clasps, combination (circumferential and bar, cast and wrought wire) clasps.

REQUIREMENTS OF A CLASP. Every clasp, regardless of its type, must satisfy certain requirements if it is to perform its designated functions. These basic requirements are:

1. Support
2. Bracing (stabilization)
3. Retention
4. Reciprocation
5. Encirclement (more than 180 degrees)
6. Passivity

These design requirements are discussed individually so that the reader will understand why each clasp must satisfy them in order to perform its designated functions.

SUPPORT. Support for any clasp assembly is provided by its associated rest, whether it is on the occlusal, cingulum, or incisal surface of the abutment tooth. The purpose of the rest is to hold the direct retainer in its designated terminal position. This is most important, because if the direct retainer is to have a predictable effect during function, its components must be held in their specifically designed position on the tooth. By holding the clasp assembly in its designated terminal position, the rest prevents the prosthesis from moving tissueward and impinging on the periodontal structures and residual ridge. The rest, because of its design and location, assists in transferring occlusal forces and the forces generated from the movement of the distal-extension base to the abutment teeth (Fig. 3-33).

BRACING. Bracing, or stabilization, for any direct retainer is provided by the rigid components on the prosthesis, such as the minor connectors and bracing arms of the clasp assembly.

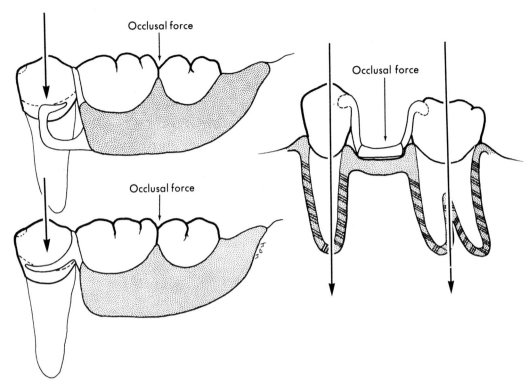

Fig. 3-33. Rest supports clasp assembly by holding it in its designated terminal position. This supporting component transfers and directs stresses to long axis of abutment tooth when an occluding force is exerted on RPD and prevents clasp assembly from moving tissueward and irritating supporting periodontal structures.

Their purpose is to resist or to transfer the horizontal or torquing forces that result from occlusion and rotational movements of the RPD base, to the supporting abutment teeth (Fig. 3-34). This is a most important aspect of prosthesis design, because it is the torquing or horizontal forces that are potentially the most damaging to the abutment teeth.

RETENTION. Retention, or resistance to dislodgement, is provided by the retentive arm of a clasp assembly's engaging an undercut area on the abutment tooth (Fig. 3-35). For a retentive arm to engage an undercut area, it must flex (or distort) as it passes over the height of contour of the abutment tooth into an infrabulge area (see Fig. 2-36).

The amount of retention a retentive arm provides is dependent on three factors: the angle of cervical convergence of the undercut area, the depth to which the retentive arm extends into the angle of cervical convergence, and the resiliency of the retentive arm.

1. Angle of cervical convergence of the un-

dercut area. The greater the angle of cervical convergence, the more the retentive arm must flex as it enters or leaves the undercut on the abutment tooth (see Fig. 2-36).

2. Depth to which the retentive arm extends into the angle of cervical convergence. The greater the depth to which the retentive arm is placed into the angle of cervical convergence, the more the arm must flex as it engages or disengages from the undercut.

3. Resiliency of the retentive arm. The resiliency of the retentive arm depends on:
   a. The diameter of the retentive arm. The smaller the diameter of the retentive arm, the more resilient it will be.
   b. The length of the retentive arm. The longer the retentive arm, the more resilient it will be. A retentive arm should never approach the undercut area in a straight line (see Fig. 2-38). The resiliency of the retentive arm

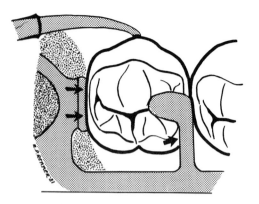

Fig. 3-34. Bracing components are minor connectors and rigid parts of clasp arm that contact prepared tooth surfaces and serve to transfer horizontal and torquing forces to supporting abutment teeth *(arrows)*. These components must contact specifically designed areas of tooth to control these potentially damaging forces.

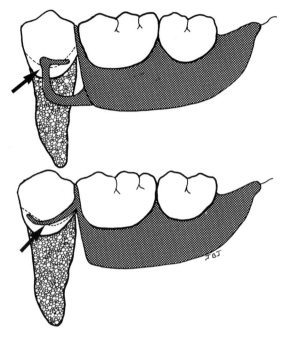

Fig. 3-35. Retentive component is flexible portion of clasp assembly. Ability of clasp assembly to resist dislodging forces is determined by its type of metal, its length, its cross-sectional form, its resistance to deformation, and its contour and by location and depth of undercut.

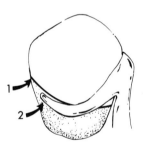

Fig. 3-36. Retentive clasp arm should be curved to increase its length. Tip should point occlusally and be round and smooth. Clasp arm should extend to mesial or distal proximal line angle of tooth. Retentive tip should be at a right angle to dislodging force. *1,* Height of contour (survey line); *2,* retentive terminal.

should be increased, whenever possible, by curving the arm to increase its length. The tip of the retentive arm should be round and smooth. It should always point occlusally; that is, the retentive tip should be at a right angle to the occlusal dislodging force and extend to the mesial or distal proximal line angle of the abutment tooth (Fig. 3-36).

c. The taper of the retentive arm. The retentive arm should taper uniformly from the body to the tip so that it is approximately half the thickness at the tip as it is at its attachment to the body of the clasp assembly.

d. The shape of the retentive arm. A round retentive arm, such as a wrought wire arm (18-gauge platinum-gold-palladium [PGP] wire), can flex in all directions, whereas a half-round retentive arm (most cast arms) will flex only in a buccolingual direction.

e. The type of metal of the retentive arm. Chromium alloys are less resilient than dental gold alloys of the same diameter because of their metallurgic properties. The retentive arm of a chromium alloy clasp assembly therefore does not need to extend as deeply into an undercut area to pro-

vide the same degree of retention as would a retentive arm made of dental gold alloy. An undercut area of 0.01 inch usually will provide adequate retention for chromium alloy clasp assemblies, whereas a 0.02-inch undercut is required for a comparable dental gold alloy retentive arm. A 0.03-inch undercut is usually required for long wrought wire (such as, 18-gauge PGP) retentive arms.

Because the retentive arm of a clasp assembly must flex when the prosthesis is inserted or withdrawn from the mouth or when it resists the variety of dislodging forces acting on the prosthesis, its resistance to deformation will transmit both horizontal and rotational forces to the abutment tooth. These forces are potentially destructive to the supporting structures if they are not adequately controlled. The dentist should make every effort to reduce, as much as possible, dependence on large amounts of clasp retention and to develop to their fullest in the prosthesis the more favorable qualities of support, stabilization, and reciprocation. These qualities of a clasp assembly tend to minimize the effect of the horizontal and rotational forces exerted on the abutment teeth by the retentive arms on the prosthesis. An RPD should therefore be designed with rigid major and minor connectors and reciprocal components. Rests should be used in sufficient numbers and locations to provide adequate support for the prosthesis. Guiding planes should be created on the abutment teeth wherever possible to develop a definite path of insertion and withdrawal of the RPD. Denture bases should be maximally extended and in intimate tissue contact so that they can use as much available support and provide as much retention for the prosthesis as possible. If these qualities are properly developed on the RPD, then a minimal amount of direct retention is usually required to resist the dislodging forces that act on it.

RECIPROCATION. The reciprocation requirement for any direct retainer is generally provided by its rigid components, such as minor connectors and bracing arms. One of their purposes is to oppose horizontal forces transmitted to the abutment tooth by the retentive tip of the retentive arm during insertion and withdrawal of the prosthesis. In reality, these forces are probably very transient because of the minimal amount of time required by the patient to insert or remove the prosthesis. In all probability, these components contribute more to bracing and stabilization than to reciprocation. A secondary function of these components,

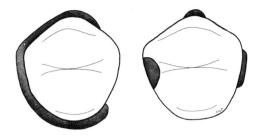

Fig. 3-37. Encirclement is provided by entire clasp assembly, which contacts tooth surface for more than 180 degrees of its circumference or by three widely separated contact points that provide tripoding effect. Encirclement prevents tooth from moving away from clasp assembly or prevents clasp assembly from slipping off tooth surface when it is subject to vertical, horizontal or torquing forces.

however, is to prevent tooth movement from overadjustment of the clasp.

ENCIRCLEMENT (more than 180 degrees). The requirement of encirclement simply relates to the amount of surface contact that a direct retainer should have with the abutment tooth. Encirclement is provided for by the clasp assembly. It is needed to prevent the tooth from moving away from the direct retainer or to prevent the direct retainer from slipping off the tooth. By having the direct retainer contact the abutment tooth for more than 180 degrees of its circumference, this requirement can be satisfied. Encirclement can also be accomplished if a minimum of three-point contact to the tooth in a tripoding effect (as in an RPI-type clasp assembly) is accomplished by the components of the direct retainer (Fig. 3-37).

PASSIVITY. Passivity is satisfied when the components of the clasp are in their terminal position and there is no active force being exerted on the abutment tooth. Any active force exerted on the tooth when the direct retainer is in its terminal position could cause damage to the periodontal ligament and possible unplanned orthodontic movement of the abutment tooth (Fig. 3-38).

POSITION OF CLASP ASSEMBLY COMPONENTS ON THE ABUTMENT TOOTH. For any direct retainer to function as designed, it must fulfill the basic requirements described above. However, the direct retainer can fulfill these requirements and function properly only if its components are properly contoured and positioned on

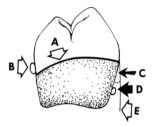

Fig. 3-38. Components of clasp assembly must be designed and placed on tooth surfaces in such a manner that when they are in their terminal position, there will be no active force exerted on abutment tooth. *A,* Height of contour; *B,* reciprocal clasp arm; *C,* angle of cervical convergence; *D,* retentive clasp arm; *E,* path of insertion. The greater the angle of cervical convergence, the more clasp arm must flex as it enters or leaves undercut.

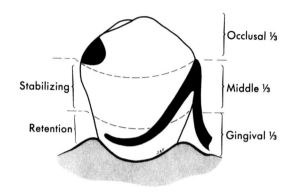

Fig. 3-39. Proper position of components of clasp assembly on tooth.

the abutment teeth (see Figs. 2-37 and 3-39). The *rest,* which provides the function of support, should be positioned on the occlusal or incisal surface or on the cingulum area of the tooth. The *bracing component,* which performs the functions of stabilization, reciprocation, and encirclement, should be positioned at the junction of the middle and gingival thirds of the abutment tooth. The *retentive component,* which performs the function of resisting minimal dislodging forces in an occlusal direction, should be located in the gingival third of the abutment tooth and positioned sufficiently away from the free gingival margin so that it will not interfere with or cause injury to the gingival tissues.

GENERAL RULES CONCERNING CLASP RETENTION

1. A clasp assembly should be designed so that only one retentive arm is used on an abutment tooth. The retentive arm should be opposed by a reciprocal component of the clasp assembly on the opposite side of the abutment tooth at a similar level.
2. An abutment tooth that has a definite taper occlusally on which the reciprocal component of the clasp assembly is located should be recontoured or restored to provide for a vertical surface to oppose the retentive arm if adequate bracing for the retentive arm is to be achieved.

3. If a buccal retentive arm is used on one side of the dental arch, it should also be used on the opposite side of the dental arch. The same principle should apply to the use of a lingual retentive arm.
4. Buccal retention on premolars is usually preferable to lingual retention, because the retentive arm can be made longer and more flexible. Either buccal or lingual retention is used on molars because of both the longer retentive arm length on molars and their surface morphologic features and axial inclination.
5. The clasp assembly design selected for an abutment tooth should be based on the location and depth of the available undercut area on the abutment tooth.
6. A retentive arm located on an abutment tooth adjacent to an edentulous area on a distal-extension RPD has varying amounts of retention, which are dependent on the amount and location of the undercut.
7. Retentive and reciprocal clasp arms should be placed as far gingivally on the abutment tooth as possible and in conformity with the height of the survey line of the tooth. They should not interfere with the free gingival margin.
8. Complicated clasp assembly designs should be avoided.

LOCATION OF THE RETENTIVE AREAS. Location of the retentive areas is probably the most important single factor in clasp selection. Location of retentive areas by surveying should precede the selection of the type of direct retainer and should be evaluated by analysis of

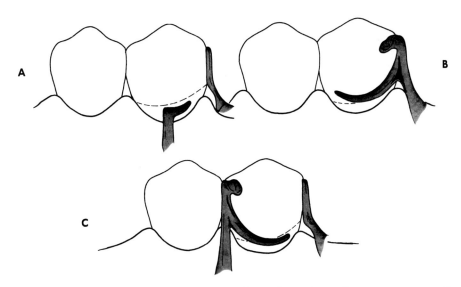

Fig. 3-40. A, Class II survey line with correct clasp relationship and contour to survey line. **B,** Class II survey line where components cannot be properly contoured or related to survey line. **C,** Class II survey line where components have been modified to relate properly to survey line with proper contour.

the different vectors and magnitudes of force that will tend to dislodge the RPD in an occlusal direction. The objective in placing retentive units is to help control the force and direction of the RPD's movement in response to reasonable dislodging forces and to do it so that the teeth, their supporting structures, and other components of the stomatognathic system will not be damaged. Some guidelines for location of the retentive area are:

1. The closer the retentive area to the edentulous area, the greater the potential of retention.
2. Retentive areas should be located as widely separated as possible throughout the remaining natural teeth in the dental arch to provide equalized retention and stability to the RPD.
3. Wherever possible, retentive areas on one side of the dental arch should be opposed by similar retentive areas on the opposite side of the dental arch (similar in depth and location on the abutment tooth surface).

Location of the retentive areas as a factor in clasp design cannot be overstressed. For example, in Fig. 3-40, the retentive area is located on the buccal surface of the abutment tooth adjacent to the edentulous area. It would be impossible to place the components of a cir-

cumferential clasp (Class I, or Akers) in their proper position on the abutment tooth if a distal occlusal rest were indicated as the tooth support unit. The bracing component of the direct retainer would be well above the junction of the middle and gingival thirds, which would induce excessive lateral or torquing stress to the abutment tooth during function. If a circumferential clasp were the clasp of choice in this situation, the dentist would have to modify its basic design so that the retentive arm could approach the undercut area from the mesial aspect of the tooth as opposed to the distal aspect. An alternative to this choice would be to modify the contour of the tooth by mouth preparation or to select a different type of direct retainer. In Fig. 3-41, the retentive area is located on the buccal surface of the abutment tooth away from the edentulous area. A better solution would be to place the components of a circumferential clasp in their proper position on the abutment tooth if a distal occlusal rest were indicated as the tooth support unit. In Fig. 3-42, the retentive area is located in the occlusal third of the buccal surface of the abutment tooth. In this situation, it would be impossible to place the components of a circumferential clasp in their proper position on the abutment tooth regardless of whether the mesial or distal occlusal rest were indicated as the tooth support unit. When the survey line does not permit use of the desired clasp form, the abutment tooth should be modified by simple selective grinding procedures or by placing a restoration to acheive the desired contours, which allow the components of the clasp to be placed in their proper location on the abutment tooth.

Having identified specific requirements that each direct retainer must satisfy if it is to function predictably, the dentist can turn to answering the question of why a particular direct retainer should be selected.

Clasp design and stress control

It was pointed out earlier in this chapter that the dentist's primary consideration in clasp se-

lection is the control of stress on the abutment teeth (Fig. 3-43). The location of the rests and the position of the minor connectors as they relate to the guiding planes are primary factors in stress control. Figs. 3-44 and 3-45 demonstrate that stresses transferred to the abutment tooth by the tissueward movement of a distal-extension RPD are controlled through the occlusal rest and the rigid minor connectors. On a direct retainer with a rest adjacent to the edentulous area, vertical forces are directed down the long axis of the tooth through the rest. Rotational stresses are directed around the dental arch by the contact of the minor connector and the guiding planes. The point of rotation occurs at the area where the minor connector breaks contact with the proximal tooth surface (Fig. 3-46). When the extension base lifts away from the supporting tissue, the retentive arm of the clasp assembly engages the retentive area and the proximal minor connector supporting the rest leans against the guiding plane or is forced to move occlusally on the guiding plane. These two activities of the components of the direct retainer assist in retaining the prosthesis against minimal dislodging forces while minimizing or controlling the stress. On a direct retainer where the rest is located on the cingulum or the incisal surface adjacent to the edentulous area and the retentive component is located on the side of the tooth adjacent to the edentulous area, a similar situation occurs.

On direct retainers (RPI type) where the rest is located on the occlusal, incisal, or cingulum surface away from the extension base area and the minor connector (in the form of a proximal

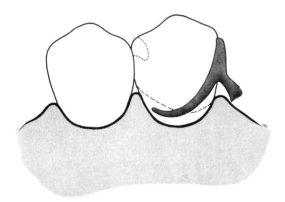

Fig. 3-41. Class I survey line with correct clasp relationship and contour.

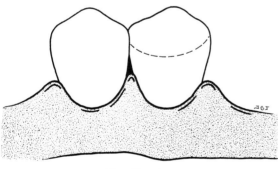

Class III undercut

Fig. 3-42. Class III survey line. It is impossible to place standard circumferential clasp assembly in proper relationship to survey line and provide proper contour without potentially exerting excessive tilting or torquing stresses on tooth.

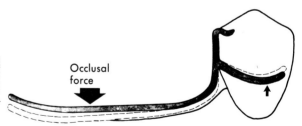

Occlusal force

Fig. 3-43. Occluding forces on extension base, resulting in stress and trauma to abutment tooth.

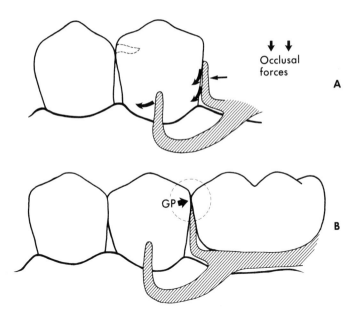

Fig. 3-44. A, Resultant movement of bar clasp assembly where only 1 mm of proximal plate contacts guiding plane. **B,** Artificial denture tooth placed so that it contacts guiding plane. Under occluding force, this contact acts as extension of minor connector and eliminates any stress release action. *GP,* guiding plane.

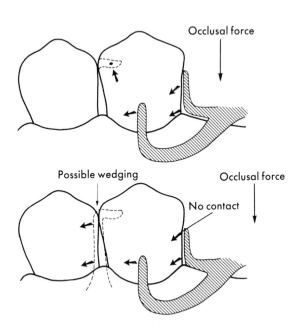

Fig. 3-45. With no contact of RPD assembly adjacent to edentulous area, horizontal and torquing forces from occlusion will be transferred to mesial rest. Wedging stresses could result, depending on amount of movement and contact of minor connector supporting rest on proximal surfaces of teeth.

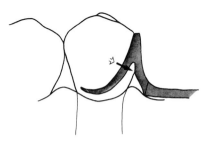

Fig. 3-46. Fulcrum (point of rotation) is relocated to area where minor connector breaks contact with prepared guiding plane.

plate) contacts the proximal surface adjacent to the edentulous base area, the amount of contact between the proximal plate and the proximal surface of the tooth determines where the rotation of the entire direct retainer is to occur. In situations where the proximal plate contacts only 1 mm of the top of the guiding plane, an occlusal force can cause the proximal plate to disengage from the guiding plane (Fig. 3-44). The retentive terminus of the retainer will move mesiogingivally, and rotation of the prosthesis will occur in the area of the mesial rest. Often, however, this stress release action is negated by the denture tooth's being ground into the abutment tooth and thus prolonging the contact with the guiding plane. To properly achieve the stress release action indicated by this direct retainer, there can be no contact of the denture tooth with the guiding plane on the abutment tooth. Incorporation of this design characteristic can result in impaction of food particles in the space created between the denture tooth and the abutment tooth and possible irritation to the underlying gingival tissues. Another problem associated with this design concept is the potential of "wedging" stresses' being transmitted to the abutment tooth by the contact of the minor connector supporting the mesial rest (Fig. 3-45). If tissue displacement or residual ridge reduction occurs in the area of the edentulous base so that the proximal plate no longer contacts the guiding plane, or if the occluding force results in the proximal plate's disengaging from the guiding plane, then rotation will occur around the mesial rest. If the minor connector supporting the mesial rest is in contact with the proximal tooth surface of the abutment tooth or the adjacent tooth, a wedging effect will be created, there will be no component of the RPD to maintain dental arch integrity, and the abutment tooth will be wedged posteriorly.

A second design philosophy is to extend the proximal plate the entire length of the proximal tooth surface with minimal relief to eliminate impingement on the free gingival margin (Fig. 3-47). If the tissue change in the extension base area exceeds the amount of relief provided, impingement on the free gingival margin adjacent to the edentulous base area can result. This philosophy provides for placing the rotation point as low as possible on the abutment tooth.

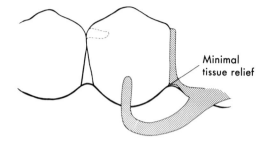

Fig. 3-47. Bar clasp assembly where proximal plate extends entire length of proximal surface of tooth on a prepared guiding plane with minimal tissue relief to eliminate impingement on free gingival margin at time of insertion of prosthesis.

Patient control is the key to implementation of this philosophy, since patient motivation and routine follow-up procedures are mandatory to prevent damage to the free gingival margin should there be any settling of the distal-extension base.

A more practical approach is the one suggested in this chapter, in which the proximal plate minor connector contacts the proximal tooth surface adjacent to the edentulous base area from just below the marginal ridge area to the junction of the middle and gingival thirds of the abutment tooth. This allows the proximal plate in the area of the gingival tissues to move in a nearly horizontal direction at an advantageous point close to the root-supported area of the tooth. Horizontal forces are transmitted through the remainder of the dental arch by virtue of arch integrity. The key to stress control is the position of the rest and the contact of the minor connector with the proximal tooth surface.

Clasp selection

The key to successful clasp selection is to select a direct retainer that will control tipping and torquing forces on the abutment teeth, provide retention against reasonable dislodging forces, and be compatible with tooth and tissue contours and the esthetic desires of the patient. These criteria are generally satisfied if the direct retainer is properly contoured and the components are properly positioned on the abutment tooth. Location of the retentive areas is the single most important factor in selecting the design of the retentive component of the clasp assembly.

The choice of a clasp cannot be made by using any general rule but by determining the amount of retention needed and where the available retentive areas are located on the abutment teeth. Additional factors to be considered are how tipping and torquing of the abutment teeth can best be avoided; how adequate stabilization can be provided; and whether the clasp design selected is compatible with the tooth and supporting tissues, esthetic demands, and the need for easy adjustment and repair. The ideal is to design a direct retainer that will provide sufficient retention to retain the RPD adequately without placing undue stress on the abutment teeth and that will be compatible with the teeth and supporting tissues, the esthetic demands, and the need for easy adjustment and repair.

Types of clasps

There have been numerous clasp assembly designs proposed for use in RPD construction. Many of these clasp assembly designs are complicated and have little practical value because they have been designed for use where the form of the abutment teeth presents a compromised situation. It is usually better to avoid the use of unusual designs by placing restorations on the abutment teeth to create favorable tooth contours that are compatible with simple clasp assembly designs. The clasp assemblies described are therefore limited to the simple and most commonly used designs, which can be divided into three basic types:

1. Circumferential clasp assemblies, where the retentive arm approaches the retentive undercut area from above the survey line (occlusal direction)
2. Bar clasp assemblies, where the retentive arm approaches the undercut area from below the survey line (gingival direction)
3. Combination clasp assemblies, which are a combination or modification of the first two types (see p. 75)

CIRCUMFERENTIAL CLASPS

CAST CIRCUMFERENTIAL (Akers, or Class I) Clasp (see Fig. 2-37)

Support: Excellent

Bracing: Excellent (bilateral)

Retention: Good (0.01- to 0.02-inch undercut)

Reciprocity: Good to excellent

Encirclement: Excellent

Passivity: Excellent

Design considerations. The cast circumferential clasp is the most logical clasp to use with a tooth-supported prosthesis where strong abutment teeth are present (Blatterfein, 1951; Steffel, 1968). This direct retainer provides a simple design that can reduce the stress to the residual ridge and more than adequately satisfy the basic requirements of a clasp. It is best suited for situations in which the retentive area is located on the buccal or lingual tooth surface away from the edentulous area. Many dentists have expressed concern regarding the stress that this clasp design places on the abutment teeth when it is used to retain a distal-extension RPD (Kratochvil, 1963, 1971; Krol, 1973a). The clasp is often pictured as traumatizing abutment teeth when used adjacent to a long-span, distal-extension edentulous area. If the minor connectors that support the rests contact the prepared guiding planes properly, the fulcrum, or rotation point, under occluding forces changes to the area where the minor connector breaks contact with the tooth (Fig. 3-47) instead of at the rest as was previously assumed. If the rest, the minor connector, and the guiding plane are properly designed, vertical stress should be transferred down the long axis of the tooth through the rest and horizontal stress transferred to the abutment tooth at the junction of its middle and gingival thirds. This horizontal stress should be dissipated throughout the dental arch. Some legitimate complaints about this direct retainer are that it covers a large area of tooth structure, thereby increasing the risk of dental caries development; that it is considered by some to be unesthetic; that it is difficult to adjust; and that its retention is somewhat less than the bar clasps. The most probable cause of failure of this type of direct retainer is improper application of its design (Fig. 3-48).

RING CLASP (Fig. 3-49)

Support: Excellent

Bracing: Excellent

Retention: Good (0.01- to 0.02-inch undercut)

Reciprocation: Good to excellent

Encirclement: Excellent

Passivity: Good

Design considerations. A ring clasp is used

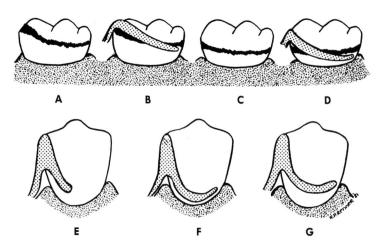

Fig. 3-48. Improper application of design for circumferential clasp. **A,** Tooth with Class III survey line. **B,** Parts of clasp assembly not in their proper positions on tooth. **C,** Survey line corrected to Class I. **D,** Correct clasp contour **E,** Straight clasp arm is less flexible and is not contoured to resist dislodging force in an occlusal direction. Curved arm is more flexible. **F,** Clasp arm is too close to free gingival tissues, which may cause food impaction. **G,** Clasp arm is properly contoured to free gingival tissue.

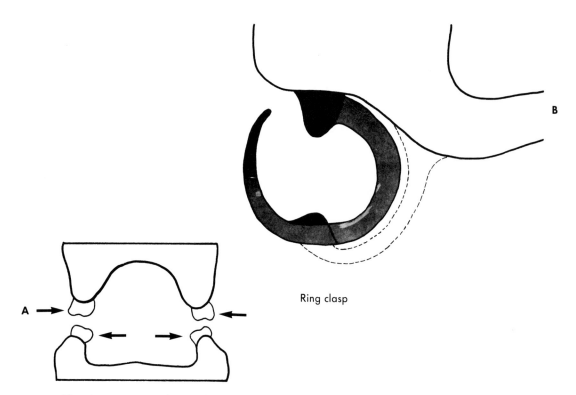

Ring clasp

Fig. 3-49. *A,* Use of ring clasp. *B,* Buccally tipped maxillary molar and lingually tipped mandibular molar.

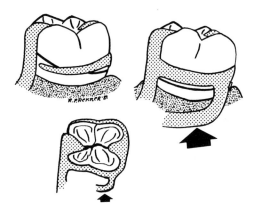

Fig. 3-50. Ring clasps can be used with or without auxiliary rest, but they should always have second minor connector attached to clasp assembly *(arrows)* to increase rigidity of clasp.

when the location of the undercut is incompatible with other types of circumferential clasp designs. In particular, this situation may arise when maxillary molars are tipped buccally or mandibular molars are tipped lingually. A ring clasp should always have a minor connector attached to the primary rest and a second minor connector attached to the clasp assembly on the opposite proximal surface of the tooth (Fig. 3-50). Failure to provide this second minor connector would leave the entire direct retainer arm unsupported and could result in uncontrolled horizontal and torquing stresses' being transferred to the abutment tooth or to fracture of the retainer arm. The ring clasp can also be used with or without an auxiliary rest, which can be attached to this minor connector. Because this direct retainer contacts a large amount of tooth surface, the abutment tooth designed to receive this type of clasp ideally should be protected with a cast restoration in an individual susceptible to dental caries.

BACK-ACTION CLASP (Fig. 3-51)

Support: Fair to poor

Bracing: Poor

Retention: Good

Reciprocation: Poor

Encirclement: Fair to poor

Passivity: Fair to poor

Design considerations. The back-action clasp is designed to be used on teeth that have either small retentive areas or excessive buccal tilting. Because of the length of the retentive arm, some dentists feel that this clasp produces a stress-breaking effect on the abutment tooth

when used with a distal-extension RPD. A close evaluation of this direct retainer demonstrates that it is similar to an unsupported ring clasp, which might easily be distorted because of the length of the clasp arm. The unsupported arm can allow excessive buccal force to be transmitted to the abutment tooth under masticatory stress. The design itself produces some additional problems in that there must be sufficient clearance between the clasp arm and the acrylic resin denture base for the clasp to function as intended. This space can easily become an area of food entrapment unless the denture tooth is hollow ground to allow the retentive arm to pass through.

The use of this clasp should be limited to natural teeth in which recontouring cannot produce the contours necessary for another type of direct retainer and in which the retentive area is located in the gingival third of the facial surface of the abutment tooth. For the clasp to function as intended by the dentist, it is necessary to maintain integrity of the dental arch by hollow grinding the denture tooth adjacent to the primary abutments.

EMBRASURE CLASP (Fig. 3-52)

Support: Excellent

Bracing: Excellent

Retention: Good to excellent (0.01- to 0.02-inch undercut)

Reciprocation: Good to excellent

Encirclement: Excellent

Passivity: Good

Design considerations. The embrasure clasp might be considered in situations in which there is a need to distribute the occlusal support, bracing, and retention to several abutment teeth. In particular, this situation arises in unilateral distal-extension RPDs in which there is a specific need for cross-arch bracing in addition to support and retention. The dentist must constantly be aware of the design problems associated with the use of this direct retainer. This design allows the use of a double rest (transocclusal rest) for increased support. However, without proper tooth preparation, the minor connector that connects to this rest may exert a wedging effect on the abutment teeth (see Chapter 5). It is also important that there be sufficient occlusal clearance with the teeth in the opposing dental arch and that the teeth that are to receive the rests are properly prepared to provide sufficient bulk of metal to

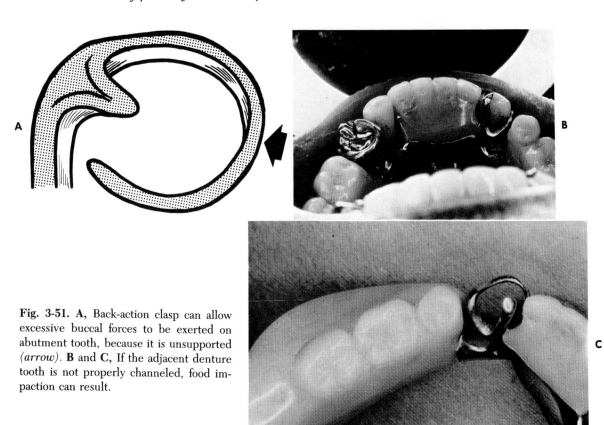

Fig. 3-51. A, Back-action clasp can allow excessive buccal forces to be exerted on abutment tooth, because it is unsupported *(arrow)*. **B** and **C,** If the adjacent denture tooth is not properly channeled, food impaction can result.

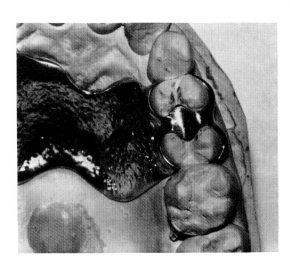

Fig. 3-52. Embrasure clasp can provide additional support through use of double rest and increased bracing because it employs two bracing arms. Retention is increased because clasp employs two retentive arms, which should be located contralaterally (both on either buccal or lingual surfaces of abutments) or diagonally (retentive arm on buccal surface of one abutment and on lingual surface of adjacent abutment).

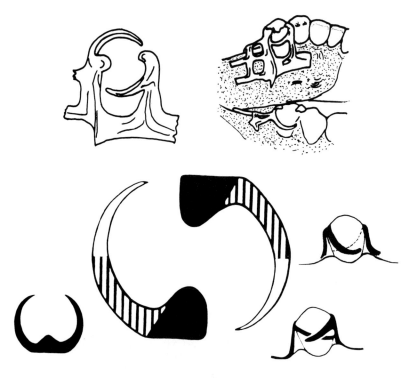

Half and half

Fig. 3-53. Half-and-half clasp is basically circumferential clasp cut in half with rest on each clasp arm assembly. This clasp can be adapted to situations where abutment tooth cannot be recontoured to receive more desirable clasp assembly.

prevent breakage. Because of the design characteristics of this direct retainer, excessive coverage of natural tooth structure may result in increased dental caries susceptibility, periodontal disease, or an esthetically unsatisfactory situation. It is often suggested that abutment teeth be protected by a cast restoration when this direct retainer is used.

The location of the retentive areas as a design consideration in the selection of the embrasure clasp is especially important, because the retentive arms of this clasp should be located so that they are either bilaterally or diagonally opposed.

HALF-AND-HALF CLASP (Fig. 3-53)
Support: Excellent
Bracing: Excellent
Retention: Good to excellent (0.01-inch undercut)
Reciprocation: Good to excellent
Encirclement: Excellent
Passivity: Good

Design considerations. This direct retainer is basically a circumferential clasp that is divided into two parts. The facial portion is identical to the facial half of a circumferential clasp, and the lingual portion originates from a minor connector and rest in the mesial and lingual embrasure of the abutment tooth being clasped. This direct retainer has often been suggested for use on isolated teeth when they cannot be made continuous with the dental arch (by placing a fixed partial denture). It is obvious that this design could create considerable torquing to the isolated abutment tooth. The dentist must be very careful to avoid trauma to the abutment tooth should this direct retainer be used for a distal-extension RPD.

MESIODISTAL CLASP (Fig. 3-54)
Support: Fair to good
Bracing: Good
Retention: Fair
Reciprocation: Good
Encirclement: Good
Passivity: Good

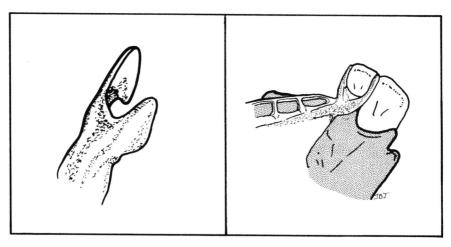

Fig. 3-54. Mesiodistal clasp has limited use because of required tooth preparation and its potentially traumatic influence on abutments for distal-extension base RPDs.

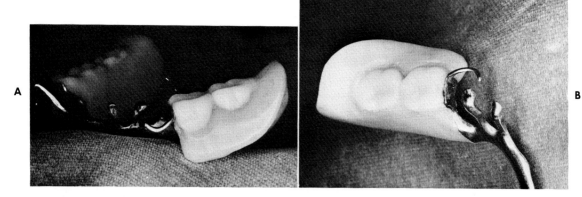

Fig. 3-55. A, Rest–proximal plate–Akers retentive arm (RPA) clasp assembly more than adequately satisfies basic requirements for use in distal-extension base situations. **B,** RPA clasp assembly.

Design considerations. This direct retainer might be considered for a tooth-borne RPD when maxillary incisors remain as the anterior abutment teeth. Although the design exhibits good supporting and bracing qualities, it may be excessively traumatic to the supporting abutment teeth when used on distal-extension RPDs. Retention for this direct retainer is gained through parallelism and frictional resistance of the clasp assembly against the natural teeth. The teeth must be prepared so that their proximal surfaces are parallel or have a slight convergence to one another. This direct retainer, like the other circumferential designs,

poses the same problems of covering excessive tooth structure and impairing esthetics.

REST–PROXIMAL PLATE–AKERS RETENTIVE ARM (RPA) CLASP (Fig. 3-55)

Support: Good to excellent

Bracing: Excellent

Retention: Good (0.01- to 0.02-inch undercut)

Reciprocation: Good to excellent

Encirclement: Good to excellent

Passivity: Good

Design considerations. The RPA clasp is a modified circumferential clasp in which the circumferential arm arises from the proximal plate adjacent to the edentulous base area. The retentive component of this direct retainer engages a retentive undercut located on the facial surface of the abutment tooth away from the edentulous area. The shoulder of the clasp arm contacts the tooth at the height of contour at the junction of the middle and gingival thirds of the tooth. This direct retainer satisfies all the requirements for use in distal-extension RPD situations. It allows for mesially oriented support, which is preferable in distal-extension RPDs (Kratochvil, 1971; Krol, 1973a). Excellent bracing is derived from the contact of the minor connector supporting the rest, the proximal plate contacting the tooth surface adjacent to the edentulous base area, and the shoulder part of the clasp arm. Acceptable retention is derived from retentive areas located on surfaces of the tooth away from the edentulous area. Requirements for adequate encirclement and passivity can easily be accommodated by this direct retainer. This type of clasp appears best suited for distal-extension RPDs where the undercut is located away from the edentulous area and for situations in which it has been determined that the tooth need not be modified to accommodate a different type of clasp.

SUMMARY OF CIRCUMFERENTIAL CLASPS. The circumferential types of direct retainers seem to satisfy the requirements of clasp design when they are properly designed and applied. Faulty application and design are the primary causes of failure within this group of clasps. In general, faulty application or design arises when:

1. The components of the direct retainer are not placed in the proper position on the abutment tooth. (This generally results from inadequate diagnosis and treatment planning.)
2. The components do not have the proper design contour.
3. The guiding planes and minor connectors are not coordinated to direct the components to and from the designated terminal position in which they will function.
4. The rests are not designed to transmit stresses to the long axis of the abutment tooth and to support the direct retainer in its designated terminal position.

All circumferential clasps have certain unfavorable design characteristics in that they cover a large amount of tooth structure and may be considered unesthetic in appearance. Patients must assume their responsibility to maintain adequate oral and denture hygiene to reduce the incidence of dental caries or periodontal disease if this type of direct retainer is to be used. Modification of the direct retainer to accommodate poor oral hygiene or esthetics may result in uncontrolled stress to the abutment teeth and reduce the effectiveness and longevity of the RPD or the abutment teeth.

BAR CLASPS. The next group of clasps to be considered are the bar, or infrabulge, clasps (Fig. 3-56). These clasps are classified by the shape of their retentive terminus (Fig. 3-57). The simplest and most commonly used bar clasps are the T-bar clasp, the modified T-bar clasp, and the I-bar clasp. Bar clasp arms originate from the denture base or the metal framework and approach the retentive area from a gingival direction. Because of the configuration of the retentive terminus, this type of clasp covers a small area of the tooth surface and is considered by some to be more esthetic than the circumferential type of clasp. These clasps, like the circumferential type, must satisfy the basic design requirements. Since the direct retainers of this group are virtually the same, with the exception of the shape of their retentive terminus, they all satisfy the requirements similarly:

Support: Excellent
Bracing: Good
Retention: Excellent (0.01- to 0.02-inch undercut)
Reciprocity: Fair to good
Encirclement: Good
Passivity: Excellent

DESIGN CONSIDERATIONS. Bar clasps (see Fig. 2-45) can provide good to excellent support, depending on whether the rest is located adjacent to or away from the edentulous area. This group of clasps does not satisfy the bracing requirement quite as well as the circumferential type, because the shoulder portion of the retentive arm does not contribute to bracing. The longer, more resilient bar-type arms, the tripping action that they produce, and the location of the retentive areas make this group of clasps more retentive than the circumferential type of direct retainers. Encirclement from this type of clasp is gained from the contact of the

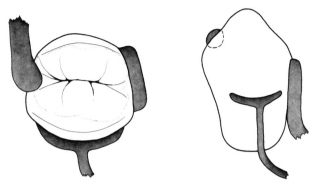

Fig. 3-56. Bar clasp assembly originates from RPD framework in edentulous area and approaches retentive area from gingival direction. These are considered to be push types of clasps and are generally designed to engage retentive areas on tooth surfaces close to extension base area.

minor connector supporting the rest, the contact of the minor connector or proximal plate, and the retentive arm when it contacts the tooth. This forms a triangulation of contact between the direct retainer and the tooth that prevents the tooth from moving away from the clasp and from slipping off the abutment tooth. As with the other clasps, this group can be designed to be passive when in its terminal position.

Bar clasps (T bar, modified T bar, and I bar) are most suitable where the retentive area is located on the side of the abutment tooth adjacent to an edentulous area. Thus, when the survey line indicates that the retentive area is located in the center or on the buccal or lingual surface of the tooth adjacent to the edentulous area, the varying configurations of bar clasps should be considered. As pointed out earlier (in design considerations of the circumferential types) the single most important factor in the selection of the clasp is the location of the retentive area.

The use of bar clasps is limited:

1. In design situations where there is a need for a great amount of horizontal bracing
2. In patients who have shallow vestibules where the minor connector supporting the retentive terminus cannot be placed in the proper anatomic relationships to the supporting soft tissues, that is, where the shape of the shoulder portion of the bar would have to be altered to accommodate the design (Fig. 3-58, *A*)
3. In situations where soft tissue undercuts or muscle attachments exist that would

cause the minor connector supporting the retentive terminus to stand away from the supporting tissues for more than 2 to 3 mm and potentially produce food entrapment (Fig. 3-58, *B*)
4. In situations where the abutment teeth demonstrate severe buccal or lingual tilting that would prevent the proper positioning of the direct retainer onto the abutment tooth (Fig. 3-58, *C*)
5. In patients who exhibit high smile lines, because the selection of a bar clasp for the maxillary canines and premolars in these patients might possibly produce an esthetically unacceptable result

Another potential problem for bar clasps is that they can easily be distorted by mishandling if improperly designed and may be difficult to repair if fractured (see Chapter 10).

If the rest, minor connector, and guiding planes of this type of direct retainer are properly designed, vertical stresses can be transferred down the long axis of the abutment tooth through the rest. Horizontal stresses can be controlled by being transferred to the abutment tooth by the proximal plate and minor connector, which contact the guiding plane at the junction of the middle and gingival thirds of the tooth.

The most probable cause of failure when this type of direct retainer is used is the improper application of its design (Fig. 3-59). Proper design for this group of clasps should be carefully executed. The retentive components should have the proper contour to resist a dislodging force in an occlusal direction and should be lo-

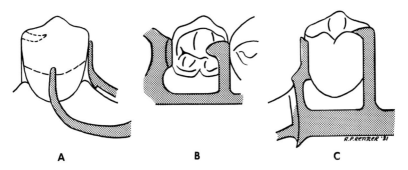

Fig. 3-57. RPI bar clasp, which one identifies by shape of its retentive tip. **A,** Buccal view of I-bar clasp assembly. **B,** Occlusal view of I-bar clasp assembly. **C,** Lingual view of I-bar clasp assembly.

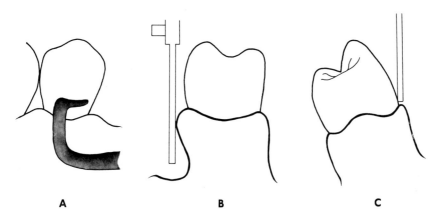

Fig. 3-58. Limiting factors in selection of bar clasp assemblies. **A,** Shallow vestibule. **B,** Severe tissue undercuts. **C,** Excessive buccal or lingual tilting of abutment tooth.

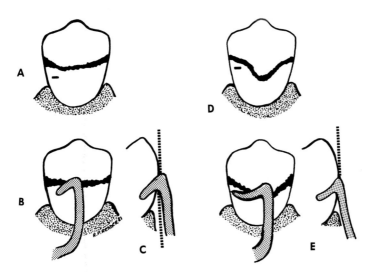

Fig. 3-59. Improper applications of design for bar clasp assemblies. **A,** Survey line is not designed for bar clasp. **B,** Retentive clasp tip is not located in gingival third of tooth. **C,** Retentive tip is improperly contoured to resist dislodging force in occlusal direction. Also, there is severe tissue undercut and shallow vestibule. **D,** Contour of tooth is altered to receive bar clasp. **E,** Correct position of bar clasp assembly.

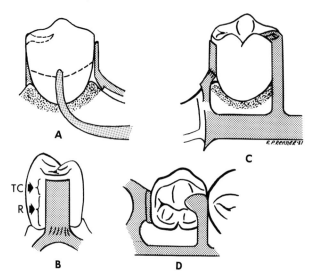

Fig. 3-60. Design characteristics of proximal plate. **A,** Buccal view. **B,** Distal view. *TC,* tooth contact; *R,* relief. **C,** Lingual view. **D,** Occusal view.

cated in the gingival third of the tooth in the designated retentive area. The retentive terminal should have a minimum of tooth contact. Dimples or grooves cut into the tooth surface to create a retentive area should be avoided, because these tend to restrict the design function of the clasp assembly. The approaching retentive arm should never impinge on the soft tissue, and the area where it traverses and covers the soft tissue should be adequately relieved.

Proximal plates used with bar clasps. Bar clasps are generally designed with a proximal plate, so the design characteristics of this proximal plate should be established first (Fig. 3-60). The proximal plate should contact the guiding plane of the abutment tooth from just below the marginal ridge and extend in a gingival direction to the junction of its middle and gingival thirds. It should contact approximately two thirds of the buccolingual width of the abutment tooth and should extend to the lingual axial line angle to provide for the bracing requirement. The proximal plate should be about 1 mm thick, with its gingival portions sufficiently relieved so as not to impinge on the free gingival margin. The proximal plate, in conjunction with the minor connector supporting the rest and the reciprocal arm and the I bar, should form a triangle to encircle the abutment tooth by more than 180 degrees.

T-BAR CLASP. The T-bar clasp derives its name from the fact that the shape of the retentive arm and its retentive terminal resemble the letter T (see Fig. 2-44). The retentive arm should contact the retentive terminal at approximately a right angle to the direction of the vertical dislodging force; however, the angles formed at this junction should be rounded. The retentive terminal should taper toward its ends, and the tips should be rounded.

The T-bar clasp is used frequently on a tooth located on either side of an edentulous space and on an abutment tooth adjacent to a distal-extension edentulous space where the retentive undercut on the tooth is located on the side of the tooth adjacent to the edentulous space (near area). It should not be used on a tooth where the retentive undercut is located on the side of the tooth away from the edentulous space (far area). It is also contraindicated where the retentive arm crosses a moderately severe soft tissue undercut or where the survey line is located near the occlusal surface of the tooth. Both of these conditions can produce an undesirable space beneath the shoulder part of the retentive arm and the underlying structures, which can cause food entrapment and irritation of the cheek or tongue.

MODIFIED T-BAR CLASP. The modified T-bar clasp assembly is a T-bar clasp with that half of the retentive terminal which lies above the survey line removed (see Fig. 2-45). It is often used instead of the T-bar clasp on maxillary canines and premolars to make the clasp assembly more acceptable esthetically.

I-BAR CLASP. The form of the I-bar clasp resembles the letter I (see Fig. 2-46). The retentive terminal of the clasp should cross the gingival margin at a 90-degree angle to engage a slight undercut (0.01 inch) on the abutment tooth. Because the retentive arm on this clasp assembly is usually shorter and more rigid than that of other bar clasps, the use of a small amount of retentive undercut will provide adequate retention for this clasp. Usually a 0.01-inch undercut is considered adequate for most chromium alloys.

The small amount of tooth-surface contact of this type of clasp makes it more acceptable esthetically than most other clasp designs and reduces the chance of dental caries occurring beneath the clasp. Its disadvantage is that unless care is used in its design, 180-degree encirclement of the tooth may not be obtained.

A modification of the I-bar clasp was advocated by Kratochvil in 1965 and later was coined the RPI clasp (see Fig. 2-47) by Krol in 1973. This I-bar hybrid clasp is advocated for use in bilateral distal-extension base RPDs. It consists of a buccal I-bar retentive arm (the I component) engaging a 0.010-inch undercut on the midbuccal portion of the abutment tooth, a proximal plate (the P component) contacting a proximal guiding plane adjacent to the edentulous area, and a mesial occlusal rest and minor connector (the R component). Advocates of this clasp assembly believe that when the proximal plate area is further modified (Krol, 1973b), the clasp will be self-releasing and will place little rotational torquing force on the abutment tooth when the distal-extension base of the RPD is placed under function. Rotation occurs around the mesial occlusal rests bilaterally while the proximal plates and I bars disengage from the abutment teeth. As with any bar clasp assembly, attention to soft tissue undercuts below the abutment tooth may preclude the use of an I-bar clasp assembly because of the potential for mucosal trauma, I-bar fracture, or food entrapment. However, the RPI clasp and the combination clasp assembly are considered by most the two direct retainers of choice for distal-extension RPDs.

SUMMARY OF BAR CLASPS. The bar clasp satisfies the basic requirements of clasp design when it is properly designed and applied. Faulty application and design are the primary causes of failure from this type of clasp. Faulty application and design arise when the components of the direct retainer are not placed in their proper position on the abutment tooth, when the components do not have the proper design contour, when guiding planes and minor connectors are not coordinated to direct the components to and from their designated terminal positions, when rests are not designed to transmit stresses to the long axes of the abutment teeth, and when rests are not designed to support the direct retainer in its designated terminal position.

Bar clasps have certain unfavorable design characteristics in that they may provide less bracing than the circumferential type and are limited in their use by soft tissue undercuts, shallow vestibules, or tilted teeth. Bar clasps, like circumferential clasps, are quite difficult if not impossible to adjust, repair, or replace if they become distorted or broken.

Favorable characteristics of bar clasps, in relation to circumferential clasps, include increased retentive capabilities because of the manner in which they function (by tripping action), longer and more resilient retentive arms, less tooth-surface contact, and better esthetics. In addition, the wide range of modifications to the design of the retentive terminal allows bar clasps to be used in a great variety of situations. The most significant factor in selection of this clasp, however, still remains the location of the retentive area.

The bar type of direct retainer, as with the circumferential type, requires the patient's acceptance of responsibility for oral hygiene maintenance. Modifications of this direct retainer to accommodate poor oral hygiene or esthetics may result in uncontrolled stresses to the abutment teeth and reduce the effectiveness of the RPD.

COMBINATION CLASPS

WROUGHT WIRE RETENTIVE ARM AND CAST CIRCUMFERENTIAL BRACING ARM

Support: Good to excellent

Bracing: Fair to poor

Retention: Good (0.02- to 0.03-inch undercut)

Reciprocation: Fair to good

Encirclement: Fair

Passivity: Fair

Design considerations (see Fig. 2-49). The wrought wire combination clasp can provide good to excellent support, depending on the location of the rest. Bracing is considerably diminished with the use of this direct retainer because of the presence of the very flexible, round, wrought wire retentive arm. Retention is satisfied through the use of an 18- or 19-gauge PGP round wire as the retentive arm (Frank and Nichols, 1981). The retentive component is completely round, so it lends itself well to retentive areas on the sides of tooth surfaces away from the edentulous area. The cross-sectional form and the length contribute to the increased flexibility of this type of retentive arm versus a cast half-round retentive arm. This direct retainer encircles the tooth more than 180 degrees. However, the flexibility of the retentive arm might allow movement of the abutment tooth away from the direct retainer in the direction of the retentive arm. In addition, the wrought wire arm may be easily distorted, allowing the remainder of the clasp assembly to be disoriented on the tooth. This direct retainer can be designed to be passive. Again, however, its flexibility allows it to be distorted easily, resulting in the direct retainer's being activated in its terminal position. This direct retainer provides a particularly advantageous design consideration in that the flexible retentive arm, being round, contacts less tooth surface, lends itself to easy adjustability, and provides for good esthetics.

There are two distinct disadvantages to the design of this type of clasp. Because of its length and cross-sectional form, it is readily subject to distortion from patient handling or from the stresses of occlusal function. Also, an additional laboratory procedure is required to solder the wrought wire retentive arm to the supporting minor connector or framework. These problems, in conjunction with the reduced rigidity and bracing properties of the wrought wire direct retainer, often limit its use. Distortion, as a limiting factor, may be reduced effectively by placing the retentive wrought wire arm on the lingual surface of the tooth and the more rigid bracing arm on the buccal or facial surface of the abutment tooth, thus reducing the opportunity for distortion by patient handling. This direct retainer should be considered for use in retaining a distal-extension RPD and in situations where a soft tis-

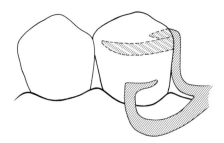

Fig. 3-61. Combination bar and cast circumferential clasp assembly.

sue undercut precludes the use of a bar clasp.

COMBINATION BAR AND CIRCUMFERENTIAL CLASP (Fig. 3-61)

Support: Good to excellent

Bracing: Fair to poor

Retention: Good (0.02- to 0.03-inch undercut)

Reciprocation: Fair to good

Encirclement: Fair

Passivity: Fair

Design considerations. The combination clasp consisting of a bar and circumferential clasp arms satisfies the design requirements indicated for both bar and circumferential clasps. In particular, use of this direct retainer is indicated by the location of the undercut. Because the retentive component is of a bar type, the retentive areas should be located on the side of the tooth adjacent to the edentulous area. The bracing requirement of this direct retainer is considerably enhanced because of the presence of the cast circumferential arm. The depth of the vestibule, tissue undercuts, and severely tilted teeth provide some of the limitations for use of this particular direct retainer.

VERTICAL RECIPROCAL–HORIZONTAL RETENTIVE CLASP ASSEMBLY (See Fig. 2-50)

Support: Fair

Bracing: Fair to poor

Retention: Good

Reciprocation: Good

Encirclement: Fair to good

Passivity: Good

Design considerations. A new clasp assembly design was introduced (Grasso, 1980) to solve the inadequacies of the reciprocal and retentive components of both the circumferential and bar clasp assemblies. The vertical reciprocal–horizontal retentive (VRHR) clasp assembly incorporates some of the desirable features of both the circumferential and bar clasp assemblies.

The components of the VRHR clasp assembly include a horizontal retentive arm, a distal occlusal rest, and a vertical reciprocating arm. A significant feature of the design is that the retentive and reciprocal clasp components make simultaneous contact with their respective tooth surfaces. Advantages of the vertical reciprocating arm are that:

1. Lingually inclined teeth can be used without modification.
2. A line or point contact is the only contact necessary between the vertical reciprocating arm and the tooth.
3. It is not necessary to make parallel surfaces for the reciprocating arm contact.
4. A survey line close to the occlusal surface of the tooth can be used.

The advantages of the horizontal retentive clasp arm concept are that:

1. Little or no recontouring of the tooth is necessary.
2. More options are available in designing the clasp assembly.
3. It permits less display of metal.
4. A longer and more flexible wrought or cast clasp may be used.

The disadvantages of this clasp, however, at this time are that:

1. The potential exists for food traps under the horizontal and vertical components.
2. The horizontal retentive arm is unable to provide bracing.

Indirect retainers

The tissueward movement of tooth-supported RPDs is prevented by the occlusal, incisal, and cingulum rests of the direct retainers. Movement away from the tissue in tooth-supported RPDs is resisted by the action of the guiding planes and retentive arms of the direct retainers. However, in distal-extension RPDs, dislodging forces tend to lift the distal-extension base, causing a displacing, rotational movement of the prosthesis about an imaginary axis of rotation (see Fig. 3-1). The imaginary axis of rotation, or fulcrum line, is established by projecting imaginary lines between rests located on the primary abutment teeth (see Fig. 2-51). As an aid in preventing rotational movement of a distal-extension RPD, the dentist can incorporate indirect retainers into the design of the prosthesis. Indirect retainers are components of an RPD that assist the direct retainers

in preventing dislodgement occlusally of the distal-extension base by exerting a leverlike action on the opposite side of the fulcrum line. An indirect retainer is composed of a rest and a minor connector. Indirect retainers are effective in proportion to their ability to provide adequate support for the prosthesis and their distance from the fulcrum line. To maximize resistance to dislodgment, indirect retainers should be placed as far from the distal-extension base as possible. To provide adequate support, they should be placed in prepared rest seats on a tooth or teeth capable of providing the support required for their function. Indirect retainers contribute an auxiliary function of providing additional vertical support and horizontal stability to an RPD.

FACTORS INFLUENCING THE EFFECTIVENESS OF INDIRECT RETAINERS. Several factors influence the effectiveness of an indirect retainer used in a distal-extension RPD. Specifically, these are the length and location of the edentulous area, the ability of the indirect retainer abutment to provide adequate support, and the type of minor connector used to connect the indirect retainer to the RPD framework.

Recent investigations suggest that indirect retainers have little effect on actual retention of the prosthesis and that the type of clasp and the contact of the minor connectors to the guiding planes exert the greatest influence of the amount of distal-extension denture base displacement (Benson and Spolsky, 1979).

However, indirect retainers play another very important role in the distal-extension RPD. Because of their position in the dental arch (ideally as far from the distal-extension base as possible), they act as primary indicators to alert the dentist for the need to reline the distal-extension RPD. When residual ridge reduction occurs and the distal-extension base adapts to the resorbed edentulous area, a lifting of the indirect retainer away from its designated terminal seat on its abutment tooth results. When observed clinically, this serves as a primary indication that the RPD should be relined or rebased to reestablish its posterior tissue support (see Chapter 10). Therefore, the use of indirect retainers in all distal-extension RPDs is recommended.

The effectiveness of an indirect retainer is determined by several factors:

1. The indirect retainer should be placed at

right angles to and as far from the fulcrum line as possible.

2. An indirect retainer should always be placed in a prepared rest seat on an abutment tooth that is capable of withstanding the stresses placed on it, preferably a canine or premolar. It should not be placed on an inclined tooth surface. Incisors, because of their inclined lingual surfaces, are not considered good abutment teeth for indirect retainers unless an incisal rest rather than a prepared lingual rest seat is used. A better location for an indirect retainer is on the first premolar or canine. Although the effectiveness of the indirect retainer may be compromised because of a somewhat shorter lever arm if these teeth are used as abutments, this disadvantage is more than compensated for by the more desirable anatomic contours and the greater amount of periodontal support that these teeth have than do the incisors. The mesial occlusal fossa of the mandibular first premolar makes an ideal location for an indirect retainer, because there is usually no opposing tooth contact in this fossa (see Fig. 2-52).

3. Direct retainers must provide positive retention for the prosthesis if an indirect retainer is to be effective. An indirect retainer, when used in conjunction with positive direct retainers, prevents rotation of the RPD around the clasp assemblies when the distal-extension base is moved occlusally. Its use moves the fulcrum line anteriorly to the abutment tooth or teeth contacted by the indirect retainer. This helps prevent the distal-extension base from lifting off the soft tissues until the retentive arms' resistance to deformation is overcome.

Indirect retainers provide several other functions in addition to controlling rotational denture base movements (indirect retention):

1. They supply additional support for the RPD and distribute the forces of occlusion over a greater number of abutment teeth.

2. They provide additional support for the major connector by helping prevent the major connector from impinging into the underlying soft tissues when the prosthesis is loaded occlusally.

3. They aid in stabilizing the RPD against horizontal forces.

4. They serve as a third point of reference for the cast RPD framework and thus are an aid in locating the correct framework position on the teeth during relining procedures or when a corrected (altered) cast impression technique is used for a distal-extension base RPD.

Connecting the retention units to the support units

If direct and indirect retainers are to function as designed, each should be maintained in its designated terminal position on the abutment tooth. The direct retainers in tooth-supported RPDs can be connected rigidly to the cast framework by major and minor connectors. Most dentists feel that this philosophy can be extended to a distal-extension RPD as long as the tissue-support areas (residual ridges) have been diagnosed as adequate to oppose the forces of occlusion and as long as they can be maintained in an acceptable state of health.

Other dentists, however, feel that in distal-extension RPDs, the tissue-supported unit (denture base) must be connected flexibly to the tooth-supported retention units (direct retainers). Their philosophy is that a flexible or semirigid minor connector between the tooth-supported retention unit and the tissue-supported unit will allow the distal-extension base to function more independently to oppose vertical occlusal forces and will reduce significantly the damaging torquing forces that could be directed to the abutment teeth.

Other dentists suggest that a flexible connector between the edentulous area and the retention unit might provide this torque reduction. Others feel that a single casting with a split major connector (see Fig. 3-19) can be designed so that tooth-supported retention units and tooth-supported edentulous areas of the RPD are connected rigidly together as another unit. The tissue-supported edentulous area of the RPD can then be flexibly or semirigidly attached to these combined support units. The combined tooth-supported units thus provide retention and cross-arch stability, but at the same time, the flexible connector allows the tissue-supported area to move tissueward without undue leverage being transmitted to the connectors. At the same time, stress accumulation and the resultant fatigue and ultimate fracture of the cast metal framework can be reduced by rounding the terminal end of the split where the two connectors join.

There are many possibilities of connecting tooth- and tissue-support units semirigidly. These include the use of bars, straps, plates, and hinges. All have some of the advantages expressed previously but also many disadvantages, such as wear, food stagnation, difficulty in relining, and fragility to patient handling and masticatory forces. However, the connection of support and retention units is best accomplished by using rigid components and connectors. As indicated earlier, proper connection of the components of an RPD is as important as any other phase of its design. Strict attention to detail must be emphasized in the selection, location, and design of the major and minor connectors. In connecting retention units to support units, the criteria for selection, location, and design are the same as those indicated for connecting the support units of an RPD to one another.

Outlining the edentulous area

The correct design of the minor connector (open latticework or mesh) covering the edentulous area must provide rigidity without creating interferences to tooth placement. This supporting component of a prosthesis is of significant importance to overall success because it provides the transport mechanism by which the forces exerted on the RPD are controlled and directed to the tooth-supporting units.

Denture base

The denture base is that part of the RPD which rests on the mucoperiosteum and underlying bone and to which the denture teeth are attached. Although the role of the denture base is to retain the artificial teeth and thus restore esthetics and masticatory efficiency, a properly designed denture base also accomplishes several other important functions:

1. It provides added retention for the prosthesis through the forces of adhesion and cohesion, which act between the tissue-fitting surface of denture base and the underlying mucoperiosteum.
2. Its tissue-fitting surface, which contacts the slopes of residual ridge, aids in stabi-

lizing the RPD against the horizontal forces transmitted to the prosthesis.
3. It provides support for the distal-extension base RPD and helps to distribute the forces of occlusion more uniformly between the natural teeth and the soft tissues covered by the distal-extension denture base.
4. Its polished surface contours, when properly developed, provide a stabilizing and retentive effect when acted on by the oral musculature.

BORDER EXTENSIONS ON DISTAL-EXTENSION REMOVABLE PARTIAL DENTURES. For the residual ridge and its mucoperiosteal covering beneath a distal-extension RPD to provide maximum support for the prosthesis, the denture base must both fit the underlying tissues accurately and cover the greatest available area within the functional limits of the border tissues. The peripheral border of a distal-extension RPD should not displace the border tissues to the extent that a complete denture does. Retention of the RPD is provided by direct retainers and intimacy of tissue contact and is not dependent on the development of a border seal as in a complete denture. Because of the elastic qualities of the border tissues, they will, if displaced, exert a continuous dislodging force on the RPD base. This force, which is transmitted through the direct retainers to the abutment teeth, can cause damage to the supporting structures of these teeth. RPD bases should therefore be extended only to the point where they contact but do not displace the border tissues to prevent food debris from collecting beneath the denture base.

The maxillary distal-extension denture base should cover the maxillary tuberosity and end in the hamular notch. Palatally, it should join the major connector on the slopes of the residual ridge. Buccally it should extend superiorly to contact the border tissues; however, it should not displace these tissues or interfere with their functional movements.

The mandibular distal-extension denture base should cover as much of the buccal shelf of the mandible (primary support area) as the buccinator and masseter muscles will permit. The denture base should extend posteriorly to cover the pear-shaped retromolar pad (or at least its anterior two thirds). The distolingual border should extend functionally to cover the retromylohyoid area from the retromolar pad to the alveololingual sulcus. The length and shape of the distolingual and lingual denture border flange should be determined by the exaggerated movements of the tongue and lingual border tissues. The most accurate method of determining these border dimensions is by means of a corrected cast impression (altered cast) of the edentulous area.

The borders of a distal-extension RPD base should be rounded and all sharp edges removed. They should be slightly narrower than the comparable borders developed on a complete denture. The anterior border of the buccal flange of a maxillary or mandibular prosthesis (see Fig. 2-53) and the distolingual border of a distal-extension RPD (see Fig. 2-54) should be thinned slightly and tapered toward the soft tissues so that the junction between the denture base and the soft tissues is as imperceptible as possible. The creation of a sharp edge should be avoided.

The buccal and lingual surfaces of the denture base should be fashioned so that they present contours that will contribute to the development of the patient's neuromuscular skills and permit the surrounding musculature to help retain the prosthesis. The mandibular lingual flange of the denture base should be made as thin as possible to maximize the tongue space and minimize the lateral forces exerted on the prosthesis by the tongue. Denture bases of acrylic resin should be smooth, well contoured, and highly polished to help prevent dental plaque and stains from accumulating on the prosthesis.

BORDER EXTENSIONS ON TOOTH-BORNE REMOVABLE PARTIAL DENTURES. Tooth-borne RPDs differ from distal-extension RPDs because the distal-extension denture base on the latter must provide support for the prosthesis, whereas support for a tooth-borne RPD is supplied by rests on the abutment teeth on each side of the edentulous space. Maximal tissue coverage of the edentulous area by the denture base is therefore not required or desirable for the tooth-borne RPD or for modification spaces (see Fig. 2-55). These denture bases should be designed so that they prevent food accumulation beneath the prosthesis, enhance esthetics, and restore only the natural soft and hard tissue contours that were lost following the extraction of the natural teeth. The borders of

these denture bases should be thin and tapered toward the tissues to make them as imperceptible as possible and without sharp edges.

Labial RPD flanges that interfere with the insertion and withdrawal of an RPD because of a severe soft tissue undercut should not be relieved on the tissue surface of the denture flange, but the denture flange itself should be shortened until the soft tissue undercut no longer prevents the prosthesis from seating intraorally. Characterization of the denture base with internal staining to enhance esthetics should be accomplished for those patients who expose the denture base during functional movements of the lips and cheeks.

Denture bases are usually made of acrylic resin, metal, or a combination of metal and acrylic resin. The excellent esthetic qualities of acrylic resin, its versatility, and its ease of fabrication and adjustment make it the most widely used material for an RPD base. A major advantage of acrylic resin is that it can be relined or rebased easily and inexpensively. The all cast metal denture base and the combination cast metal and acrylic resin denture base can be relined or rebased only with difficulty if at all. The acrylic resin denture base is therefore considered the base of choice for most distal-extension RPDs, because this type of prosthesis usually requires relining or rebasing periodically as a result of tissue changes that accompany residual ridge resorption.

The all cast metal denture base is used in selected instances because it is more hygienic, can be cast with greater accuracy, and has a higher thermal conductivity, which tends to promote a better mucosal response to coverage by the denture base than does acrylic resin. However, because relining is made very difficult or impossible, the use of the cast metal denture base should be limited to Kennedy Class III RPDs, where future relining or rebasing procedures are not anticipated (Fig. 3-62).

An all cast metal denture base (see Fig. 2-56) may be indicated in tooth-supported RPDs with short edentulous spans or when there is insufficient vertical space to properly position and retain the denture teeth to an acrylic resin base. The denture base should be kept thinner than comparable acrylic resin denture bases, but sharp margins must be avoided, especially at the borders. All cast metal denture bases should not be used to treat patients when

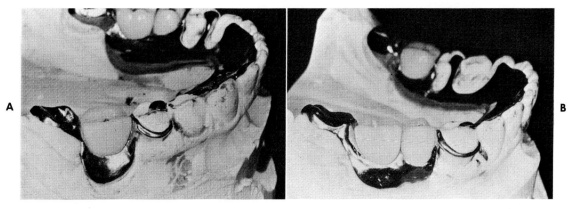

Fig. 3-62. A, All cast base for tooth-supported partial denture. **B,** Tube tooth placed on the site of mandibular first molar.

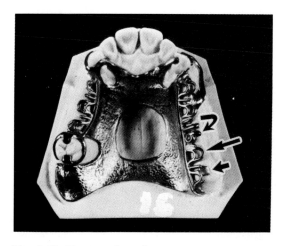

Fig. 3-63. Design of acrylic resin retention area is dependent on presence of at least 1 mm of relief and tissue stops and on position of acrylic resin retentive section.

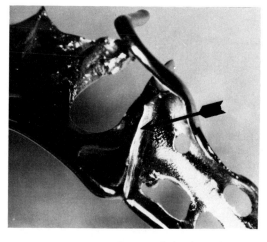

Fig. 3-64. Location of internal finishing line *(arrow).*

edentulous areas have not previously been subjected to the stress of a distal-extension RPD. It has been reported (Carlsson and Persson, 1967) that within the first 60 months following edentulation the greatest rate of residual ridge reduction in the patient's mucosal and skeletal height occurs during the first 12 months. Therefore, a distal-extension RPD placed over the residual ridge during the first 12 months would require relining sooner than an RPD inserted 12 months after the teeth were extracted. Since the all cast metal denture base RPD is not easily relined, it is recommended that patients not be treated with it until they have worn an acrylic resin denture base for at least 12 months.

The combination cast metal and acrylic resin

denture base consists of a cast metal base, which fits over the residual ridges, and acrylic resin, which is processed to the metal to enhance esthetics, restore lost tissue contours, and retain the artificial teeth. Inasmuch as the metal covers the residual ridge, the advantages and disadvantages of its use are the same as for the all cast metal denture base. Its use is therefore primarily limited to the Kennedy Class III RPD or to a modification space where the residual ridge is well healed.

DESIGN CONSIDERATIONS FOR THE DENTURE BASE. Adequate bulk and strength in the metal at the junction of the framework base and the minor connectors are essential (Figs. 3-63 and 3-64). The minor connectors should be raised at least 1 mm from the tissue to allow the framework to be adequately embedded in the acrylic resin and to provide strength to support the acrylic resin. Tissue stops should be used on a distal-extension RPD framework to hold its end in the proper position while the framework is being processed with acrylic resin. The top brace of the open lattice–type retentive section of the framework should extend either to the buccal or lingual of the crest of the residual ridge with loops placed over the residual ridge. The main brace of the open lattice should not be placed over the crest of the residual ridge, because it may interfere with proper denture tooth placement. If a meshwork type of retention is to be used, an anticipated difficulty will be placement of a tin foil substitute on the master cast through the mesh if the framework is to be held in the lower half of a denture flask during processing.

FINISHING LINES. Finishing lines should be provided on all RPD frameworks wherever denture base acrylic resin and the metal join (see Figs. 3-31, 3-32, and 3-64). A finishing line allows the acrylic resin to terminate in a butt joint to produce a smooth surface. An internal finishing line is located on the internal, or tissue, surface and is formed while relief is being placed in the master cast. An external finishing line is located on the polished surface of an RPD and is formed in the wax pattern. Saliva and debris will accumulate between the denture base acrylic resin and the metal if the acrylic resin ends in a thin edge. The acrylic resin will also fracture if left too thin in this area.

To facilitate relining procedures, *internal maxillary finishing lines* should be placed close to the point at which the vertical and horizontal planes of the palate meet. To minimize stress concentration and the potential for fracture, the external finishing line should never be placed directly over the internal finishing line. It may be placed superior to the internal finishing line so that a minimum amount of denture base acrylic resin is used on the lingual aspect of the denture teeth.

Internal and external mandibular finishing lines are placed immediately posterior to the distal abutment tooth. They should incline slightly posteriorly from the gingival margin of the abutment teeth. They should not incline anteriorly, or the denture base acrylic resin

will lie below the abutment teeth. Anterior finishing lines are made when anterior teeth are missing. These are placed mesial to the remaining teeth and incline slightly in a mesial direction.

A palatal major connector should have a specially prepared seal along the border of the connector where it contacts the soft tissues (see Fig. 3-21, *C* and *D*). This seal is formed from a beading placed at the border of the major connector that will displace the soft tissues very slightly. Its purpose is to prevent food from collecting under the maxillary major connector. This bead is made approximately 3/4 to 1 mm deep and the same width as the edge of the design of the maxillary major connector. The groove must fade out at least 6 mm away from the gingival tissues to prevent tissue displacement of the marginal gingiva. It also may fade out over the center of the cast when a hard midline suture or maxillary torus is present.

SURVEYING

To ensure that the supporting, retaining, and connecting components of the RPD can be directed to and maintained in their designed position, the dentist, when placing clasps on teeth, must locate and delineate their contour and position on the abutment teeth and other associated oral structures as they relate to one another. In other words, the dentist must identify a basic position or path of placement that puts the teeth and associated tissues in the most advantageous position for their preservation. The dentist determines the basic position for the RPD by surveying the cast with a dental surveyor. This establishes a baseline for all planning, design, and construction of the RPD.

The dental surveyor

A dental surveyor consists of two basic parts, a platform and vertical tool-holding arm to which surveying instruments can be attached and an adjustable surveying table that holds a dental cast. The surveying table holds a dental cast in a definite predetermined position (Fig. 3-65). The analyzing rod indicates the parallelism or lack of parallelism of tooth planes or surfaces to the predetermined cast position and the relative parallelism of the teeth to each

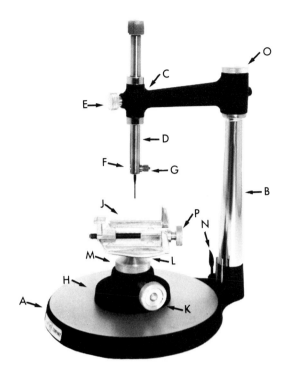

Fig. 3-65. Ney surveyor. Parts description: *A,* Horizontal surveyor base; *B,* upright column; *C,* cross arm with spindle bearing; *D,* vertical spindle; *E,* spindle tightening screw; *F,* tool holder; *G,* tool holder locking nut; *H,* survey table; *J,* tilt-top and model clamp; *K,* locking screw of tilt-top; *L,* ball pivot; *M,* ball retaining ring; *N,* rack for accessories when in use; *O,* storage compartment for tools (undercut gauges, analyzing rod, carbons, wax trimmer); *P,* model clamp adjusting screw. (Courtesy The J.M. Ney Co.)

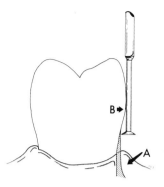

Fig. 3-66. Surveying identifies soft tissue *(A)* and tooth structure that require modification by mouth preparation to accommodate proper positioning of RPD components *(B).*

other. This gives the dentist a positive evaluation of how each tooth is positioned relative to the basic cast position and how each tooth is positioned in relation to the other remaining tissues and teeth. Tissue undercuts that are inconsistent with the path of placement of the prosthesis and that might influence the RPD design are also demonstrated using this instrument.

Purposes of surveying

The ultimate goal in surveying a dental stone cast is to establish a position that will facilitate control by transferring stress through the components of the RPD to the long axes of the abutment teeth and the primary supporting area of the residual ridges (Hanson and associ-

ates, 1975). This position is considered to be the *most advantageous position* for the design of the RPD. In accomplishing this goal, several important diagnostic facts are established relative to the design of the RPD. Surveying identifies areas of the mouth that may require alteration by surgical or restorative procedures to accommodate the proper position of RPD components (Fig. 3-66). The RPD most suitable for each patient's existing set of circumstances can then be constructed. The dentist can identify soft or bony tissue undercuts that would interfere with the proper positioning of major or minor connectors and the denture base. Surveying also enables the dentist to identify the height of contour (survey line) of the proposed abutment teeth. When the height of contour of all of the remaining teeth is known, it is easy to note the tooth surfaces that are parallel to each other and those that are not. Proximal tooth surfaces that are parallel to one another can act as guiding planes to assure a definite path of placement for the RPD. When the height of contour indicates a lack of parallelism of the proximal tooth surfaces, these areas can be modified by selective grinding or restorative procedures to make them parallel (see Chapter 5). Parallel guiding planes should be located on all tooth surfaces adjacent to edentulous areas and on all tooth surfaces where minor connectors are indicated to have tooth contact.

Surveying also serves to locate and measure areas of the teeth that may be used to retain the RPD. The surface areas of the teeth that lie below the height of contour (survey line) delineate the areas that can be used by the direct retainer to provide retention (Fig. 3-67). Undercut gauges can be used with the surveying instrument to positively measure the depth of undercut areas that may be used for retention (Fig. 3-68). Structurally, retention is provided by the tip of the retentive arm's engaging a specific amount of undercut in the gingival third of the tooth. When a dislodging force acts on the RPD in an occlusal direction, the flexible retentive tip of the direct retainer (clasp assembly) is forced to deform as it passes over the height of contour of the abutment tooth. The amount and the location of the undercut and the resistance of the metal to deformation determine the amount of retention, or the designated degree of resistance to displacement (Fig. 3-69). Retention should always be the minimum necessary to resist reasonable dislodging forces. Surveying can also be used to delineate the height of contour of abutment teeth and to locate undercuts that may be excessive and may need to be corrected or blocked out before duplication (Fig. 3-70). Surveying can also be used to record for future reference the dental stone cast position in relation to a selected path of insertion and withdrawal of the prosthesis (Fig. 3-71).

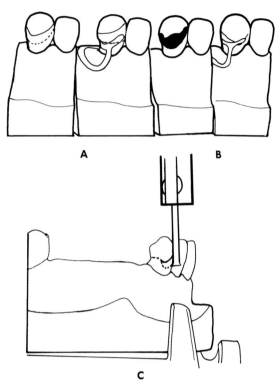

Fig. 3-67. A, Solid line represents height of contour on abutment tooth at most advantageous position. Dotted line represents desirable height of contour to locate components of clasp assembly optimally. **B,** Optimal height of contour can be achieved by reducing axial contour of tooth. This can be accomplished by selective grinding, providing that dentine is not exposed. **C,** Tooth will require preparation and restoration if dentine is exposed. Indicated tooth reduction is marked on stone cast to serve as blueprint for mouth preparation.

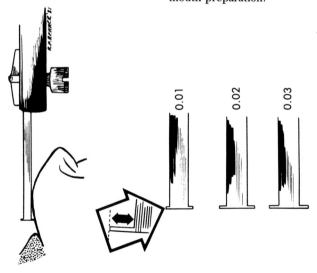

Fig. 3-68. Undercut gauges. Three gauges supplied with surveyor provide three exact amounts of horizontal undercut. Silver color, 0.01 inch; copper color, 0.02 inch; and black color, 0.03 inch. Measurements are of distance from shank of gauge to rim of gauge head.

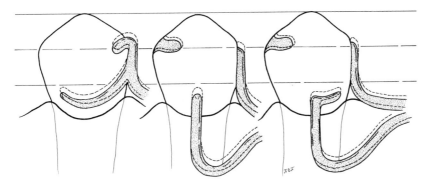

Fig. 3-69. Retention is provided by flexible portion of clasp assembly. It is ideally located in gingival third of tooth crown. When force acts to dislodge RPD in an occlusal direction, retentive tip is forced to deform as it passes from its location in undercut area over greatest contour of abutment tooth. Amount and location of undercut—as well as type of metal, its taper, cross-sectional form, length and contour—determine amount of retention provided by retentive clasp arm.

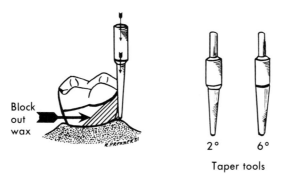

Block out wax

2°   6°

Taper tools

Fig. 3-70. Tapering instruments for blocking out undesirable undercuts.

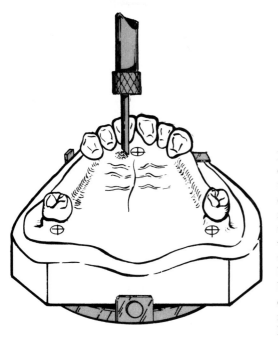

Fig. 3-71. Tripoding. After most advantageous position of cast has been determined, it is necessary to record that position in relation to surveyor for future reference. Method of recording relation of cast to surveyor is known as tripoding. Carbon marker is placed in vertical arm of surveyor, and arm is adjusted to height at which cast can be contacted in three divergent locations. Vertical arm is locked in position, and cast is brought into contact with tip of carbon marker. It is best to have these three points located on immovable or hard tissue, because tissue displacement during impression procedures could produce error in reestablishing recorded position. Reorientation of cast to surveyor is accomplished by tilting cast on surveying table until analyzing rod again contacts the three points.

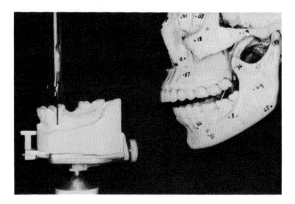

Fig. 3-72. Most advantageous position of cast simulates anatomic position.

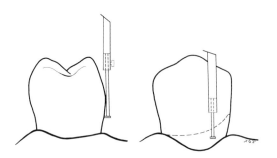

Fig. 3-73. Retentive areas are located and recorded on cast.

Procedure for surveying
Placing the diagnostic cast on the surveying table (Fig. 3-72)

Wherever possible, the diagnostic cast should be surveyed with its occlusal plane as parallel as possible to the base of dental surveyor and perpendicular to the analyzing rod so that the path of placement and withdrawal of the prosthesis will be vertical to the occlusal plane. Most patients will tend to insert an RPD by biting it into place, although this is not advisable because of its potential for damage to the prosthesis; if the path of placement is other than vertical to the occlusal plane, such seating may permanently deform the clasps.

Placing the surveying table and diagnostic cast under the surveying instrument (see Fig. 1-8)

With the analyzing rod in place, the parallelism of the potential tooth surfaces to be used for guiding planes is checked. (Guiding planes are located on all tooth surfaces adjacent to edentulous areas and on all tooth surfaces where minor connectors are indicated to join rests to the major connectors.) Slightly altering the anteroposterior tilt of the surveying table will identify the most acceptable potential guiding planes on the diagnostic cast or indicate the mouth preparation procedures needed to establish the guiding planes at the most advantageous position of the cast.

The retentive areas on the proposed abutment teeth are checked with the undercut gauge for equal amounts of undercut and for their proper location in the gingival third of the crowns of the teeth. Undercuts should be bilaterally opposed and as widely spaced as possible. Altering the mediolateral tilt of the surveying table will determine the most equitable distribution of undercuts for the clasp assemblies. Undesirable soft tissue undercuts are located by using the analyzing rod. The components of the framework and denture base must pass over these undercut areas.

Locating and measuring the depth of the retentive areas (Fig. 3-73)

An appropriate undercut gauge is placed in the vertical instrument holder of the surveying instrument, and the amount of undercut present (0.01 to 0.03 inch) is measured and its location determined on each proposed abutment tooth. When no retentive area exists, abutment tooth contours can be altered to provide the necessary contour for retention. If an excessive retentive area exists, the teeth can be recontoured to remove the excessive undercuts. It must be remembered that the retentive area should be located at the desired depth (0.01 to 0.03 inch) in the gingival third of the tooth crown.

Recording the diagnostic cast position to permit its reorientation (tripoding) (see Fig. 3-71)

After the mouth preparation procedures necessary to establish guiding planes and retentive areas are identified, the analyzing rod is locked in position on the surveying instrument with a set screw. The analyzing rod is replaced with a carbon rod and sheath, and the surveying table and diagnostic cast are moved about the plat-

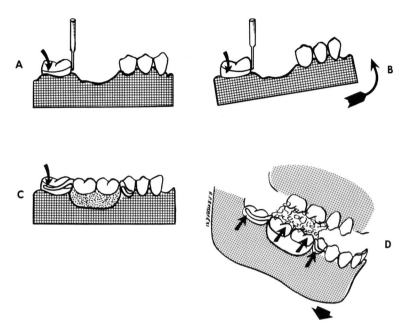

Fig. 3-74. A, Retentive area is insufficient to resist a reasonable dislodging force when cast is surveyed at its most advantageous position. **B,** Tilting cast creates positional, or false, tooth contours, which are present only in relation to surveying rod. **C,** Clasp is in false retentive area. **D,** Retentive area is not in path of displacement when RPD is subjected to dislodging forces in an occlusal direction.

form. Three widely spaced points are marked on the dental stone cast with the carbon marker (one anterior and two posterior on hard-tissue structures, teeth, or bony landmarks). If desired, the subsequent master cast can be grooved on the side to provide tripod points for reproduction in the refractory cast for later reorientation during the framework wax-up procedure.

Determining a treatment plan for mouth preparation (see Chapter 5)

A blue pencil is used to mark areas that have been identified for tooth preparation and alteration by selective grinding on the diagnostic cast. It must be remembered that the dentist's objective is to create, through mouth preparation, a situation in which each components of the RPD can be located in its ideal position as it relates to the teeth and the soft tissues. If guiding planes or undercuts are not properly located on the teeth or do not have the proper relationship to each other, such situations can be controlled by altering the contour of the teeth by selective grinding or by placing a res-

toration. It has been suggested that tilting the diagnostic cast on the surveying table can produce the most advantageous position with a minimum of mouth preparation. Tilting of the cast on the dental surveyor to alter the location and amount of undercuts on the abutment teeth in relation to the path of insertion for the purpose of using a more desirable type of clasp, improving esthetics, or minimizing food impaction can create an impression of positional, or false, tooth contours (Hanson and associates, 1975). These positional tooth contours will be present only in relation to the surveying rod not in relation to the path of displacement during function (Fig. 3-74). A tilt of the diagnostic cast of no more than 10 to 15 degrees from the horizontal is the maximum allowable before the dentist begins to create false tooth contours.

Surveying the master cast

After the mouth preparation has been completed as planned by the diagnostic survey and recorded in the patient's record, an impression is made and a master cast fabricated. The most advantageous position for insertion and withdrawal of the prosthesis can then be reproduced on the dental surveyor and checked to ensure that the mouth preparation has been accomplished correctly. Tripoding of the master cast can now be done and the exact position of the retentive areas noted. The final design can be drawn in detail on a duplicate master cast. This, along with the master cast and a detailed written dental laboratory prescription (work authorization), can be sent to the dental laboratory for fabrication of the framework.

SUMMARY

The systematic approach to design identifies two types of support: tooth and tissue support. Available tooth support can be achieved through the design and placement of rests. Selection of tooth-supported units is based on periodontal health, crown-root ratio, crown and root morphologic features, previous response to stress, and the patient's age. Rest placement is determined by the teeth that remain their relationship to each other, and their relationship to the edentulous areas. Tissue support is achieved by the type of impression made, noting that corrected or altered cast impressions are indicated to adequatley provide for tissue support in distal-extension RPDs.

Once the mechanism for support is identified and the location and design determined (or the method of achieving the support determined) the next step is to connect the support units. Connection of the support units is accomplished by selecting and designing major and minor connectors. Major connectors are selected on the basis of their ability to provide support and rigidity and to distribute stress between the support units. Minor connectors (struts, plates) are selected on the basis their ability to stabilize the abutment teeth and to serve as a mechanism by which stresses can be controlled and transmitted between the support units. The contour of their design should be such that they promote rather than interfere with the health of the supporting soft tissues.

The third step in the systematic approach to design is to select the components of design for retention of the RPD. The key to successful clasp selection is to select a direct retainer that will control tipping and torquing of the abutment teeth, provide retention against reasonable dislodging forces, be compatible with tooth and tissue contours, and satisfy the esthetic desires of the patient. The criteria are generally satisfied if the direct retainer is properly contoured and if its components are properly positioned on the prepared abutment teeth. Location of the retentive areas (undercut) is the determining factor in the design of the retentive component of the direct retainer.

The next step in the systematic approach to design is to connect the retention units to the major connector by properly designed and positioned minor connectors. Again, their function is to contribute stability and to control and transmit to the rests and supporting tissues of the edentulous areas stresses resulting from attempted vertical dislodgement.

The last step in the systematic approach to design is to outline the edentulous areas of the RPD and design them so that they will retain the denture base and not interfere with proper tooth positioning.

Most technical failures of an RPD service result from errors in design: rests that are not properly located or contoured; direct retainers that are not designed with their components properly contoured and positioned on the abutment tooth; major and minor connectors that are not contoured and placed in the proper relation to the tooth surfaces or the soft tissue; or edentulous areas and finishing lines that are not properly contoured and positioned.

Proper placement and contour of the components of design can be achieved only through an adequate survey and well-planned mouth preparation. The components of the RPD must be selected to control stress to the abutment teeth and the tissues caused by forces of occlusion and the movements of the distal-extension bases. Alterations in design may be dictated by the patient's age or previous response to stress or by the dentist's prudent judgment. Compromising the ideal in the location and design of components, however, may jeopardize the potential success of the prosthesis.

4 Examination, diagnosis, and treatment planning

INTRODUCTION

Careful planning by the dentist is a fundamental factor in successful prosthodontic treatment. For each dental patient, a unique *treatment plan* must be developed on the basis of an analysis of the patient's problems and needs. This analysis, or *diagnosis,* is made during the course of a number of *examination* procedures. Routine examination procedures commonly include an assessment of the patient's health status, one or more intraoral and extraoral examinations, an analysis of the patient's radiographs, a study of the mounted diagnostic casts, and, if applicable, an inspection of any existing dental prostheses. In addition, questions designed to explore the patient's dental history and his or her psychologic state must be a part of the examination process.

Comprehensive treatment plans for partially edentulous patients are usually more complicated than are treatment plans formulated for completely edentulous patients or for patients who do not require the replacement of missing teeth. For the dentist to plan the treatment that best meets the special needs of a patient, a number of decisions must be made:

1. Will this person's needs best be met with a fixed partial denture, a removable partial denture (RPD), a complete denture, a combination of these treatments, or with no prosthodontic treatment at all?
2. If an RPD is necessary, what will be the best design for it, or what design features must be incorporated in it to obtain the best possible function, comfort, and esthetics?
3. What additional dental treatment is indicated to restore the remaining dentition and the oral tissues to the best state of health obtainable, considering the patient's circumstances?

4. What special treatment is required to prepare the mouth for the acceptance of the prosthesis?
5. What is the most logical sequence of treatment to follow in accomplishing all of the planned procedures?

The answers to these questions may be derived in a logical and systematic manner. An orderly sequence of examination and diagnostic procedures is described in this chapter. The diagnostic significance of various examination findings is also discussed. Finally, the integration of this information into the development of a comprehensive plan of treatment for a partially edentulous patient is presented.

EXAMINATION PROCEDURES AND DIAGNOSTIC INFORMATION
Conduct of the examination
Get-acquainted interview

Unless the patient is already well known to the dentist, some time should be spent in getting acquainted with the patient and in reviewing the patient's personal data (Plainfield, 1969). Certain key items, such as the patient's age and occupation, often have diagnostic significance. For example, the patient's age gives the dentist a general indication of his or her ability to adapt to wearing a prosthesis. Younger patients generally adapt easily to new situations, whereas older persons tend to have more difficulty in learning to wear removable dentures. General health, resistance to injury, and the healing response are also generally related to a person's age. Younger patients are often chiefly concerned about esthetics (Fig. 4-1). Persons in the "prime of life" have major concerns about function and comfort as well as esthetics, whereas many older patients are primarily interested in the comfort of their dentures (Fig. 4-2).

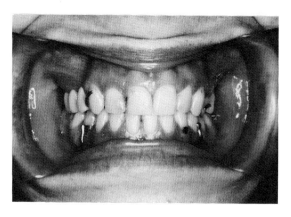

Fig. 4-1. Maxillary and mandibular RPDs in mouth of young patient. Maxillary right posterior denture teeth are placed against residual ridge to eliminate buccal flanges for esthetic reasons.

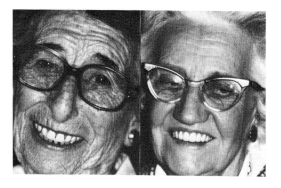

Fig. 4-2. Chronologic versus biologic age. Both patients are same chronologic age, but patient on left appears older biologically. (From Renner, R.P.: Complete dentures: A guide for patient treatment, 1981, p. 27. Copyright © by Masson Publishing USA, Inc., New York.)

For patients of any age whose occupations require them to deal with the public, appearance is usually a primary consideration. The ability to speak naturally and easily may be extremely important to a teacher or a preacher. A retired person often has more time to "play with" his dentures and to find minor problems with them. Thus, knowing the patient's occupation often helps the dentist to predict the type of response to treatment that may be expected.

From the very beginning of the interview and examination processes, the patient may provide significant clues regarding his attitudes toward dental health and dental treatment (Schole, 1959). The dentist should be alert for

this information and should note his or her impressions in the patient's clinical record as the interview proceeds.

To introduce the examination, a dentist may ask "Why did you come to see me?" or "What brings you to the dentist?" This directly opens the way for patients to tell of their problems and needs, as they see them. Patients will often express their desires regarding treatment at this time. If, however, this is not readily communicated, the dentist may ask "How can I help you with your problem?"

Occasionally, patients will have very definite ideas about what they want, and it is important for the dentist to determine if their expectations are realistic. "What do you expect that this treatment will do for you?" is a stimulating inquiry. The patient's expectations regarding appearance, comfort, and function need to be well explored. "How do you think that you will get along with a denture (or a "bridge," etc.)?" is another question that will often elicit additional clues regarding the patient's concept of prosthodontic treatment.

It is an extremely valuable practice for the dentist to *record* the patient's answers and key remarks as they are expressed. Either an examination form or plain paper may be used. As much as possible, the patient's own words should be recorded by the dentist.

Dental history

"Tell me about your previous dental treatment" is a good way to lead the patient into his dental history. It is essential that the dentist determine how the patient has accepted and adapted to past dental treatment. The patient's past attitudes will tend to persist throughout future treatment. It is especially important for the dentist to note indications of dissatisfaction with previous dental care or complaints regarding previous dentists (Figs. 4-3 and 4-4). These "red flags" may alert the dentist to unsolvable problems, untreatable patients, or potentially unsatisfied patients (Bliss, 1951).

The reasons for the loss of the patient's missing teeth are significant and should be elicited by questioning. A history of severe dental caries raises suspicions of current as well as past neglect or nutritional problems. The extraction of teeth because of advanced periodontal disease not only suggests a history of neglect but also is predictive of continued alveolar bone or

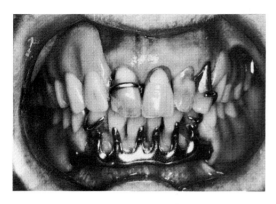

Fig. 4-3. Maxillary and mandibular RPDs are unesthetic because too much of cast metal framework is visible.

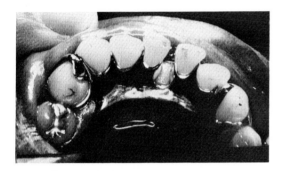

Fig. 4-4. Patient has diastema between teeth number 24 and 25. Discontinuous lingual plate was designed to circumvent this space so that a minimum amount of metal is observed from labial side.

residual ridge resorption as a result of systemic factors.

The loss of teeth as a result of traumatic injury or surgical excision of malignant tissue is important for the dentist to note. The side effects of trauma and surgery are often long lasting and must be considered in the diagnosis. The reasons for the loss of teeth, as well as the manner in which the patient describes the losses, are keys to the patient's attitude toward his teeth and his "dental IQ" (Plainfield, 1969).

Health and medical history

The patient's health and medical history are of great importance in making treatment decisions and predictions because of the dependent relationship of oral health to systemic health. Every dentist, like every physician, is required to be fully informed of the patient's physical and emotional condition before beginning treatment (Bliss, 1951).

It is a common practice in many dental offices to have the patient fill out an abbreviated health questionnaire at the time of registration. This record may be adequate for some dental treatment regimens, but it is the dentist's responsibility to explore thoroughly any suspicious or provocative responses. Complete, reliable medical histories are sometimes not obtained without persistent questioning, since dental patients commonly do not relate general systemic conditions or medical problems to their dental treatment. For patients whose initial health survey suggests the existence of multiple medical or emotional problems, a more comprehensive questionnaire, such as the Cornell Medical Index (Bolender, 1979), may provide additional useful information.

A comprehensive medical history will at times reveal problems for which a patient's physician should be consulted before a diagnosis is made and a treatment plan formulated. Chronic degenerative or dysfunctional diseases such as diabetes, arthritis, obesity, hypertension, and osteoporosis usually compromise treatment results. Women who are going through or who have passed through the menopause may have special physical and psychologic problems that make their treatment more challenging. The limitations to success imposed by these conditions must be explained to the patient at the time of the presentation of the treatment plan.

Medication history

Surveys have shown that a large number of the patients who typically require prosthodontic treatment are taking from one to several types of medication. Many drugs that patients use adversely affect the oral tissues. Because of the effects of many drugs on oral tissues and because of occasional complications of drug interactions, it is imperative for the dentist to record the patient's medication regimen. The dentist must then intelligently analyze this information and carefully consider the problems that may result not only from the patient's diseases themselves but also from the drugs that the patient is taking for them.

Dietary patterns

A patient's dental and general health problems are often complicated by nutritional inadequacies (Perry, 1961). The dentist may gain important clues to dietary imbalances or deficiencies by asking a few simple questions, such as : "What do you eat for breakfast?"; "What do you eat for lunch?"; "What do you eat for dinner?"; and "What kinds of foods do you especially like?" Any significant variation from a normal, balanced nutritional intake signifies the need for a more definitive dietary evaluation (Massler, 1979a and b; Perry, 1961). Instructions for a diagnostic dietary survey are presented in the nutrition counseling section of this chapter.

Subjective evaluations

During the course of the preliminary interview and history-taking, an observant dentist will make valuable subjective evaluations of the patient's physical condition, muscular control, facial expressions and tooth display, speech patterns, mental capacities, and dental IQ.

Importance of a written record

It is most important for the dentist to make written notes of all pertinent observations and of all diagnostic information obtained during the course of the interview. This information will be needed at the treatment planning phase, and it will be impossible for the dentist to remember all of the details of the interview without a written record. The notes also constitute an important legal transcript and should remain a permanent part of the patient's dental record. This principle applies equally to the information obtained from the clinical examination of the patient. Its importance is emphasized repeatedly (Maison, 1959).

Clinical examination of the patient

This section of the chapter outlines a logical and comprehensive sequence of visual and digital examination procedures. It also discusses the diagnostic significance of each procedure's findings. The suggested sequence divides the procedures into a restorative-oriented examination, a periodontally oriented examination, an examination of the mucosal and bony tissues, and an occlusion-oriented examination. Although the idea of four examinations sounds complicated at first, practice reveals this system to be practical and efficient. When followed, it ensures that no important diagnostic information is overlooked.

Good lighting, a clear mouth mirror, a sharp explorer, and a calibrated periodontal probe are required for the examination. Appropriate charting and recording forms are also essential.

Oral hygiene status

The dentist observes and notes in the clinical record whether the patient follows excellent, fair, or poor oral hygiene practices, as evidenced by the presence of food, bacterial plaque, or calculus. When an RPD is inserted, it is especially important that the patient's remaining natural teeth and tissues receive consistent and meticulous cleaning in order for an acceptable degree of health to be maintained. The patient's oral hygiene status before prosthodontic treatment provides reliable evidence of the importance that the patient attaches to this critical factor.

If inadequate oral hygiene practices are evident, the treatment plan must provide for a program of oral health care instruction. Control of dental plaque (Strategman and Shannon, 1974) is so critical to the success of RPD treatment that unless the patient is willing to cooperate in an effective plaque control regimen, the prognosis for the proposed treatment will be seriously compromised. The locations of unusual accumulations of calculus, plaque, or food debris should be recorded so that these areas may be rechecked at subsequent examinations.

INTERPROXIMAL FOOD IMPACTION. There are two types of interproximal food impaction: *vertical* food impaction (Fig. 4-5), which is the forceful wedging of food against the gingival tissues and into the interproximal spaces through occlusal pressure, and *horizontal* food impaction, which is the forcing of food between the teeth by the tongue, lips, and cheeks. The dentist should note whether food impaction between two particular teeth is the result of faulty marginal ridge relationships, faulty contact areas, or a plunger cusp in opposing dentition.

CARIOUS LESIONS AND MISSING TEETH. Beginning with an inspection of the maxillary right posterior teeth, the dentist records all detectable carious lesions and defective restorations. At the same time, missing teeth are also recorded on the chart. After the maxillary right quadrant is inspected, the maxillary left quadrant is examined, followed by the mandibular left quadrant, and finally the mandibular right quadrant. Areas of erosion or unusual abrasion should be checked at this phase of the exami-

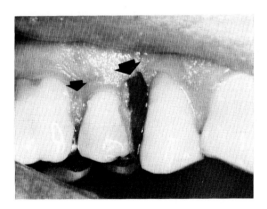

Fig. 4-5. Inadequate contact areas between teeth may result in vertical food impaction *(arrows)*.

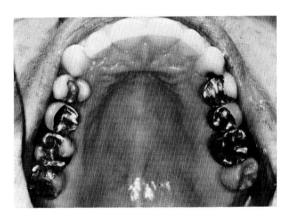

Fig. 4-6. Teeth of patient with rampant dental caries have been restored with amalgam or cast restorations.

nation, and those areas that will require restoration should also be recorded.

The extent of dental caries activity shown in the patient's mouth is of great diagnostic importance. The dentist should evaluate the degree of caries susceptibility, and record an assessment of this critical factor. If dental caries has been a significant problem, basic decisions will depend on the potential ability of the patient to control this disease.

All carious teeth must be restored before prosthodontic treatment is started (Fig. 4-6). A treatment plan for a caries-prone patient should include participation in a caries control program. Plaque control instruction and dietary counseling are usually needed. After the elimination of all active carious lesions, an observation, or "trial," period is recommended if the treatment schedule permits. During the trial period, the patient's oral hygiene practices and susceptibility to disease are reevaluated before prosthodontic treatment is begun.

Periodontal health

The general color of the gingival tissues should be examined. Healthy gingivae are pink, translucent, and have a dull stippled appearance (varying degrees of melanin pigmentation may be present in dark-skinned or Oriental persons) (Beube, 1953). The color changes slightly at the line of demarcation between attached gingival tissue and the movable alveolar mucosa (Fig. 4-7). Red, smooth, shiny gingivae may indicate the presence of gingivitis (Fig. 4-8). The marginal gingiva may turn red

and the alveolar mucosa may become bluish-red when these tissues are congested as a result of infection. A pale, smooth appearance to the gingiva suggests the presence of anemia or circulatory deficiencies.

The texture of the zone of attached gingiva next to the teeth is examined. The attached gingiva is normally stippled. It forms a firm, resilient cuff around each tooth. The band of attached gingiva should be several millimeters wide, and it is especially important that the patient have an adequate zone of this keratinized tissue around teeth that are potential abutments for an RPD (Fig. 4-9).

Blunting and thickening of the marginal gingiva may be observed. Pronounced "festooning" of the gingiva creates problems if clasps or other components of an RPD framework must pass over them. The festoons also tend to trap debris and hinder the cleaning of tooth surfaces in the gingival area.

Gingival clefts are occasionally associated with the loss of attached gingiva. This may indicate the presence of periodontal pockets that require therapy before prosthodontic treatment. Any clefts or areas of gingival recession that extend apically farther than the cementoenamel junction of any tooth should be noted in the clinical records (Fig. 4-10).

Following the same orderly sequence as described in the caries examination, the dentist measures and records the depths of the periodontal pocket that exist around all of the remaining teeth (Fig. 4-9, *A*). The base of each gingival sulcus and periodontal pocket is

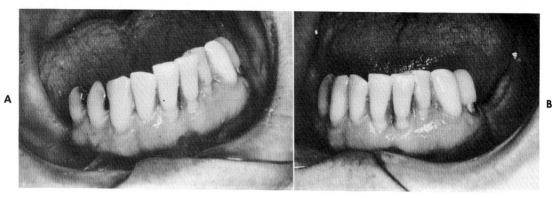

Fig. 4-7. A, Right side of patient's mouth. Tissues appear normal in that gingivae are light pink, translucent, and have a stippled surface. There is deep red color at line of demarcation between mobile mucosa and firmly attached gingivae. Periodontal disease is under control. **B,** Left side of patient's mouth is similar to right side.

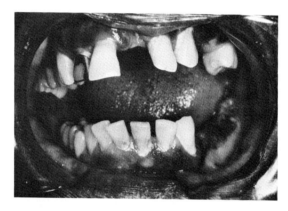

Fig. 4-8. Patient with abnormal periodontal tissues. There is change in pink gingival color. Patient had poor oral hygiene and motivation and was not willing to cooperate in keeping her teeth clean and tissues healthy after repeated instruction and demonstrations.

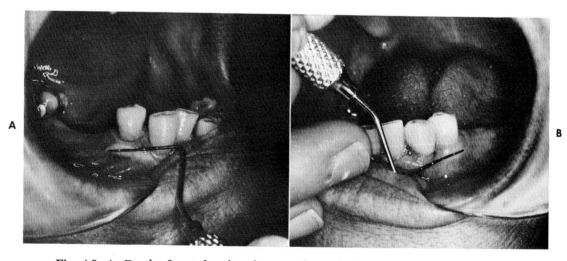

Fig. 4-9. A, Depth of periodontal pocket must be probed. At least eight recordings are made: three on buccal, three on lingual and one each on mesial and distal surfaces of each tooth. Level of epithelial attachment is measured with periodontal probe. There is lack of attached gingiva on tooth number 21. **B,** There is lack of attached gingiva on tooth number 28.

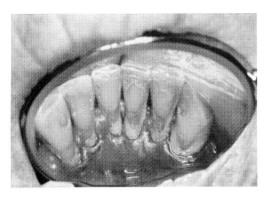

Fig. 4-10. Gingival recession accompanied by pocket formation has occurred on lingual side of natural teeth.

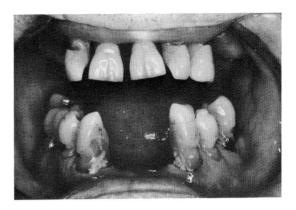

Fig. 4-11. Patient with extreme tooth erosion and periodontal disease. Decision must be made whether mouth can be restored before treating patient with RPD.

probed at three points on the buccal surface and three points on the lingual surface. By charting the depths of the pockets, the dentist produces a "map," or outline, of the pockets. This record is essential in determining the type of periodontal therapy, if any, that may be required (Fig. 4-11). Any existing periodontal disease must be controlled before prosthodontic treatment is begun (Gomes and associates, 1980).

The degree of mobility of all mobile teeth should be recorded (Grant and associates, 1972). Normal physiologic movement of a healthy tooth is barely, if at all, discernable. A scale commonly used for classifying mobility is given below.

Class 1: a tooth demonstrates greater than normal movement, but less than 1 mm of movement in any direction.

Class 2: a tooth moves 1 mm from normal position in any direction.

Class 3: a tooth moves more than 2 mm in any direction, including rotation or depression.

A change from normal physiologic movement may indicate traumatic occlusion or periodontal disease. Teeth exhibiting a mobility of Class 3 have an extremely poor prognosis and usually will require extraction.

Oral mucosa

The mucosa of the palate, edentulous ridges, tongue, cheeks, floor of the mouth, and vestibules should be examined. The location and appearance of any ulcerations, areas of inflammation, or suspicious lesions are recorded. Ir-

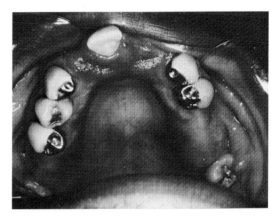

Fig. 4-12. Highly inflamed, red granular area under existing maxillary RPD. As part of diagnosis, culture must be taken to rule out or confirm presence of *C. albicans*.

ritations caused by rough teeth or by an existing prosthesis should be noted.

Unusual white or red lesions anywhere in the oral cavity must be diagnosed. A biopsy may be required in order to verify the diagnosis. Appropriate treatment must be planned.

Candidiasis (Fig. 4-12) is a fungus infection frequently seen in the mucosa underneath existing dentures, especially in the maxilla. Antimycotic antibiotic therapy is required to control the infection before additional prosthodontic treatment is begun. *Candida albicans* infection is frequently associated with the presence of papillary hyperplasia of the palate (Bauman, 1977; Budtz-Jorgensen, 1978a, 1981; Renner and associates, 1979).

RESIDUAL RIDGE. The edentulous ridges are visually inspected and palpated with the fingertips. The size and shape of the ridges and the height and location of the adjacent muscle and soft tissue attachments are noted. The ridges may be described in the clinical record as "high," "flat," "narrow," or "wide."

The firmness of the overlying mucosa is determined by palpation. Areas of flabby, movable tissue over the denture-bearing regions of the residual ridges are observed. Pressure is exerted with the fingertips on several areas of the ridges to observe the patient's response. Areas that are sensitive to digital pressure should be noted. Also the top (crest) and sides of the ridges should be palpated to detect the presence of sharp spines or ledges of bone (Fig. 4-13).

The capability of the residual ridges to tolerate the pressure and friction of a tooth-tissue–borne RPD needs to be carefully assessed if an accurate prognosis for the outcome of prosthodontic treatment is to be made. The completed prosthesis will be considered unsuccessful if the denture-supporting tissues cannot, with reasonable comfort, bear the load placed on them.

An atrophic mucous membrane is frequently found overlying the residual ridges of elderly or malnourished patients. This abnormal mucosa appears to be thin, smooth, and transparent, somewhat resembling a layer of plastic food wrap. The color of such tissue may range from pale pink to red, but it will blanch readily under moderate finger pressure.

An atrophic mucous membrane sometimes burns or hurts spontaneously. It is usually sensitive to pressure, intolerant of pressure from dentures, easily bruised, and slow to heal following injury. If the examination reveals this type of tissue covering potential denture-bearing areas, special note should be made in the examination record so that these factors will not be overlooked when the treatment plan is presented to the patient.

Medical and nutritional therapy, as described later in this chapter, often bring about improvement in patients with an abnormal mucous membrane (Barone, 1965). It is not wise for the dentist to institute prosthodontic treatment until he or she is satisfied that the denture-bearing mucosa has been brought to the best obtainable state of health.

Ideally, denture-bearing residual ridges should be wide, smooth, rounded, and covered with tough, firmly attached, keratinized mucosa (Atwood, 1973). Ridges that are flat, narrow, sharp, sensitive, or covered with flabby tissue will not function well as areas of support (Fig. 4-14). If any of these undesirable conditions exists, compromises in denture comfort and function must be anticipated, and the patient must be counseled accordingly. Mandibular residual ridges tend to exhibit these undesirable characteristics (Fig. 4-13) more frequently than do maxillary residual ridges.

Enlarged, hyperplastic tuberosities are frequently encountered in the maxillary arch. If these structures are flabby or spongy or if they intrude into the interridge space, they should be described on the clinical record so that surgical reduction may be planned.

TORI. If palatal or lingual tori are present, the dentist should record their locations and note whether surgical modification of the tori should be considered in treatment planning (Fig. 4-15, *A*). Generally, small tori do not have to be removed when a patient is treated with an RPD. The major connector of the RPD can usually be designed around these anatomic anomalies. If the tori are very large or mushroom shaped, or if they will otherwise interfere with comfort, function, or speech, they should be surgically removed before prosthodontic treatment is instituted (Fig. 4-15, *B*).

Occlusion

CENTRIC RELATION. To observe the contacts of the teeth in the centric relation, the dentist should ask the patient to touch the teeth together *slowly and lightly* until the *first* contact is felt and then to "close all the way." Demonstration of a "slide" between the initial contact and the position of maximum intercuspation indicates that there is a discrepancy between closure of the jaw in centric relation and the centric occlusion position. This variance may be normal for the patient or it may be traumatic.

The need for occlusal equilibration should be diagnosed at this time. The recontouring or restoration of teeth to make the centric relation and centric occlusion positions of the jaw coincide is sometimes but not always required. Certainly, premature contacts in normal closure and deflective occlusal contacts that cause protrusive or lateral slides must be corrected. The location of any abnormal deflective occlu-

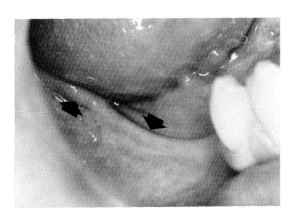

Fig. 4-13. Sharp angular shelflike or spinelike irregularities of residual ridge can be painful to patient if thin layer of mucoperiosteum is trapped between bone and denture base.

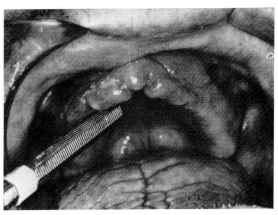

Fig. 4-14. Hyperplastic tissue of anterior maxilla results from anterior hyperfunction. Patient had porcelain maxillary anterior denture teeth in maxillary complete denture and seven mandibular natural anterior teeth and was not wearing mandibular distal-extension RPD.

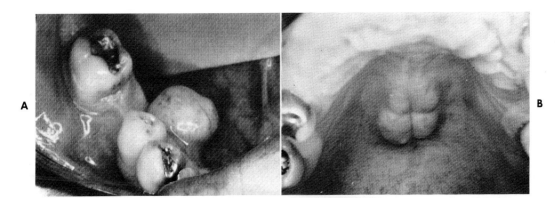

Fig. 4-15. A, Mandibular lingual tori must be surgically removed before patient can be treated with RPD. Tori usually interfere with placement of maxillary or mandibular major connector. These tissues are easily abraded because of their thin mucoperiosteum, and RPD is generally uncomfortable. **B,** Patient with torus palatinus that should be surgically removed. If it cannot be removed, it should not be covered by RPD.

sal contacts or prematurities should be determined and recorded on the clinical chart.

Many dentists accept a discrepancy between centric relation and centric occlusion positions, frequently seen in "normal" patients, if the following conditions are met:

1. The jaw closes smoothly and consistently into the centric occlusion position.
2. There are multiple, simultaneous, stable occlusal contacts in the centric occlusion position.
3. There is no evidence of a slide following the initial occlusal contact.

4. There are no symptoms of dysfunction.

Many partially edentulous patients exhibit abnormal patterns of closure caused by deflective occlusal contacts. Deflective contacts develop as a consequence of the drifting of the remaining teeth following the loss of teeth. Gross occlusal irregularities must be corrected before treatment with removable prostheses is initiated to avoid the perpetuation of the imbalances by the RPDs (Gilson, 1958). On the other hand, precise equilibration can often be completed only after the RPDs are inserted to complete the occlusal scheme (Henderson, 1972).

CENTRIC OCCLUSION AND PLANE OF OCCLUSION. The dentist should hold the patient's jaws together lightly in maximum intercuspal occlusion and observe the occlusal relationships of the remaining teeth (Beck, 1972b). Simultaneous examination of the articulated diagnostic casts is very helpful at this stage. The presence of teeth that have supraerupted into opposing edentulous spaces so that they disrupt the continuity or the orientation of the occlusal plane of the dental arches (Fig. 4-16) should be noted especially. Also the interridge space between the maxillary tuberosity and the mandible (retromolar area) should be reevaluated for adequacy of denture base coverage and extension.

Reestablishment of a relatively regular, straight plane of occlusion is critical to the success of the prosthodontic treatment. Extruded teeth, if untreated, usually prevent restoration of a nontraumatic, harmonious pattern of occlusion. Correction of this problem eventually requires one of the following treatment alternatives, depending on the severity of supraeruption:

1. Selective grinding of the cusps
2. Restoration with a crown at the proper height
3. Gross reduction and restoration, often involving endodontic treatment
4. Extraction of the offending tooth

A "deep" or excessive anterior vertical overlap (overbite) (more than 3 mm) should be noted. Severe vertical overlap of the anterior teeth often results in problems in the design and fitting of RPDs. Excessive anterior vertical overlap may also be a sign of posterior occlusal collapse, with its accompanying loss of interarch space.

Abnormal horizontal overlap (overjet) (Fig. 4-17) relationships should also be noted if observed. Excessive anterior horizontal overlap, or "open bite," may be diagnostic of abnormal swallowing or tongue thrust habits. Either of these conditions creates difficulties in wearing RPDs.

ECCENTRIC OCCLUSAL AND TRAUMATIC OCCLUSAL CONTACTS. The dentist should have the patient move the jaw laterally from the centric occlusion position and should observe the tooth contacts that provide guidance in the left and right excursions. If strong, immobile natural teeth are not providing guidance for jaw movements, compromises in function and comfort with removable prostheses may be expected. Problems of retention and stability of an RPD will certainly occur if the stresses of mandibular guidance fall onto the replacement denture teeth of the prosthesis.

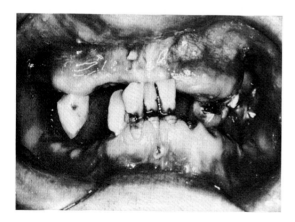

Fig. 4-16. Maxillary and mandibular teeth have extruded into edentulous areas. Clinical judgment is necessary to determine whether teeth should be extracted, recontoured, or restored or whether endodontic and periodontic treatment is necessary before any prosthodontic intervention.

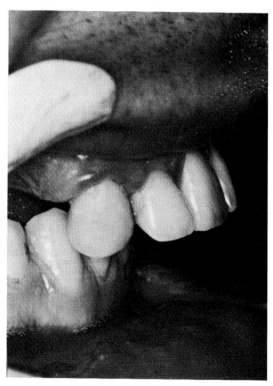

Fig. 4-17. Skeletal Class II jaw relationship that demonstrates protruding maxillary anterior teeth.

Often, the loss of some of the teeth, followed by some drifting of the remaining teeth, results in malposed teeth and traumatic occlusion, with mandibular guidance being forced upon weak teeth (Fig. 4-18). Common signs of traumatic occlusion are mobile teeth or excessive attrition of the occlusal surfaces. Teeth that exhibit abnormal mobility during lateral jaw movements often have an unfavorable prognosis.

The dentist should also at this time look for evidences of bruxism or clenching. Mobile or chipped teeth or severely worn opposing facets are suspicious signs of these parafunctional habits. A person who clenches or grinds his or her teeth subjects them, their supporting structures, and any prosthesis worn to destructive forces. If a parafunctional habit is verified or even strongly suspected, the patient must be counseled regarding the effects of the habit.

Existing prostheses

If the patient has been wearing an RPD, a great deal of useful information may be gleaned from an examination of this prosthesis. Factors that should be especially noted include the adequacy of the design, possible harmful effects resulting from poor adaptation, the size and type of denture teeth, and the occlusal scheme of the denture. Notes should be made of changes that need to be made in a new prosthesis. However, the dentist must be careful not to change good features of the existing prosthesis to which the patient has adapted but only to modify unsuccessful features.

Tongue

The size of the patient's tongue should be observed in relation to the space available within the dental arches. If the lateral borders of the tongue protrude outward through the edentulous spaces, or if the tongue "overflows" the occlusal table of the remaining mandibular teeth, problems with the tongue's adapting to the presence of a new prosthesis may be anticipated (Kessler, 1955) (Fig. 4-19).

Temporomandibular joint

Any abnormalities of joint function, such as clicking or "catching," detected during the course of the oral examination should be noted on the clinical record. In addition, comments by the patient regarding the temporomandibular joint (TMJ) should be recorded (Zarb and associates, 1978). Complaints of pain, tenderness, or swelling in the area of the TMJ should receive careful consideration. The treatment of the varied disorders of the TMJ and its musculature are beyond of the scope of this book, but the importance of further diagnostic tests and appropriate therapy, if they are indicated, is emphasized (Boucher, 1962).

Muscle tone

The tonicity of the muscles of the face and lips is an important factor in the success of prosthodontic treatment. In patients who have had a loss of occlusal vertical dimension and facial support because of long-standing edentulism or inadequate prosthodontic replacement of missing teeth, loss of muscle size and muscle

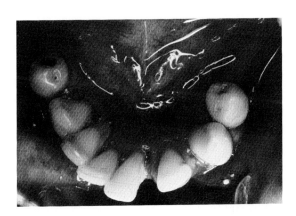

Fig. 4-18. Decision should be made concerning disposition of malposed teeth.

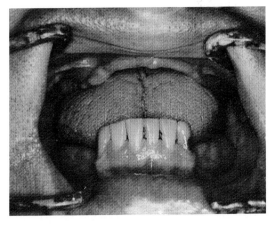

Fig. 4-19. Patient has an enlarged tongue that will resist adaptation to dentures.

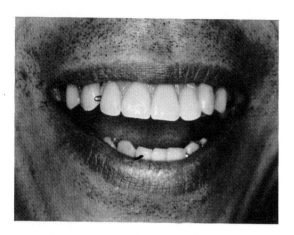

Fig. 4-20. Patient with esthetic maxillary RPD replacing four anterior teeth.

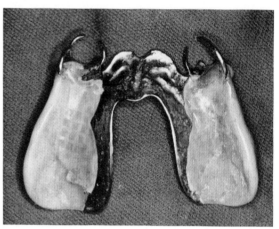

Fig. 4-21. Maxillary RPD that is improperly designed to approximate gingival tissues. Maxillary major connector is *not* placed at least 6 mm away from gingival margins.

tone is evident. Thin, soft lips, narrow vermillion borders, drooping corners of the mouth, and pronounced facial wrinkles are diagnostic signs. It should be noted on the clinical record whether the muscle tone is good, fair, or poor.

Problems of esthetics and function are often complicated by the loss of muscle strength and tone. On the other hand, with the provision of adequately constructed prostheses, a redevelopment of the tone and power of the muscles of facial expression and mastication may sometimes occur (Fig. 4-20).

Pulp vitality tests

Pulp vitality tests are recommended for teeth with suspicious carious or radiographic lesions or for any teeth whose vitality is questioned. Electrical or thermal stimulation may be employed. The results of the tests should be recorded to make later comparisons possible.

Oral or systemic evidence of reduced tissue tolerance

The problem of reduced tissue tolerance is related to the systemic health of the patient. When oral or systemic conditions are not favorable, the added stress of an RPD on the abutment teeth and associated supporting tissues will be too great for these tissues to withstand (Jones, 1976). Thus, when the supporting tissues deteriorate, the RPD becomes unstable and there is an increase in the destructive forces on the remaining intraoral tissues. The amount of remaining alveolar bone previously lost through systemic or local factors has a per-

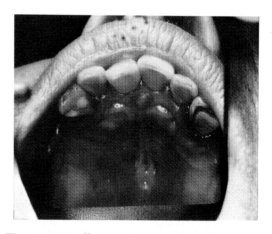

Fig. 4-22. Maxillary RPD caused breakdown of gingival tissues around all remaining natural teeth. Prognosis for remaining canine teeth is questionable if they are to be used as abutments for another RPD.

tinent bearing on whether the remaining dentition should be retained or extracted. The patient who cannot biologically replace bone elements as fast as they are used has a poor chance of retaining the remaining teeth when they are used as abutments for an RPD (Figs. 4-21 and 4-22).

A patient's systemic condition and ability to provide a normal metabolic function are important factors in the success or failure of an RPD. Some systemic conditions that have intraoral manifestations and that can influence prosthodontic treatment are included in Table 4-1.

TABLE 4-1
Systemic changes in the RPD patient important to the general practitioner

Systemic condition	Clinical signs and symptoms	Mucosal alterations	Bony alterations	Muscle and central nervous system alterations	Prosthodontic considerations
Pernicious anemia	Dryness of mouth, disturbance of taste sensation	Susceptibility to denture trauma	—	—	Constant monitoring of denture stability and occlusion is required to minimize pressure areas. Poor denture retention results from lack of saliva.
Vitamin or nutritional deficiencies	Dryness of mouth, loss of appetite, decline in taste sensibility, capillary fragility, weight loss, general weakness	Difficult regeneration, susceptibility to RPD trauma, thinning, easy abrasion (dry mucosa adheres to RPDs and is easily abraded), reduced resistance to infection	Osteoporosis with severe alveolar destruction with low Ca intake and Ca/PO$_4$ imbalance, low protein and vitamin intake	Muscle weakness; fatigue and depression	Dietary counseling and supplementation are needed when eating habits cannot be changed. Monoplane occlusal scheme, as advocated by Jones (1972), should be used. Proper base extension and stability are needed to prevent mucosal irritation.
Hypertension	Breathlessness on exertion, angina on effort, palpitation, epistaxis, headache, dizziness	—	—	—	Avoidance of hypertensive episodes is important. Premedication should be used when necessary. Appointments should be short and stressless. Dentist should have a reassuring and considerate attitude.
Diabetes	Dryness of mouth; tendency to obesity; increased thirst, hunger, and urinary output; weakness and weight loss	Susceptibility to RPD trauma, reduced tissue tolerance to RPDs, mucosal hyperemia and swelling, burning palate	Reduced bone tolerance to RPDs, rapid bone loss with elevated blood glucose levels	—	Borders should not be overextended. Patient's mouth is prone to sore spots that become secondarily infected. Patient must maintain good tissue hygiene. Tissue rest should be maximized. Dentist should recall patient frequently to correct occlusion and monitor bone stability.

Continued.

Adapted from Renner, R.P., Complete dentures: a guide for patient treatment, New York, 1981, Masson Publishing USA, Inc.

TABLE 4-1
Systemic changes in the RPD patient important to the general practitioner—cont'd

Systemic condition	Clinical signs and symptoms	Mucosal alterations	Bony alterations	Muscle and central nervous system alterations	Prosthodontic considerations
Osteoporosis	Decrease in skeletal mass and radiographic decrease in bone density; earlier onset in females than in males as a result of normal aging	—	Marked alveolar ridge resorption with advancing age, generalized osteoporosis of maxilla and mandible during sixth decade and beyond	—	Patient has tendency to narrowing of maxillary ridge and broadening of mandibular ridge, leading to posterior tooth crossbites. Dentist should avoid reducing interocclusal distance. Possibility of pathologic fracture exists. Occlusion should be well balanced, and maximum coverage of residual ridges should be provided for support.
Dermatologic diseases					
Lichen planus	Mucosal inflammation and pain, hyperkeratosis	Epithelial erosion, ulceration, mucosal plaque formation	—	—	Severe cases of erosive lichen planus or pemphigus may prevent the comfortable wearing of RPDs.
Fungal infections	Easily removed milk curdlike lesions	Inflammation, milk curd lesions, papillomatosis			Dentist should eradicate fungal lesions with antimycotic antibiotic therapy before RPDs are fabricated.
Postradiation therapy	Dryness of mouth, osteomyelitis, necrosis, trismus of muscles of mastication	Susceptibility to RPD trauma, necrosis from radiation-induced vascular changes	Necrosis of bone from radiation-induced vascular changes	Muscle trismus	Dentist must correct sore spots rapidly. Overextensions should be avoided so that they do not become secondarily infected, leading to osteoradionecrosis. Xerostomia reduces patient's ability to wear dentures. Vertical dimension of occlusion is reduced because of muscle trismus.
Climacteric	Tendency to gag, burning sensation, dryness of mouth, vague areas of pain, taste alterations	Glistening, reddening, and edema; susceptibility to RPD trauma; burning tongue and palate; serous-filled blisters; epithelial sloughing; loss of keratin from mucosa	Generalized osteoporosis	Psychologic changes and emotional instability	Longer adjustment phase to RPDs is required because of mucosal and psychologic changes.

Examination, diagnosis, and treatment planning 103

Chronic pulmonary diseases (such as emphysema and chronic bronchitis)	Shortness of breath, wheezing, increased respiratory rate, persistant cough	—	—	Decreased muscle tone, lowered sensitivity to stimuli, low cough reflex	Patient has little pulmonary reserve and poor reaction to stress. Dentist should keep appointments short. Vertical dimension of occlusion is difficult to record because of patient's tendency to mouth breathe.
Salivary gland disorders	Xerostomia, painful and burning mucosa	Mucosal sensitivity, plaque retention, mucosal abrasion and ulceration from denture base	—	—	Wearing the RPD becomes intolerable because of pain, burning, and frictional abrasion of the oral mucous membrane from tissue-fitting and polished surfaces.
Neurologic disorders Bell's palsy	Facial paralysis with mouth drawn over to opposite side, saliva runs from angle of mouth	Numbness in affected side, inability to feel collected food in buccal sulcus	—	Inability to retract corner of mouth or to whistle	Dentist should not overstretch the angle of mouth and should add sufficient bulk to buccal surface contour of maxillary RPD to support flaccid muscles.
Parkinsonism	Impaired movement, muscular rigidity, tremor, slowness, limited range of movement	Soft, hypokeratinated mucosa, denture stomatitis	—	Speech difficulty, increased salivation, difficulty in mastication because of muscle tremors	Dentist should teach careful oral hygiene, use tissue conditioners, balance occlusion, and use nonanatomic teeth. Retention is impaired from increased salivation. Maximum peripheral extension decreases denture retention. Patient lacks muscular coordination to control RPDs. Judgment of vertical dimension of occlusion is difficult because of tremor and hypertonicity of muscles.
TMJ disturbances	Pain and tenderness of joint with crepitation on movement; leveling of joint surfaces; sclerosis; reduced distance between articular eminence and condylar head	—	—	Limited range of motion of the mandible in all dimensions	Danger of subluxation exists during dental procedures. Mandibular excursive movements are painful, and there is reduced capacity for maximal mouth opening. Impressioning is difficult, and special trays are required. Maxillomandibular relations are difficult to record and reproduce. Frequent occlusal adjustments are necessary.

Radiographic examination and diagnosis

A panoramic radiograph is of great diagnostic value and should be made whenever possible. Anatomic relationships of the teeth, supporting tissues, and the jaw bones are more readily visualized in a panoramic radiograph. Periapical radiographs of the remaining teeth may also be required in order to supplement the panoramic radiograph. Teeth that have a questionable prognosis or that will probably require surgical, endodontic, or restorative treatment should be shown on individual periapical films, because resolution of detail is better on these films. When a panoramic radiograph is not available, a full mouth series of periapical radiographs should be made. It is necessary to make the radiographic exposures before the examination appointments so that the radiographs may be processed and mounted before the examination time. The mounted radiographs must be examined on a well-lighted viewbox.

In the radiographic examination, special consideration is given to the diagnostic factors discussed below.

Carious lesions

Initial carious lesions and recurrent caries adjacent to existing restorations should be noted. Deep lesions or extensive restorations in teeth that are potential abutments for prostheses should receive special scrutiny. Obvious indications for endodontic therapy or for cast restorations should be recorded.

Alveolar bone resorption

In most partially edentulous patients some loss of alveolar bone will be evident, and in many patients the bone loss will be severe, as judged on the radiographs by the height of the alveolar crest shadows around the roots of the remaining teeth (Fig. 4-23).

Both the quantity and quality of the bone support for potential abutment teeth are critical factors in the long-term success of an RPD, so a careful evaluation of these factors must be made at this time. Abutment teeth will be called upon to withstand greater than normal vertical, horizontal, and torquing forces applied to them by the prosthesis. A tooth that has lost one third or more of its alveolar support may not be strong enough to bear these unusual loads.

The radiographic crown-root ratio is a com-

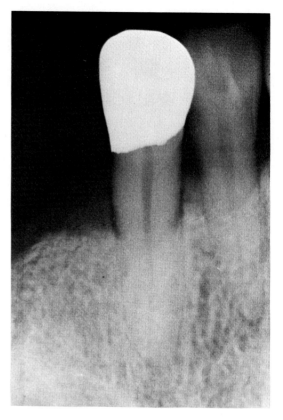

Fig. 4-23. Alveolar bone loss around maxillary cuspid is caused by added stress of traumatic occlusion.

monly used index for classifying the degree of support existent for teeth being evaluated as probable abutments. The length of the tooth crownward from the crest of the alveolar bone is compared with the length of the tooth root apically from the alveolar crest, and the comparison is expressed as an approximate ratio.

A tooth with normal, undiminished alveolar support will have a crown-root ratio of approximately 1:2. A tooth that extends as far above its supporting alveolus as its root extends into the alveolar bone is said to have a crown-root ratio of 1:1 (see Fig. 3-5).

As a general diagnostic guide, a tooth with a crown-root ratio of more than 1:1 is considered to have an unfavorable prognosis as an abutment tooth. However, the clinical mobility and periodontal health of the tooth must also be considered when treatment planning decisions are made.

Bone density

The relative radiographic density of the bone around the remaining teeth, particularly in the

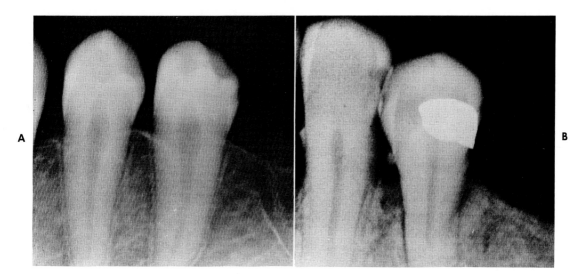

Fig. 4-24. A, The lamina dura appears as radiopaque white line around radiolucent dark line of periodontal ligament on dental radiograph. This patient's tooth has dense lamina dura and should withstand applied functional stress. **B,** This patient's tooth does not have evidence of dense lamina dura and may not respond favorably to applied stress.

vicinity of potential abutment teeth, should be closely observed. Areas of bone around teeth that have been subjected to unusual lateral or occlusal stresses have been referred to as "bone index areas." The response of the bone to heavy functional loads, as demonstrated in the "index areas," is diagnostically significant.

An increased degree of trabeculation and condensation of the bone close to stressed teeth is a favorable sign. Bone that is radiologically translucent, with sparse trabeculae and thin laminae dura, suggests a guarded prognosis for the teeth in question.

The density of the bone in residual ridge areas is likewise of diagnostic importance. Heavy trabeculation and thick cortical plates signify a favorable prognosis for the supportive capacity of the residual ridge. Areas of bone that are relatively radiolucent and poorly trabeculated and that exhibit a thin or interrupted superior cortical plate may be expected to undergo comparatively rapid and severe resorption (Atwood, 1962; Tallgren, 1970; Wical, 1974a and b). They are poorly suited for the support of a removable prosthesis.

Root configuration

The size and shape of the roots of potential abutment teeth, as shown in the radiographs, are of value in determining the resistance of the

teeth to the additional forces to which they will be subjected. Abutments with long, multiple, and divergent roots will have a favorable prognosis, because the forces transmitted to them will be distributed to a larger number of periodontal ligament fibers and to a greater area of supporting alveolar bone. Teeth with short, conical, or fused roots will have an unfavorable prognosis because of their decreased resistance to the forces of function (see Fig. 3-6).

Periodontal ligaments and the lamina dura

The width of the periodontal ligament around the roots of the teeth is of significance in evaluating the stability of the teeth (S. Miller, 1950). A thin, uniform ligament space is a more favorable sign than is a widened, irregular space.

The lamina dura is a thin plate of bone that surrounds the root of each tooth and provides attachment for the periodontal ligament. On a radiograph, it appears as a radiopaque line outlining the alveolus (Fig. 4-24). A thin, irregular, or interrupted lamina dura may indicate the presence of traumatic occlusion, periodontal destruction, or systemic bone disease. Abnormal areas, if observed, should be noted. It must be remembered, however, that radiographs do not show the relationship between periodontal pocket depth and alveolar bone resorption (Fig. 4-25).

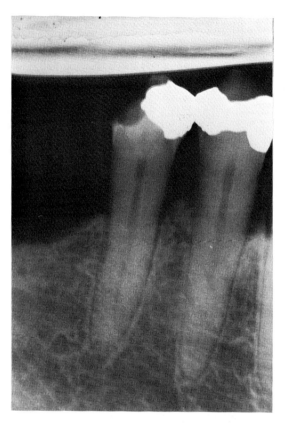

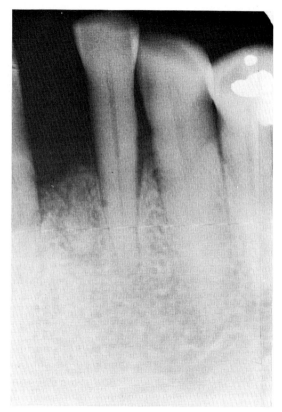

Fig. 4-25. Edentulous area that may not withstand normal occlusal loading. Clinical judgment must be used to determine whether splinting of abutment teeth will counteract some of destructive forces directed to residual ridge. Patient has not worn RPDs for approximately 8 years.

Fig. 4-26. Nonpathologic retained root in area number 24 that need not be surgically removed. To remove the nonpathologic retained root, excessive amount of alveolar bone would be lost through surgical procedure.

Radiolucent or radiopaque lesions

The presence of cysts, abscesses, embedded teeth or roots, or foreign bodies should be noted so that appropriate surgical diagnosis and treatment may be planned. Buried root tips or impacted teeth that show no sign of pathosis and are encapsulated by normal-appearing bone need not always be surgically removed (Fig. 4-26).

Analysis of the diagnostic casts

It is essential that accurate casts of the dental arches be available at the time of the diagnostic examination. They must be mounted in centric relation on a suitable dental articulator. A face-bow registration and a centric relation record are required for a reliable mounting (Fig. 4-27). The procedures described in Chapter 7 may be used to obtain these mounting records.

Before the examination appointment, impressions must be made and poured for diagnostic casts and the mounting records must also be made.

Criteria for the acceptability of diagnostic casts include the following:

1. Anatomic details of the dental arches should be accurately reproduced, including the teeth, gingival tissues, frenum attachments, and residual ridges.
2. There should be no dental stone nodules, voids, or artifacts in critical anatomic areas of the casts.
3. The bases of the diagnostic casts should be between 10 and 15 mm thick at the thinnest areas.
4. The bases of the casts should be approximately parallel to the occlusal plane of the dental arch.

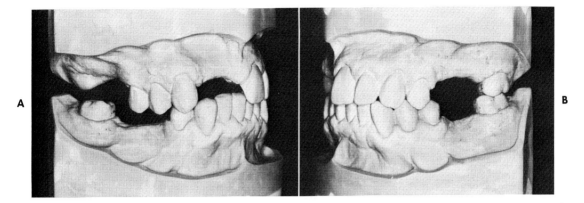

Fig. 4-27. Mounted diagnostic casts in centric occlusion. **A,** Right lateral view. **B,** Left lateral view.

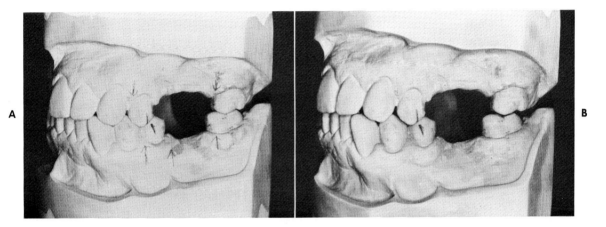

Fig. 4-28. A, View of mounted diagnostic casts in centric relation. **B,** View of mounted diagnostic casts in centric occlusion.

5. The sides of the diagnostic cast should be neatly trimmed perpendicular to the base and a few millimeters outside of the depth of the vestibular tissues.
6. The "tongue space" of the mandibular cast should be clear of unnecessary dental stone, with a flat "floor" approximately level with the depth of the lingual vestibules.

Evaluation of the mounted diagnostic casts
Occlusal relationships

Normal and abnormal occlusal contacts between opposing teeth may often be studied more easily with mounted diagnostic casts than is possible in the patient's mouth. Deflective occlusal contacts, or interferences between centric relation and centric occlusion positions, are critical factors to assess (Fig. 4-28).

Plane of occlusion

The plane of the occlusal surfaces of the teeth should be evaluated very carefully. For the occlusal surfaces of the teeth to function together in harmony with the movement of the TMJ, they must occlude on a plane that is relatively even and level (Sheppard and Sheppard, 1968). In partially edentulous mouths, the drifting and extrusion of the remaining teeth tend to create uneven or irregular occlusal planes. The resulting malocclusion is traumatic to the teeth, their supporting structures, and to the TMJ. Extruded or tipped teeth that violate the regularity of the occlusal plane require modification by means of selective grinding or placement of cast restorations. Severely malposed teeth may require extraction (see Fig. 4-18).

It is desirable for the posterior height of the

mandibular plane of occlusion to be near the level of the center of the retromolar pad. Occlusal planes that have been grossly disoriented because of the extruded teeth or because of enlargement of the maxillary tuberosities must be corrected (Kelly, 1972).

Abutment teeth contours

The contours and axial inclinations of potential abutment teeth should be studied to determine whether the fitting of a fixed or a removable partial denture may be practical. Teeth used as RPD abutments often require recontouring to reduce undesirable undercuts and to enhance contours favorable for clasping (Figs. 4-29 through 4-31). Teeth that have inclinations unfavorable for clasping or that have bulk or contours inadequate for rest seats, guiding planes, or retentive areas require cast restorations.

Rest seat areas

The occlusal contacts of the anterior and posterior teeth at sites where rest seats are desired must be carefully evaluated (Fig. 4-32). Rest seats on maxillary anterior teeth must be placed in areas that will not interfere with the occlusion of the mandibular anterior teeth.

Embrasure-type direct retainers require occlusal clearance for the occlusal rest seats and for transocclusal extensions of the rest preparations (Fig. 4-33). Occasionally, the casts will reveal the necessity of reducing an opposing cusp tip to obtain the required clearance for an occlusal rest or an embrasure clasp.

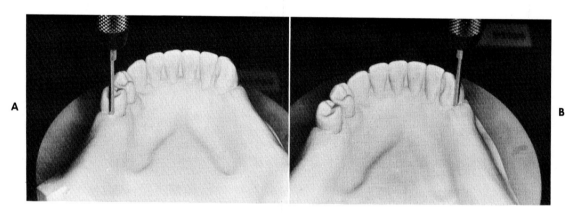

Fig. 4-29. A, Diagnostic cast should be tilted slightly anteriorly and posteriorly to determine most favorable path of insertion and withdrawal. Guiding planes are located on tooth number 20. **B,** Path of insertion and removal and guiding plane are located on tooth number 27.

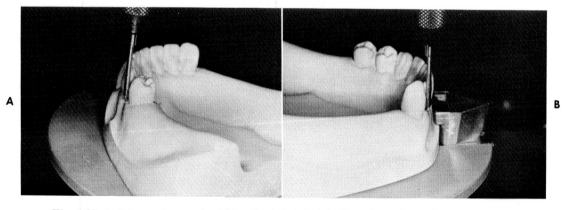

Fig. 4-30. A, Diagnostic cast should be tilted slightly labially or buccally to determine retention on tooth. Retentive area is determined on tooth number 20. **B,** Retentive area is determined on tooth number 27.

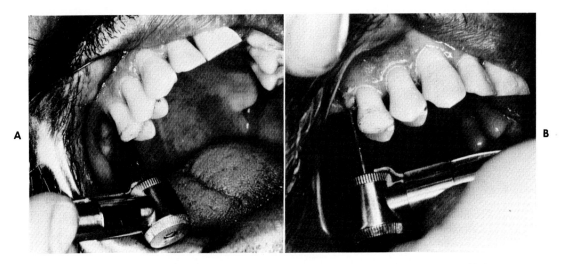

Fig. 4-31. A, "Mouth surveyor" may be made by cementing carbon marker onto old fissure bur. Height of contour of tooth is marked and areas that need recontouring are observed. B, Note height of contour of tooth after recontouring procedure.

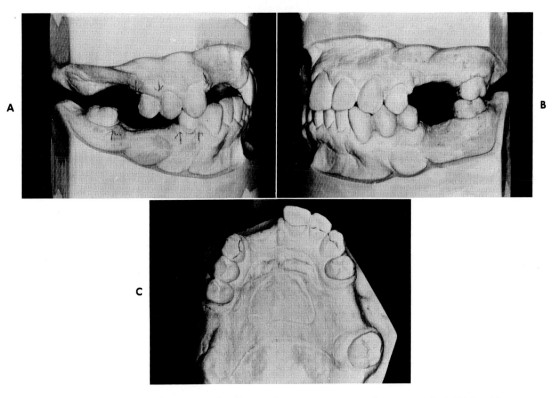

Fig. 4-32. Arrows are drawn on side of cast where rest seats may be prepared. A, Right side. B, Left side. C, Occlusal contacts of anterior teeth are evaluated by line's being drawn on lingual surfaces of maxillary anterior teeth where mandibular anterior teeth make contact.

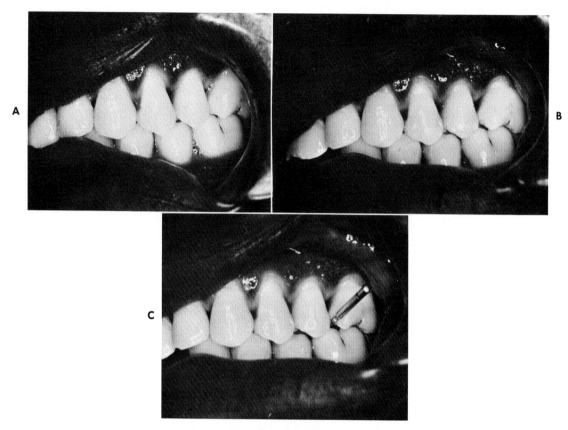

Fig. 4-33. A, Embrasure clasps need occlusal clearance and transocclusal extension of rest preparations, which is more difficult to achieve in patient with extremely tight occlusal contacts. B, Occlusion after rest preparation has been made on maxillary first molar. C, Occlusal clearance is checked with tapering diamond stone.

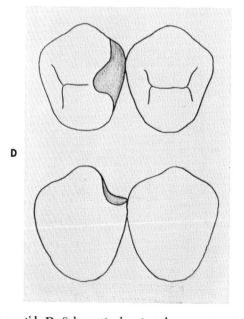

Fig. 4-33, cont'd. D, Schematic drawing shows rest seat preparation.

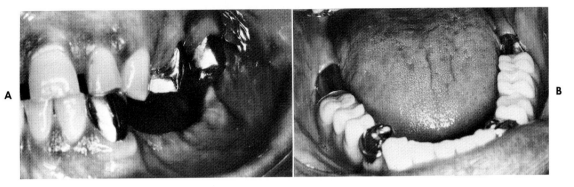

Fig. 4-34. A, When patient is examined for interridge distance, there should be 2 mm of clearance between tooth and residual ridge to prevent breakage of acrylic resin. This patient has less than 2 mm of interridge clearance. **B,** Very thin metal denture base extension was constructed on RPD between tissues and opposing teeth.

Interarch space (interarch distance)

The space available between opposing residual ridges or between the teeth of one arch and the residual ridge of the opposing arch is of diagnostic significance. Insufficient space for the components of a proposed prosthesis or for the establishment of an acceptable plane of occlusion is a problem requiring correction (Fig. 4-34). Surgical reduction of enlarged tuberosities is frequently indicated to allow for the placement of RPD bases or for the creation of a favorable plane of occlusion.

Ridge relationships

The horizontal, as well as the vertical, relationship between the opposing arches is important, and it is more easily observed on the diagnostic casts than in the patient's mouth. The need to consider cross-bite occlusal relationships will be revealed by observing the relationship of the mounted diagnostic casts.

Tissue contours

Some soft tissue contours and undercuts are often more clearly demonstrated on the diagnostic casts than in the patient's mouth. On the diagnostic casts, the size and shape of bony tori are evident (Fig. 4-35). Ledges and sharp exostoses that may interfere with the placement of an RPD are also easily seen. Sharp or severely undercut mylohyoid ridges, which may require surgical recontouring, should be noted.

Evaluation of the patient's psychologic status

Personal and psychologic factors are often more significant to the success of prosthodontic

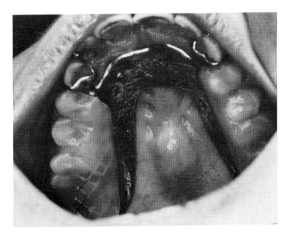

Fig. 4-35. Maxillary RPD designed to circumvent maxillary torus. Caution must be exercised when this design is used because major connector may be too flexible and cause tissue damage.

treatment than are the patient's physical conditions. Before proceding with definitive treatment planning, it is critical that the dentist accurately assess the patient's attitudes toward his or her oral health and dental treatment. By the end of the interview and examination, the dentist must form an opinion as to whether the patient's emotional makeup is likely to make treatment easy, difficult, or impossible.

Each individual has distinct personality traits that, when evaluated, may help to predict the course of prosthodontic treatment. A system for classifying dental patients may help the dentist anticipate the response of an individual patient. One useful classification describes four types of patients: (1) philosophic, (2) emotional, (3) exacting, and (4) indifferent.

Philosophic patients are rational and well balanced. They realize the importance of a healthy mouth. They do not expect perfection but rather a reasonable degree of esthetics, comfort, and efficiency in their prostheses.

Emotional patients are nervous or temperamental. Their dental history reveals neglect and fear of dentists. They are pessimistic about their ability to wear a dental prosthesis successfully. They tend to be suspicious of the dentist's ability and intentions. They exaggerate symptoms and problems.

Exacting patients are perfectionists and demand unrealistic degrees of perfection from the completed treatment. These patients are unwilling to accept changes in their oral hygiene and eating habits. They will expect the same efficiency in chewing that they had with their natural teeth. They are critical of the minutest details of esthetics, fit, and function. They usually are critical of previous dentists, and they often request written guarantees.

Indifferent patients are unconcerned about their appearance and their oral health. They have neglected, unhealthy mouths. They exhibit little patience or perseverance in adapting to a prosthesis, and will often remove it for the least excuse. Because they offer no opinions or suggestions during the examination and treatment, they lead the dentist to believe that treatment will be easy. After a prosthesis is completed, however, they often prove to be uncooperative and difficult patients.

A patient's past experience with dentists and with dental treatment, as explored in the initial interview, provides some of the best clues to the patient's attitude and motivation. The dentist's assessment of these factors must be recorded, since they must be considered in establishing a treatment plan, a prognosis, and a fee for the services that will be prescribed.

Evaluation of the patient's economic priorities

It is important for the dentist to determine, before planning definitive treatment, the patient's economic priorities and limitations. The success of any prosthodontic treatment will likely be jeopardized if the patient is not convinced that the benefits, as the patient sees them, are worth as much as the treatment costs or if the patient feels that he or she cannot really afford the treatment. The patient's prac-

tical financial limitations should be respected and given a reasonable rank among the factors involved in the planning of treatment.

PROSTHODONTIC TREATMENT CHOICES

All significant items of information from the interview, the oral examination, the radiographic survey, and the examination of the diagnostic casts can now be correlated to complete the diagnosis for the partially endentulous patient. When the patient's problems and needs have been analyzed, the dentist may begin answering the five basic questions introduced at the beginning of this chapter. The answers to these questions are incorporated in the *treatment plan*.

The first question is "What type of prosthodontic treatment will best serve this patient's needs when all of the relevant factors or viewpoints are considered?" These factors include:

1. *The patient's systemic and oral health.* A healthy patient may have a healthy mouth, and this combination speaks well for successful treatment. However, a sick person cannot have a healthy mouth, and the treatment's success will be limited in such an individual. Complicated, heroic, or risky treatments are not usually indicated for patients with chronic health problems.

2. *The patient's age.* The age of an older patient may only be important as it affects the patient's physical and mental health and economic status. The age of a young patient, though, is very significant in prosthodontic treatment planning when the extraction of teeth is contemplated. The extraction of teeth (with the exception of nonfunctional third molars) generally brings the start of degenerative changes in the jaws (residual ridge reduction) and face that may be described as manifestations of premature aging.

3. *Physiologic and mechanical considerations.* These factors are discussed in detail later.

4. *The desire of the patient.* The desire of the patient to save or to lose his or her teeth, for whatever reasons are important to the patient, must be considered. This may sometimes be a minor influence that

is easily modified. At other times it may be the overriding factor in determining the plan of treatment. It must not be forgotten that a responsible patient has the right to decide the fate of his or her own oral health.

5. *The patient's psychologic status.* The ability of the patient to understand, accept, adapt to, and appreciate the treatment should be a major consideration (Heartwell, 1970; Cinotti and associates, 1972).

6. *The economic status and priorities of the patient.* It is important for the dentist to remember that the patient may have a value system that is entirely different from that of the dentist, and the difference in cost between different plans of treatment may be a dominant factor in the choice of treatment. Financial factors and the benefits and limitations of dental insurance are becoming increasingly significant in the treatment choices available to the patient.

Fixed partial denture

It has been claimed that, when it is indicated, a fixed partial denture (Fig. 4-36; see also Fig. 1-6) is most nearly the ideal prosthetic restoration. Its advantages include the fact that it is similar in feel and function to the natural teeth that it replaces. It can be worn without concern for removal or loss. It is often a very attractive and natural-appearing prosthodontic replacement. A fixed partial denture may be the restoration of choice when the following conditions are met (Coelho, 1957):

1. The edentulous span is short enough and straight enough that the requirements of rigidity and strength of the fixed partial denture will not be compromised.

2. There are strong, well-supported abutment teeth at each end of the edentulous space.

3. The patient's hygiene habits and dexterity will ensure reasonable efforts to clean the hard-to-reach crown margins and the tissues beneath the fixed partial denture pontics.

4. The reduction of tooth structure for the construction of abutment crowns is accepted by the patient or is required for restoration of the teeth in any event because of dental caries or injury.

5. The forces of mastication can be directed along the long axes of the abutment teeth.

Combinations of fixed and removable partial dentures

Certain situations call for the use of a combination of fixed and removable partial dentures (Fig. 4-37; see also Figs. 1-7, *E* and *F*). For example, missing anterior teeth with minimal alveolar bone loss should be replaced by a fixed partial denture even when posterior teeth are to be replaced by an RPD for the following reasons:

1. The fixed partial denture eliminates the unfavorable leverages that exist when re-

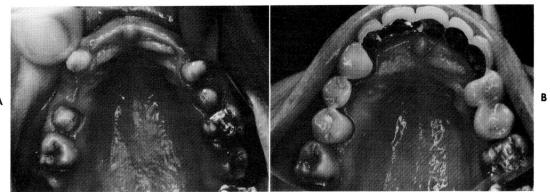

Fig. 4-36. Ideal treatment, when indicated, for replacement of teeth is fixed partial denture.
A, Patient before treatment. **B,** Patient after treatment with fixed partial denture.

placement denture teeth are attached to the RPD anterior to the fulcrum line.

2. Patients will be more apt to remove the RPD at night to rest the tissues if anterior esthetics is not compromised in doing so.

3. Esthetics will not be a consideration if the posterior RPD has to be repaired or replaced.

A fixed partial denture should also be used for splinting an isolated posterior tooth that is to be a terminal abutment for an RPD. Lone-standing mandibular second premolars occasionally present this situation following the loss of the first premolar. Standing by itself, the second premolar is very vulnerable to unfavorable leverages placed on it by a distal-extension RPD. Splinted to the adjacent canine by a fixed bridge, the second premolar may function well as an RPD abutment tooth.

When only two canines remain in the dental arch, a cross-arch tissue (splint) bar between

cast restorations placed on canines (Fig. 4-38) may be used to provide support and retention for an RPD. The tissue bar provides a favorable distribution of forces transmitted to it, dividing them between the two splinted teeth.

Removable partial denture

An RPD (Fig. 4-39; see also Figs. 1-2 and 1-4) is the restoration of choice under the following conditions:

1. When there are no posterior terminal abutment teeth present, so that a distal-extension base is required to support the prosthesis.

2. When the edentulous spaces are too extensive or too curved to be successfully restored with a fixed partial denture (Figs. 4-40 and 4-41) (Zarb and MacKay, 1981).

3. When there is a need to provide replacement for missing hard and soft tissues with an acrylic resin denture base in order to restore normal tissue contours and lip support.

4. When the cross-arch splinting provided by an RPD will be helpful in supporting and preserving periodontally weakened teeth.

5. When potential abutment teeth have not fully erupted, so that treatment with a fixed partial denture is not feasible. This situation is not uncommon among young patients.

6. When only periodontally weakened anterior teeth remain to provide anchorage for a prosthesis. Special design adaptations, such as the swing-lock partial denture (Fig. 4-42) (Antos and associates, 1978), a flexible major connector (Fig. 4-43) (Bick-

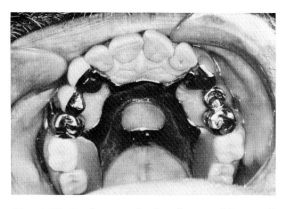

Fig. 4-37. Combination fixed and removable partial denture for distal-extension base is treatment of choice both esthetically and functionally.

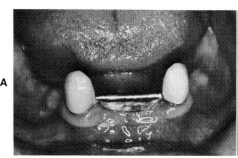
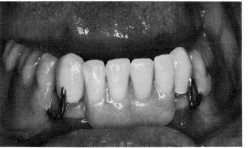

Fig. 4-38. A, Patient was treated with splint bar (tissue bar) by joining of two mandibular canines with straight round bar with labial guiding planes. **B,** Mandibular RPD in place.

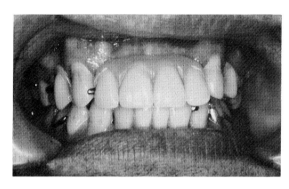

Fig. 4-39. Maxillary and mandibular RPDs are alternate form of treatment.

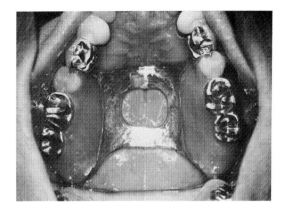

Fig. 4-40. Maxillary distal-extension RPD.

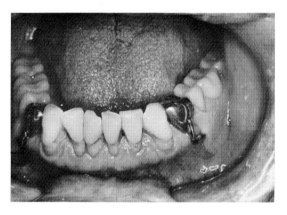

Fig. 4-41. Bilateral distal-extension mandibular RPD.

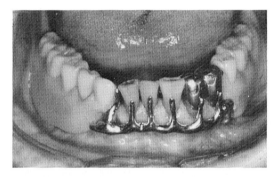

Fig. 4-42. Swing-lock attachment* was used to help stabilize periodontally compromised mandibular anterior teeth.

───────────

*Idea Development Co., Dallas, Texas.

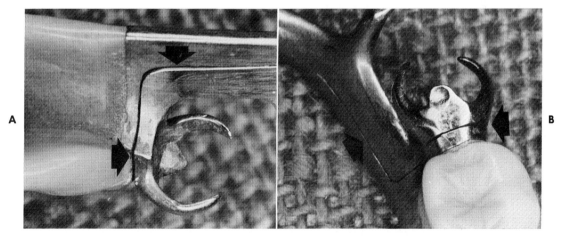

Fig. 4-43. A, Split lingual bar may be used to reduce stress on weak abutment teeth *(arrows).* This is tissue-fitting surface view of RPD. **B,** Occlusal view of same RPD *(arrows).*

ley, 1969), or a removable partial overdenture (Fig. 4-44) (Strohaver and Trovillion, 1976) may be employed to reduce stress on the weak abutment teeth. The progression to an overdenture or a complete denture may thus be postponed.

7. When it is anticipated that additional teeth will be lost sometime after the fabrication of the prosthesis. Additional denture teeth may be added to an RPD that has been designed with this contingency in mind. A tooth-supported RPD may even be converted to a distal-extension RPD by the addition of a denture tooth and an appropriate denture base (Fig. 4-45).

8. When the difference in cost between

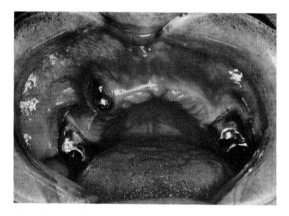

Fig. 4-44. When root can be saved, treatment of choice is to use it to support RPD.

RPD treatment and extensive fixed partial denture treatment may be a significant deciding factor for a patient with limited finances.

In making a choice between treatment with a fixed or removable partial denture, the dentist should consider the advantages of an RPD:

1. An RPD can replace lost supporting tissues in addition to missing teeth. Normal contour, appearance, and facial support may be restored with the acrylic resin denture base material where bone and alveolar tissue have been lost.

2. An RPD can use soft tissue areas of the mouth for support in addition to using the teeth, so an RPD may function successfully when the teeth alone cannot support a fixed partial denture.

3. An RPD may help the patient maintain a more acceptable level of oral hygiene. Because it may be removed conveniently, it enables the patient to clean both the prosthesis and the remaining natural teeth more efficiently (Fig. 4-46) (Applegate, 1958a; Zarb and MacKay, 1981).

4. An RPD may be designed to splint and stabilize weakened abutment teeth and to prevent the loosening, drifting, or extrusion of retained teeth (Antos and associates, 1978). The cost of cast restorations and the problem of unhygienic soldered splints may sometimes be avoided when an RPD is used.

5. An RPD may be designed to distribute the forces of mastication to many support

A 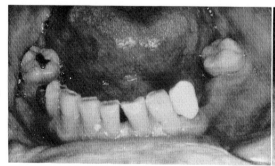 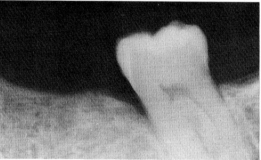 B

Fig. 4-45. A, A tooth-bounded edentulous area in patient with weak posterior abutment tooth (number 17) who requires treatment with RPD. **B,** Radiograph of tooth (number 17) that may require extraction at a future time after patient is treated with RPD. This possibility must be considered in diagnosis, treatment plan, and design of RPD.

areas and to multiple abutment teeth to prevent the overloading of only two or three teeth.

Complete dentures

In spite of the recognized advantages of saving natural teeth when it is possible to do so, there are a number of legitimate indications for treating patients with complete dentures (Renner, 1981). These include:

1. Significant involvement of the remaining teeth with advanced periodontal disease, manifested by excessive mobility of the teeth or severe loss of supporting alveolar bone
2. The presence of uncontrolled, rampant dental caries
3. Totally and habitually inadequate patient oral hygiene practices
4. The presence of too few salvageable teeth capable of serving as abutments for an RPD or overdenture.
5. Severe malocclusion or misalignment of the remaining teeth or a severely disoriented occlusal plane, which makes functional restoration of the dental arches physically or economically impractical
6. The opportunity to obtain a superior cosmetic result by replacement of malposed or unsightly teeth with a completely new dentition rather than by restoration of the natural teeth

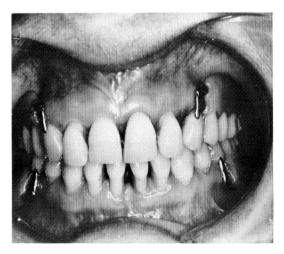

Fig. 4-46. Oral hygiene of this patient is excellent after periodontal therapy and treatment with RPDs.

7. The better comfort, esthetics, retention, and stability that often can be achieved by the use of a maxillary complete denture rather than a large, complicated maxillary RPD that does not have sufficient abutment tooth support
8. Economic factors that may make a complete denture more feasible for a patient than a fixed or removable partial denture, which requires an additional cost for treating and restoring the remaining natural teeth that may far exceed the fee for the prosthesis itself, making the total fee for conservative treatment more than the patient can afford to pay

In choosing between treating a patient with an RPD or a complete denture, the dentist should remember the following additional points:

1. Retention of teeth preserves alveolar bone. Early extraction of teeth, particularly in young patients, may prematurely hasten the destructive resorption of essential supporting bone (Atwood, 1979; Tallgren, 1970; Carlsson and associates, 1965).
2. A mandibular RPD is generally more stable and functional that is a mandibular complete denture; thus it is easier for most patients to learn to wear. For these reasons, it is advisable to retain, whenever possible, strategic mandibular teeth to support an RPD or overdenture (Brewer and Morrow, 1980; Strohaver and Trovillion, 1976).

Combinations of complete and removable partial dentures

Quite often, the maxillary and mandibular arches are restored with different types of prostheses, because the indications for treatment for the separate arches may vary. For example, a clinical situation encountered very frequently is an indication for a complete denture in the maxillary arch occluding with an RPD in the mandibular arch (Kelly, 1972). This combination of prostheses is usually successful, providing that proper support of the mandibular RPD is maintained throughout the life of the prostheses.

A mandibular complete denture opposed by natural teeth in the maxillary arch is less well tolerated. The patient's well-supported maxillary teeth can exert much more force on the mandibular denture than the edentulous mandibular ridges can withstand, and therefore the tissues beneath the mandibular denture are constantly traumatized. The consequences are continual soreness and accelerated resorption of the mandibular residual ridge. Again, this situation emphasizes the importance of retaining even a few mandibular teeth (for an RPD or overdenture) to aid in withstanding the forces of mastication.

TREATMENT PLANNING

Following the diagnostic review, if it has been determined that the needs of the patient will best be met by treatment with an RPD, the next decision in the sequence is "What will be the most functional design for the RPD?" The design process begins with the selection of the teeth for use as abutments.

Selection of the abutment teeth

Diagnostic evaluations of potential abutment teeth were made during the examinations of the mouth, of the radiographs, and of the mounted diagnostic casts. In choosing the specific teeth, it must be remembered that abutment teeth must withstand unusual vertical, horizontal, and torquing forces that are transmitted to them by the RPD in function.

In review, the teeth selected as abutments should have the following characteristics:

1. Adequate support for the roots. Factors of support discussed previously include the crown-root ratio, the quality of the alveolar bone surrounding the root or roots, the size and shape of the roots, and the thickness of the periodontal ligament. Minimal mobility is desirable.
2. Healthy periodontal tissues, including an adequate zone of attached gingiva. The presence of minimal periodontal pockets is a favorable factor.
3. Healthy coronal structure, or the tooth's capability of being restored so that its coronal portion is strong enough to serve as an abutment.
4. Coronal morphologic features that are favorable for the preparation of rest seats for support and of guiding planes for guid-

ance of the RPD during insertion and removal.
5. Axial alignment that permits a reasonable path of insertion and allows the forces of occlusion to be directed vertically along the axis of the roots
6. Coronal morphologic features that are favorable for clasping, with reference to the most logical path of insertion.
   NOTE: Characteristics 3, 4, 5, and 6 can often be enhanced with the placement of cast restorations.
7. A position in the dental arch that facilitates the favorable distribution of stress. Teeth that are in contact with other teeth in the arch are better able to withstand stress than are isolated teeth.
8. The absence of pulpal or periapical pathosis.

Design of the removable partial denture

When the abutment teeth have been evaluated and chosen, a tentative design for the RPD should be carefully drawn on the diagnostic cast (Blatterfein, 1952a). The dentist develops the design, following the essential principles of support, retention, bracing, guidance, and stress control. The sequence of steps involved in surveying the diagnostic cast and designing the RPD is described in detail in Chapter 3.

Responsibility of the dentist

It must be emphasized that the *dentist should design the RPD* (Morse and Boucher, 1969). Only the dentist who has performed the examination of the patient and who is familiar with all of the relevant factors is in a position to determine which design features of an RPD are physiologically acceptable. The dentist receives a fee for assuming this responsibility and is the person best qualified to ensure that the design will meet the important requirements of preserving the remaining natural teeth and tissues and providing the best obtainable function, comfort, and appearance.

Preeminence of the removable partial denture treatment plan

Most patients for whom RPD treatment is indicated will also require other treatment, such as operative dentistry and periodontal therapy. The fitting of an RPD is usually only the last phase of the total treatment plan.

It cannot be emphasized too strongly that whenever a patient is to receive an RPD, *the prosthodontic treatment plan is the key plan with which all other treatment plans must be coordinated.* The design of the RPD will determine to a great degree the types of surgical, periodontic, and operative dentistry treatments that will be required for the optimal degree of rehabilitation. Therefore, it is vital to plan the RPD first.

If this principle is violated, the dentist may discover, following the completion of other treatment, such situations as improperly contoured abutment crowns or teeth that have been restored to previously existing malpositions. Without proper preplanning, expensive and time-consuming endodontic and periodontic procedures may often be performed on teeth that later will have to be extracted to permit treatment with an RPD.

The dentist may avoid these frustrating situations by determining in advance of the supporting treatment the requirements for the RPD. Even though the prosthodontic treatment is commonly done last, it must be planned first, because its success depends to a great extent on the degree to which other treatments complement it.

Complementary dental treatment planning

For optimal function and comfort to be achieved with RPD treatment, the patient's oral tissues must be brought to the best possible state of health before the RPD is constructed. Various surgical, periodontic, and operative dentistry procedures are commonly required to complement the prosthodontic treatment. The sequencing of these procedures should be planned in advance to ensure efficient management of the patient's comprehensive treatment. Although in practice the order of treatment may vary, a logical sequence for planning is suggested below.

Surgical procedures

Surgical procedures should be scheduled early so that postoperative healing may proceed as quickly as possible. Final impressions for the construction of RPDs are usually postponed until optimal surgical healing has occurred. Decisions regarding teeth that require extraction because of extrusion, periodontal disease, or malalignment should be made as early as possible.

The removal of tori or exostoses is planned if it appears that they will interfere with the design or wearing of the RPD. Enlarged maxillary tuberosities are surgically reduced if they extend below the desired plane of occlusion or if they interfere with the placement of the maxillary or mandibular denture bases.

Other surgical procedures occasionally indicated may include frenectony, modification of high muscle attachments, or excision of flabby tissue from the edentulous residual ridges.

Oral hygiene and plaque control instruction

The effective control of dental plaque is one of the most significant factors in the success of RPD treatment. The need for plaque control instruction varies widely among patients, but early emphasis on this aspect of treatment, when it is indicated, is desirable. The response of the patient to this instruction will often influence the course of future treatment. In addition, the early adoption of improved oral hygiene practices is an advantage when periodontic treatment procedures are also required (Derry and Bertram, 1970).

Periodontal treatment

The periodontal health of the retained teeth is one of the most critical considerations, so periodontal therapy, when required, must be given high priority (Beyron, 1973). The goals for periodontal therapy include the elimination of deep periodontal pockets, the elimination of infection and inflammation, and the restoration of optimal gingival architecture. The preservation or provision of an adequate zone of attached gingiva around all abutment teeth is also desired.

Endodontic therapy

When they are indicated, endodontic procedures are usually planned so that they may be done simultaneously with the surgical and periodontal procedures. Both pulpal and periapical lesions may be treated routinely. Teeth that have been successfully treated endodontically may be used as RPD abutments if they meet the criteria listed previously.

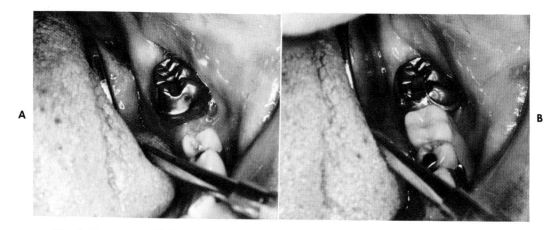

Fig. 4-47. A, Lingual ledge is placed in cast gold restoration that acts as long rest and guiding plane. **B,** Mandibular RPD viewed intraorally. Lingual reciprocal clasp arm is confined within tooth contour.

Occlusal equilibration

Premature centric contacts, deflective occlusal contacts, or undesirable slides during closure should be eliminated before restorative dentistry procedures are performed so as to avoid reproducing the abnormal occlusion pattern in the restorations. In practice, definitive selective grinding for patients with long-standing malocclusions must often be accomplished in stages, as functional occluding surfaces are restored and the jaw is allowed to revert to more normal patterns of function. Several adjustments may be necessary over the course of treatment.

Operative dentistry procedures

One of the primary factors for the dentist to consider when planning restorative dental treatment is the importance of achieving a reasonably straight, even occlusal plane. It is nearly impossible to eliminate traumatic contacts during functional movements of the jaw if an irregular occlusal plane is preserved. Treatment with an RPD that has an occlusal table that is "swaybacked" to accommodate opposing extruded or malposed teeth is a compromise that usually leads to failure of the treatment. For this reason, cast restorations are frequently required in order to restore a proper plane of occlusion. Sometimes when existing cast restorations are retained it may be necessary to modify the opposing RPD.

The restoration of RPD abutment teeth with cast metal or porcelain-fused-to-metal crowns is frequently indicated. The contours and anatomic features of abutment castings are critical to the success of prosthodontic treatment (Fig. 4-47).

The RPD design should be established and recorded on the mounted diagnostic cast before any abutment crown preparations are made. This is a very important concept, based on the principle that the dentist must know in advance where the rest seats and guide planes will be placed in order to create adequate space for these features during tooth reduction. For example, extra occlusal reduction is required in areas where rest seats are to be placed in order to allow for an adequate thickness of metal under the rest seat.

All carious lesions must, of course, be treated and restored before the construction of an RPD is started. The use of silver amalgam restorations in abutment teeth is generally accepted, provided that modern, high-strength alloys are used (Fig. 4-48). Existing silver amalgam restorations that have seen years of service should be examined critically if they are present in abutment teeth. Replacement of old restorations is usually indicated if rest seat preparation will involve the restorations.

Modifications to natural tooth surfaces

The preparation of the natural teeth for reception of an RPD follows in sequence in the treatment plan. Guiding planes and rest seats are the usual modifications to be considered. The artificial creation of undercuts and the re-

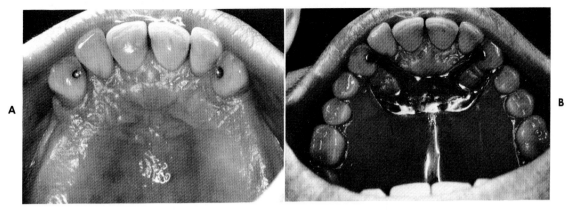

Fig. 4-48. A, Mesial alloy rest may be placed in maxillary or mandibular canines in lieu of fabrication of cast restoration. Mesial alloy rests are shown in maxillary cuspids. **B,** Completed maxillary RPD.

duction of undesirable undercuts are other alterations to teeth that may be planned. These procedures are described in detail in Chapter 5. Again, it is emphasized that the dentist must be guided in these modifications by the design that has been established on the diagnostic cast during the planning phase of treatment.

Construction of the removable partial denture

Any unusual design or construction features that affect the complexity or cost of the prosthesis should be noted. Examples of commonly employed variations are the use of mechanical attachments or all cast metal denture bases (Fig. 4-49).

Postinsertion maintenance

Notes regarding unusual maintenance requirements, such as an anticipated need for frequent recall appointments (Roberts, 1980) or for an early relining, should be included in the record so that they will not be overlooked later (Morstad and Petersen, 1968) (Fig. 4-50).

Importance of a written treatment plan

A sequential list of all of the anticipated clinical treatment procedures culminating with the completion of the prosthodontic treatment should be outlined in writing. A written treatment plan enables the dentist to:
1. Plan the time and appointment schedule necessary for the treatment and provide this information to the patient

2. Accurately estimate the professional fees for the treatment
3. Coordinate the schedule for dental laboratory procedures with the patient's clinical appointments
4. Provide the patient with a copy of the treatment plan, an advisable practice in all cases in which misunderstandings could occur
5. Meet the legal requirements of informed consent

Occasionally, modifications to the treatment plan will be found necessary as treatment progresses. It is important that notes of these changes be added as supplements to the original treatment plan record in order to prevent later misunderstandings.

MEDICAL CONSULTATIONS

Dentists must assume responsibility for recognizing medical problems that require the attention of a physician when these conditions manifest themselves in the mouth. A number of systemic diseases, including diabetes, anemia, osteoporosis, and gastrointestinal disorders, may exhibit signs and symptoms in the oral tissues. If signs suggestive of systemic problems are detected during the oral examination, a consultation with the patient's physician should be obtained. When required, proper medical treatment may be instituted before the dental treatment or concurrently with the dental appointments.

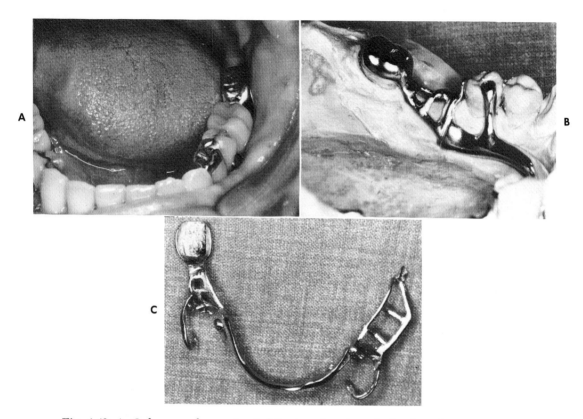

Fig. 4-49. A, Onlays may be constructed for tipped molars. Occlusal overlay RPD viewed intraorally. **B,** Occlusion is restored with chrome cobalt overlay. **C,** Underside of overlay is part of RPD.

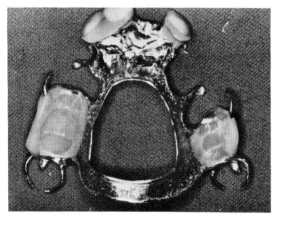

Fig. 4-50. Maxillary RPD of patient illustrated in Fig. 4-12 shows presence of dental plaque on tissue side of its acrylic resin and metal components.

NUTRITION COUNSELING

Surveys have demonstrated that a high percentage of prosthodontic patients have dietary patterns that contribute to nutritional deficiencies. Whenever the medical history, the interview, or the examination raises questions regarding the adequacy of a patient's diet, the dentist should give serious consideration to dietary evaluation, diet counseling, or nutritional therapy (Barone, 1965).

Oral signs that are suggestive of nutritional imbalances include atrophic mucous membrane, excessive resorption of alveolar bone, high rate of dental caries, and excessive deposits of salivary calculus.

Patients who have systemic diseases or oral conditions for which inadequate nutrition is a contributing factor cannot be restored to health until their nutritional problems are corrected. An effective plan of rehabilitation for these patients may require the use of therapeutic dietary supplements during periods when their masticatory ability is impaired. Patients with less than desirable eating habits should also have guidance and encouragement in establishing better long-term dietary practices.

Dietary evaluation

When a detailed dietary evaluation is indicated, the patient is asked to keep a record of everything he or she eats and drinks for a period of 5 to 7 days. The completed diet diary is then evaluated at a subsequent appointment. A comparison of the patient's recorded dietary intake with the recommended intakes of food that constitute a balanced diet is the basis for a practical and useful evaluation. A recommended diet (Dairy Council of California, 1975) includes:

1. Two to four servings a day of foods from the dairy or milk group
2. Two or more servings a day from the meat or protein group
3. Four or more servings a day from the vegetable and fruit group
4. Four or more servings a day from the whole-grain cereal group
5. A minimal but reasonable intake of refined carbohydrates

Significant variances from a balanced diet that show up in the patient's diet history indicate the need for counseling. Provision for this should be made in the treatment plan.

Making dietary recommendations that will be effective yet acceptable to patients of various backgrounds and habits requires some knowledge of nutrition, foods, and eating patterns. Instructions regarding specific techniques of dietary counseling are beyond the scope of this chapter, but this information is available from other sources. Dental practitioners should be encouraged to learn to provide these valuable services in their own offices.

In many areas, it is possible to refer patients to a registered dietitian for dietary counseling. In these situations it is important that the consulting dietitian, when planning diets and menus, recognize the handicaps faced by a patient with impaired masticatory ability.

PRESENTATION OF THE TREATMENT PLAN

The treatment plan prepared for presentation to the patient should describe the therapy that, in the judgment of the dentist, best meets the needs of the patient. The goals to be sought are the preservation of the remaining teeth and oral tissues, the restoration of the best obtainable function and appearance with an RPD, and the maintenance of maximum comfort.

The course of treatment and the results that can realistically be expected should be explained as completely as possible. Visual aids, including diagnostic casts, pictures (Roraff, 1971), and radiographs, can be freely used in helping the patient to understand the goals and the possibilities of treatment. Estimates of the time and costs involved should be given clearly. The patient should be encouraged to ask questions, because the better the patient understands the treatment, the easier it will be for him or her to accept it.

Alternate treatment plans are necessary in some situations. Adequate, if less than optimal, treatment may be considered because of factors such as age, limited finances, or the patient's personal desires. It is the patient's decision to accept or reject any of the plans presented once he or she has been fully informed of the choices. Even in "ideal" plans of treatment, compromises are sometimes necessary (Carlsson and associates, 1965). The patient must be informed of the limitations of treatment that result from the patient's own health and oral conditions.

In the discussions of the proposed treatment and its results, enthusiasm, optimism, and encouragement should be shared. Even salesmanship has an effective and proper role, but the dentist must be careful not to give overenthusiastic promises or guarantees of success. The dentist must emphasize, in a kindly and positive manner, that the success of the treatment is as much a responsibility of the patient as it is of the dentist.

PROGNOSTIC AIDS FOR REMOVABLE PARTIAL DENTURE TREATMENT

Because successful RPD treatment depends on many physical and mental variables, it is advisable for the dentist to use a checklist to ensure that all of the conditions that influence treatment have been examined. A checklist is important because it enables the dentist to estimate the prognosis for the treatment and the difficulties to be expected. The following prognostic aid form for RPDs will help fulfill this aim.

PROGNOSTIC AIDS FOR REMOVABLE PARTIAL DENTURES

Patient _____

History

Sex and age of patient: _____

Occupation: _____

Systemic conditions: _____

Nature of complaint: _____

Clinical findings	Significance
1. Systemic evidence of reduced tissue tolerance:	
☐ Favorable	Good prognosis.
☐ Unfavorable	Added stress on abutment teeth will result in their loss.
2. Quality of oral hygiene:	
☐ Excellent	
☐ Good	Start oral hygiene program.
☐ Poor	Start oral hygiene program; patient must show willingness to cooperate.
3. Anatomic anomalies:	
☐ Tori	If large, surgical removal required.
☐ Ledging	Surgical removal required if involved with denture base.
☐ Other	Note anomalies of teeth and residual ridge.
4. Tension habits:	
☐ No	Good prognosis.
☐ Yes	Bruxers and clenchers develop abnormal destructive forces on teeth and residual ridges.
5. Muscle tone:	
☐ Tense	Extensions critical.
☐ Average	Slight overextension possible.
☐ Flaccid	Maximum extension possible.
6. Surgical and periodontal tissues:	
a. Color:	
☐ Pink	Normal.
☐ Red	Gingivitis, traumatic occlusion.
b. Form and surface:	
☐ Gingival edema	Glossy appearance.
☐ McCall's festoon	Traumatic occlusion or toothbrush injury.
Stillman's cleft	Ulceration extending to labial or lingual surface.
☐ Stipling	Normal velvety surface.
c. Thickening of periodontal space:	
☐ Uneven	Added stress or abnormal occlusal wear.
☐ Even	
d. Calcareous deposits:	
☐ Supragingival	Scaling required.
☐ Subgingival	Root planing and curettage required.
☐ Materia alba	Patient education required.
e. Gingival recession:	
☐ Recession apically to cementoenamel junction	Periodontal surgery required.
f. Level of epithelial attachment:	
☐ Pocket depth 1 to 3 mm	Good prognosis.
☐ Pocket depth 3 to 5 mm	Periodontal surgery required.
☐ Pocket depth more than 5 mm	Periodontal surgery required.

PROGNOSTIC AIDS FOR REMOVABLE PARTIAL DENTURES—cont'd

Clinical findings	Significance
7. Information about the teeth:	
a. Vitality:	
☐ Vital	Good prognosis.
☐ Nonvital	Endodontic therapy may be required.
b. Dental caries or recurrent caries:	
☐ Caries susceptible	All teeth must be restored before starting RPD.
c. Mobility:	
☐ Less than 1 mm	Excellent abutment.
☐ 1 mm movement	First discernable movement.
☐ More than 1 mm movement	Tooth may have to be extracted.
☐ May be depressed	Tooth should be extracted.
d. Extruded teeth:	
☐ Slight	Reduction (by grinding) and use of long occlusal rest required.
☐ Medium	Onlay required.
☐ Extreme	Endodontic therapy or extraction required.
e. Condition of existing restorations:	
☐ Restoration inadequate	New restoration or crowns may be required.
f. Abrasion and erosion:	
☐ Present	Must be restored before starting treatment.
g. Shape and length of crowns:	
☐ Insufficient length	Electrosurgery may be required.
☐ Lacks undercut	Restoration (Class V, crown, etc.) required.
h. Abnormal inclinations:	
☐ Slight	Reshaping and recontouring of tooth required.
☐ Medium	Restoration required.
☐ Extreme	Endodontic therapy or extraction may be required.
i. Length of time since missing teeth were extracted:	
☐ 1-5 years	May indicate osteoporosis, abnormal masticatory habits, poor attitudes of patient, etc.
8. Radiographic examination:	
a. Lamina dura:	
☐ Absence	Indicates periodontal disease or bone destruction.
☐ Uneven	Tooth tilted and needs restoration.
☐ Thinning	Indicates periodontal disease.
☐ Uninterrupted	Good prognosis.
b. Residual roots/teeth:	
☐ Impacted, no pathologic conditions	Patient should be informed.
☐ Impacted, pathologic conditions	Surgery required.
☐ Impacted third molars	Patient should be informed and tooth retained in younger patients for development of tuberosity, ridge form, and possible support at later date.
c. Maintenance of normal bone support in areas of more than average stress loads (bone index):	
☐ Positive bone factor	Areas in the radiograph in which teeth are known to have assumed a more than normal work load should be observed. Bone normally is maintained.
☐ Negative bone factor	Bone has not been maintained, and more work load will cause loss of abutments

Continued.

Clinical findings	Significance
d. Shape and length of roots:	
☐ Conical	May need splinting.
☐ Small	May need splinting.
☐ Multirooted	Good prognosis.
9. Residual ridge area:	
a. Irregularity in size and form:	
☐ Full rounded	Good support.
☐ Narrow	Poor support.
☐ Low or flat	Poor support.
☐ Low tuberosity	Surgery required.
b. Hyperplastic tissues:	
☐ Present	Tissue conditioning, oral surgery, or both required.
c. Sharp, spine-like irregularities:	
☐ Sharp mylohyoid ridge	Surgery or lingual denture flange that stops short of ridge required.
d. Interarch space:	
☐ Inadequate	Surgery required to obtain enough space for acrylic resin and artificial teeth.
☐ Adequate	Ideal.
10. Esthetics:	
a. Lips:	
☐ Normal	Two mm thick anterior flange.
☐ Thick	Anterior flange made thin.
☐ Thin	Flange is critical.
☐ Short	Tooth selection critical.
☐ Long	One mm of incisal edge must be observable.
☐ Protruding anterior teeth	May require orthodontic therapy.
☐ *Important:* Record esthetic desires of patient here	
b. Shade selection (record here):	
c. Diastema between anterior teeth	Metal of major connector must not show.
11. Patient's past experience with RPDs:	
☐ Satisfied	Usually no problem.
☐ Not satisfied	Reason for dissatisfaction should be determined.
☐ Never satisfied	Patient may not be able to adapt and is a poor risk.
12. Occlusion:	
☐ Normal	
☐ Centric occlusion not in harmony with centric relation	No occlusal equilibration required unless there is damage to the oral tissues.
☐ Traumatic	Occlusal equilibration should be accomplished before treatment, during treatment, and when prosthesis is inserted.

PROGNOSTIC AIDS FOR REMOVABLE PARTIAL DENTURES—cont'd

Clinical findings	Significance

13. Interocclusal space:
    - ☐ Sufficient
    - ☐ Insufficient   Areas of abutment teeth that are to receive rests must be examined critically to evaluate space available and to estimate space that will need to be provided.

14. Temporomandibular joint dysfunction:
    - ☐ Normal
    - ☐ Clicking   Usually followed by pain and degenerative changes.
    - ☐ Pain and tenderness   Clenching or grinding of teeth. Muscle spasm from yawning or extended dental treatment.

15. Tongue size and mobility:
    - ☐ Large   Caused by lack of replacement of posterior teeth. May cause mandibular RPD to lift posteriorly.

16. Selection of abutments:
    - ☐ Molars and cuspids   Best abutments for stability and strength.
    - ☐ Bicuspids   Better claspability than cuspids.
    - ☐ Incisors   Poor abutments.
    - ☐ Isolated teeth   Poor abutments.
    - ☐ Tipped tipped   Long occlusal rest or crown required.

17. Patient's attitude toward a new RPD:
    - ☐ Philosophic   Ideal type. Realizes importance of a healthy oral cavity. Does not expect perfection; dentures will provide a reasonable degree of comfort and efficiency.
    - ☐ Emotional   Nervous and temperamental. Dental history reveals neglect and ill health. Feels that he or she can never wear dentures or improve on existing dentures.
    - ☐ Exacting   Perfectionist. Will not change living habits, especially in regard to eating. Will expect same efficiency and esthetics as to shape, color, size, and arrangement as with natural teeth. Will want a written guarantee.
    - ☐ Indifferent   Unconcerned with appearance. Has neglected, unhealthy mouth. After dentures are completed will have no patience or perseverance. Offers no suggestions, but by unwillingness to adjust to dentures, will be the most difficult postinsertion patient. Usually has been forced by a relative to come to the dentist.

18. Crowns are to be constructed:
    - ☐ Tooth preparations
    - ☐ Guiding planes, retention on surveyor, crown waxed for rest
    - ☐ Precementation on surveyor

5 Mouth preparations for removable partial dentures

Successful removable partial dentures (RPDs) do not just happen; they evolve from a methodical, well-planned sequence of events. The mouth is rarely, if ever, ideally suited to receive an RPD. The dentist must alter certain oral structures or conditions to prepare the mouth to receive the prosthesis. Mouth preparations for RPDs are identified as those procedures that are accomplished to prepare the mouth for the reception of the prosthesis. More specifically, they are those procedures that change or modify existing oral structures or conditions to: (1) facilitate the placement and removal of the prosthesis, (2) facilitate its efficient physiologic function, and (3) enhance its long-term success.

Generally speaking, all dental procedures executed to accomplish the above purposes can be classified as mouth preparations for RPDs. This broad classification can be divided into: (1) prosthodontic mouth preparations and (2) nonprosthodontic mouth preparations. Nonprosthodontic mouth preparations include procedures in oral surgery, orthodontics, periodontics, endodontics, restorative dentistry, fixed partial denture prosthodontics, behavioral sciences, and occlusion, although many dentists would classify those procedures related to occlusion and restorative dentistry as prosthodontic mouth preparations. This chapter does not discuss nonprosthodontic mouth preparations other than to identify them and make some applicable comments on occlusion.

Mouth preparations constitute an important and essential phase of RPD service. The care and attention with which mouth preparations are planned and executed by the dentist have a direct bearing on the ease of treatment, the level of success that is achieved, the longevity of the prosthesis, and the preservation of the remaining oral structures (Glann and Appleby, 1960; Johnston, 1961; McCracken, 1956; Schorr and Clayman, 1954). Too many RPDs have failed because the mouth preparations were improperly executed or, even worse, omitted (Schwartz and Barsby, 1980). The latter circumstance is a sinful omission for which there is no excuse. Mouth preparations are professional responsibilities and should be planned and executed by the dentist.

BROAD OBJECTIVES

The broad objectives in planning mouth preparation for removable partial dentures are:
1. To establish a state of health in the supporting and contiguous tissues
2. To eliminate interferences or obstructions to the placement, removal, and function of the prosthesis
3. To establish an acceptable occlusal scheme
4. To establish an acceptable occlusal plane
5. To alter natural tooth form to accommodate the requirements of form and function of the prosthesis

For specific objectives to be accomplished, they must first be identified.

PLANNING MOUTH PREPARATIONS: HOW THEY EVOLVE

When the need for the placement of an RPD is identified or suspected as a preferred choice of treatment, an orderly, sequential plan of action should be triggered in the dentist's mind. This plan of action should include:
1. A thorough examination of the patient, including familial, general health, and dental histories
2. A thorough examination of the oral structures, including vitality testing, mobility records, and a periodontal evaluation
3. A complete roentgenographic survey

4. The making of accurate diagnostic casts and their mounting on a suitable dental articulator in centric relation (retruded contact relation)
5. Diagnosis and evaluation of the data gathered from the examinations
6. Surveying of the diagnostic casts
7. The formation of an orderly, sequential treatment outline to meet the patient's specific needs; this outline includes the design of the RPD

As the final design of the RPD evolves, the need for specific mouth preparations is identified and recorded in an appropriate manner.

The final design of the RPD is the product of:

1. The dentist's concepts of the basic principles of RPD design
2. The biologic data obtained from the clinical evaluation of the patient's intraoral and extraoral structures
3. The mechanical factors obtained from an analysis of the diagnostic casts using a dental cast surveyor

Often the final design of the RPD is a compromise between the mouth preparations needed for an ideal treatment plan and those mouth preparations that can be executed practically to achieve an acceptable treatment plan. As the final design of the RPD is established, the mouth preparations necessary for its success can be identified. The mouth preparations that evolve should be recorded in a manner that: (1) clearly identifies the procedures to be accomplished and (2) lists the sequence in which they are to be performed.

EVALUATING DATA: OCCLUSAL CONSIDERATIONS

The basic principles, concepts, and practice of occlusion relative to diagnosis and treatment planning are treated elsewhere in this text (see Chapter 7). Only those occlusal considerations affecting the mouth preparations for the RPD are addressed here.

Early in the diagnosis and treatment planning effort, the dentist must evaluate the patient's occlusion. Basically, the dentist must determine:

1. The type of occlusion (group function, canine guidance, balanced occlusion, etc.) that the patient has

2. Whether there is a need to change or modify the patient's existing occlusion
3. Whether the intercuspal position is in harmony with the patient's centric jaw relation (retruded contact relation)
4. The status of the plane of occlusion and of the occlusal curve.

Type of occlusion

The type of occlusion that the patient has should be identified and the intended occlusal scheme clearly envisioned while the dentist is developing the treatment plan. To coordinate all restorative and fixed partial denture procedures with the intended occlusal scheme, the dentist must have specific treatment objectives in mind. Having evaluated the patient's occlusion, the dentist must decide whether there are changes that could or should be made in the occlusion that would enhance the prognosis. Some other factors to be considered are occlusal adjustment, orthodontics, fixed partial denture prosthodontics, RPD prosthodontics, and, occasionally, surgical orthodontics. The important point for the dentist to realize here is that the objectives of the occlusal scheme should be identified early in the diagnostic effort and that all nonprosthodontic and prosthodontic procedures should then be executed in a manner that will provide the type of occlusion intended.

Occlusion and maxillomandibular relations

The dentist should determine whether harmony exists between the patient's intercuspal position (centric occlusion) and the retruded contact position (centric jaw relation). If not, the dentist must decide whether to synchronize the patient's intercuspal position with the retruded contact relation.

There is no general agreement within the prosthodontic discipline as to whether this synchronization should be accomplished routinely in the absence of pathologic disturbances that are usually attributed to improper occlusion. Hence, in these instances, the dentist will base the decision on his or her own personal philosophy of occlusion. In the absence of a strong personal philosophy, a dentist might base the decision on the degree of difficulty involved in attempting to synchronize the intercuspal position with the retruded contact position. For example, when only a few tooth contacts are involved, it would appear reasonable to accomplish the task. However, when numerous contacts are involved and considerable effort would be required, it might be prudent, in the absence of recognizable pathosis, to use the patient's intercuspal position. The rationale for this decision is that the more tooth contacts involved in the task of synchronizing the patient's occlusion with centric jaw relation, the greater the possibility of creating tooth awareness on the part of the patient. Tooth awareness may, in turn, trigger parafunctional habits, such as bruxism, and invite the problems attendant to them. In other words, the more numerous the tooth contacts, the more involved it becomes to accomplish the task without creating tooth awareness and triggering occlusally related pathosis. Clinical practice has shown that unless the examination reveals a clear indication to change the patient's existing occlusal relation, it is generally best not to do so. When occlusal adjustment is indicated, it should be accomplished before restorative, fixed partial denture, and RPD therapy. When there are insufficient tooth contacts to provide a stable intercuspal position, it is reasonable to adjust the occlusion to achieve harmony between the retruded contact position and the intercuspal position in the finished RPD. The occlusal scheme of the finished RPD should then provide some freedom for tooth contacts in the intercuspal position.

Occlusal plane

The occlusal plane should be evaluated on the mounted diagnostic casts and intraorally. If the restorative effort involves treating the patient with a maxillary complete denture opposed by a mandibular RPD, the occlusal plane should be as good as practical. In these instances, it is beneficial to use an occlusal template* to evaluate the existing occlusal plane or occlusal curve on the diagnostic cast. Using an appropriate template (flat or curved), the location and magnitude of discrepancies in the occlusal plane are easily identified (Fig. 5-1). Plans for correcting the defects are noted and recorded as a part of the treatment plan.

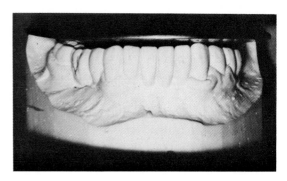

Fig. 5-1. Curved 20° occlusal template* is used to analyze irregular occlusal curve on diagnostic cast. Location and magnitude of discrepancies in occlusal curve are noted and recorded. Occlusal adjustments needed will be accomplished early in sequence of mouth preparations.

Occlusal overlays

Occlusal overlays and onlay rests (see Chapter 3) can be used as a part of the RPD framework to eliminate infraocclusal defects. An ideal occlusal plane or occlusal curve can be provided for an opposing maxillary complete denture by the use of occlusal onlays (Fig. 5-2) or onlay rests (Fig. 5-3). When the involved teeth have to be restored with a cast restoration for any reason (such as to provide adequate undercuts, to restore enamel defects, to splint teeth, or to shorten the clinical crown), the requirements for the desired occlusal scheme should be incorporated into the design of the cast restorations (Fig. 5-4).

If the treatment plan involves only one RPD, the occlusal plane in the opposing dental arch should be evaluated and, if necessary, modified to provide the desired occlusal plane before the construction of the RPD is undertaken.

If the treatment effort does not involve a maxillary complete denture, then the occlusal plane does not need to be ideal to be physiologically acceptable.

Supererupted teeth

Supererupted (extruded) teeth pose defects in occlusal plane and most often are encountered in the posterior dental arch segments. Such teeth should be treated in relation to the

---

*Trubyte 20° or 0° posterior template, Dentsply International, York, Pa.

*Dentsply International; York, Pa.

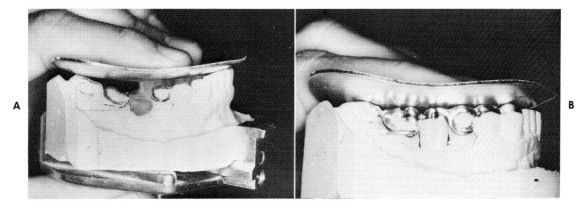

Fig. 5-2. A, Ideal occlusal curve is planned to aid in development of balanced occlusal scheme for opposing maxillary complete denture. Teeth 27, 28, 29, and 31 will receive cast occlusal onlays. **B,** Acceptable occlusal curve is achieved using occlusal onlays as component of RPD. Onlay rest on mandibular second molar also functions as: (1) major connector, avoiding need for lingual bar to extend to distal of molar, and (2) minor connector, from which clasp arms originate.

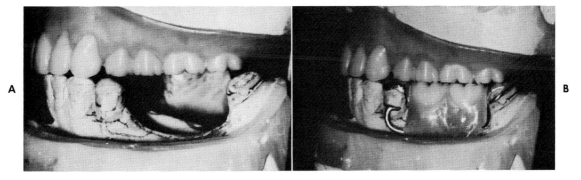

Fig. 5-3. A, Corrections of irregular occlusal curve are needed to provide acceptable plane of occlusion for maxillary complete denture. Maxillary complete denture is carried through wax try-in stage before fabrication of mandibular RPD. Acceptable occlusal curve is established by waxed denture occlusion. In this patient, 0° teeth were used in curved occlusal scheme. **B,** Occlusal plane has been improved using onlay rests on mandibular molar and premolar. Occlusal curve is completed with mandibular denture teeth.

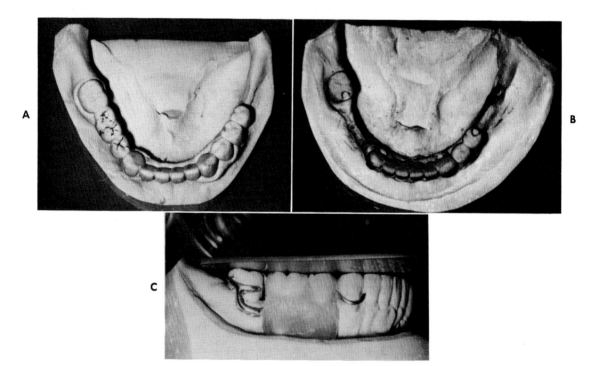

Fig. 5-4. A, Diagnostic cast of patient with nonserviceable fixed bridges and irregular occlusal plane is illustrated. In newly devised treatment plan, mandibular right premolar pontics will be replaced as component of RPD because of questionable bony support of right mandibular molar. During reconstruction, acceptable occlusal curve will be established to provide stable occlusion for maxillary complete denture. **B,** Contours and occlusal morphologic features of restored abutment teeth provide ideal occlusal curve on which to arrange denture teeth for maxillary complete denture. **C,** Sagittal view of occlusal curve established with new cast restorations and completed with denture teeth of RPD.

magnitude of the problems they create and the importance of the teeth to the success of the RPD. The problems enountered by posterior supererupted teeth are usually: (1) insufficient space in positioning the opposing prosthetic teeth and (2) their potential for causing occlusal trauma. Extruded teeth in the anterior dental arch segment pose an additional problem of esthetics. Generally, the severity of the problems created by extruded teeth and the amount of treatment required are in direct proportion to the degree of extrusion. For purposes of effective dialogue Table 5-1 presents a classification of supereruption of posterior teeth that is related to the degree of extrusion and the probable treatment needed.

A Class I supererupted tooth poses no appreciable problems in positioning the prosthetic replacement teeth in the opposing dental arch and has no potential for creating occlusal trauma. Hence, no treatment is needed.

A Class II extruded posterior tooth poses definite problems, but their magnitude is moderate and they can be successfully managed by selective grinding of the tooth cusps (enamoplasty).

In a Class III extruded posterior tooth, there are moderately severe problems that cannot be successfully managed without altering the tooth to such a degree that the enamel is penetrated, thus requiring the placement of a restoration (usually a cast restoration). In Class III(E), the degree of tooth reduction needed will cause pulpal exposure, necessitating endodontic therapy in addition to a complete cast crown restoration.

In Class IV, the tooth is severely extruded. If the tooth is considered nonessential to the success of the RPD, it may be extracted. When a Class IV(E)extruded tooth is considered nonessential for retention but essential for support in eliminating a distal-extension RPD situation, it may be treated endodontically and used as an overdenture abutment (Firtell and associates, 1979; Bolender and Becker, 1981; Strohaver and Trovillion, 1976). On occasion, even a single hemisected molar root may be so treated to considerable advantage. In Class IV(O), when the extruded teeth are considered to be essential for the retention, bracing, and support of the RPD, surgical orthodontics might be considered as a mechanism for repositioning the tooth and alveolus. The age, financial status, health, and mental attitude of

TABLE 5-1
Classification of supererupted posterior teeth

Classification	Degree of extrusion	Probable treatment required
Class I	Slight	None
Class II	Moderate	Enamoplasty to reduce height of clinical crown (incisal edge, cusp tips)
Class III	Moderately severe	Complete cast restoration
Class III(E)*	Moderately severe	Endodontic therapy and complete cast restoration
Class IV	Severe	Extraction is permissible if tooth is nonessential or useless to success of RPD
Class IV(E)*	Severe	If tooth is nonessential for bracing or retention but desirable for support, endodontic therapy is indicated and tooth may be used as abutment for removable partial overdenture
Class IV(O)†	Severe	If tooth is considered essential for bracing, retention, and support, its repositioning by means of surgical orthodontics is indicated
Class V	Moderate to moderately severe	None (because of tooth's position in dental arch, interridge space, or degree of disclusion of posterior teeth in eccentric excursive movements)

*Endodontic therapy required.
†Orthodontic therapy required.

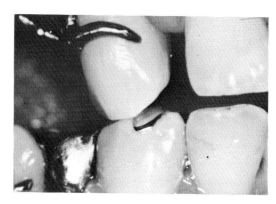

Fig. 5-5. Incisal hook rest on mandibular canine is illustrated creating occlusal interference during right lateral eccentric movement of mandible.

the patient and the position of the tooth in the dental arch are important considerations for such procedures. When such procedures are deemed desirable, the tooth and its bony support can be repositioned to an acceptable position.

Class V extruded teeth pose moderate to moderately severe problems relative to an ideal plane of occlusion and space relation but cause no occlusal trauma, either because of: (1) their location in the dental arch or (2) disclusion of posterior teeth during eccentric mandibular movements provided by anterior canine guidance. In such cases, the spatial relationships pose moderate inconveniences, but they can be successfully managed. Class V situations are most often seen when the maxillary molars have extruded into the mandibular edentulous space. When there are no mandibular molars distal to the extruded tooth, the potential for occlusal trauma is not great, because of the location of the extruded tooth in the dental arch. Under these circumstances, there is no reason for the dentist to severely alter the "bilevel occlusal plane." Shortening the cusp tips by means of selective grinding is usually satisfactory to provide acceptable interarch space. When mandibular molars extrude into an edentulous maxillary space adjacent to a mesially positioned maxillary tooth, the potential for occlusal trauma is significant and must be carefully evaluated. However, it is not uncommon for occlusal trauma to be avoided because of

significant cuspid guidance. When there is sufficient space to place the prosthetic teeth, there is no reason to change the plane of occlusion other than the personal desire of the dentist to achieve a more conventional occlusal plane.

Infraerupted teeth

Infraerupted teeth pose defects in the plane of occlusion that can usually be successfully managed by one of three methods:

1. Orthodontic repositioning
2. Placement of a cast restoration on the tooth to increase the clinical crown
3. Use of an occlusal onlay as a part of the RPD or as an onlay rest (see Fig. 5-3, *B*) to restore the clinical crown to the plane of occlusion.

The degree of tipping, the dental caries index, economics, the presence or absence of enamel defects, and the degree of necessity of the tooth in question for providing retention will influence the choice of treatment.

Occlusal interferences from components of the removable partial denture

Certain components of an RPD framework have the potential for introducing occlusal interferences; notable among these are:

1. Occlusal rests
2. Incisal rests (Fig. 5-5)
3. Clasp assembly shoulders
4. Lingual ledge and cingulum rests

5. Minor connectors on maxillary anterior teeth

When completing the RPD design, the dentist must give careful consideration to the position of these components. These metal parts require bulk for strength and must be partially or totally confined within the normal tooth contour to avoid occlusal interferences. Provision must be made to ensure that the mouth preparations to accommodate these metal parts will provide the space required for adequate bulk. Other parts of the RPD that may cause occlusal interferences are minor connectors, proximal plates, metal pontics, occlusal overlays, and prosthetic teeth. These parts must be formed to harmonize with the planned occlusal scheme. The dentist must envision the intended occlusal scheme and keep its objectives clearly in mind in planning and executing those treatment procedures affecting the occlusion. Failure to do so will often result in occlusal discrepancies that will adversely affect the prognosis of the treatment.

Tipped molars

Because tipped molars occur with considerable frequency and pose a variety of problems in RPD design, they deserve some special comments. Not only do they offer significant possibilities for interferences with the placement of major and minor connectors (particularly a mandibular lingual bar), but they also present problems of clasp assembly placement and often create food traps. The magnitude of the problem presented by a tipped molar is directly proportional to the degree of its tip and its relation to the planned path of placement and withdrawl of the prosthesis (Fig. 5-6).

Although they might be tipped in any direction, tipped molars are most often mesially inclined and conventionally provide a high survey line on their mesial surface. In addition to the mesial tilt, maxillary molars often have a buccal tilt, whereas mandibular molars most often have a lingual tilt. The design requirements for the RPD can usually be met by moderate selective grinding procedures when the degree of the tilt is moderate (5° to 10°). Molars with severe tilts (15° or more) require a more careful appraisal. Such molars are best repositioned orthodontically. This provides a better opportunity for the forces from the RPD to be distributed along the long axis of the tooth and

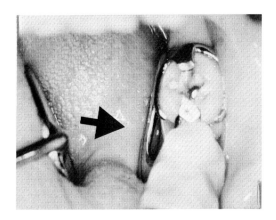

Fig. 5-6. Lingually inclined mandibular molar creates lingual interference and compromises position of mandibular lingual bar major connector. Note marked relief for major connector *(arrow)*.

eliminates the possibility of interferences from the clasp assemblies and major and minor connectors. Severely tipped molars that are not to be repositioned orthodontically deserve careful appraisal, since they will require significant tooth alterations to meet RPD design requirements. Although severly tilted molars in either dental arch present significant interferences, mandibular tilted molars offer the greatest opportunity for problems in RPD design.

The predominantly mesially located undercuts on tilted molars suggest a clasp assembly design that traditionally approaches the undercut on the tipped molar from the distal side. Severely tipped mandibular molars with a lingual tilt offer considerable possibilities for interferences from a lingual bar major connector during placement and removal of the prosthesis when the lingual bar is to be extended to the distal surface of the tooth to support a clasp assembly. In such instances, when the RPD framework is fully seated there will be a significant space between the lingual bar and the alveolar mucosa (Fig. 5-6). A major connector so placed will interfere with tongue function, present a great potential for food entrapment, and in general be annoying to the patient. In such instances, it is best for the dentist not to extend the major connector to the distal surface of a tilted mandibular molar. Attempts to do so will require tooth modifications of an extreme magnitude if the lingual interferences are to be avoided. Tooth modifications of this magnitude are generally not practical without penetrating the enamel, which will require the dentist to place a cast restoration on the tooth. If the tooth requires the placement of a cast restoration for any reason, the tooth can be reshaped to meet RPD design requirements. It is usually possible to eliminate the need for the mandibular lingual bar to extend to the distal surface of a severely tilted molar by "design management" even when retention is a requirement of the clasp assembly. Ring clasps, modified ring clasps, or onlay rests (see Fig. 5-2, *B*) can be successfully employed to manage the problem with only moderate tooth alterations. An occlusal overlay used in this way will:

1. Correct the defect in the plane of occlusion
2. Serve as a minor connector that may carry the retentive arm into the mesial undercut
3. Eliminate the necessity for a lingual bar to be extended to the distal surface of the tipped molar.

Tipped molars with enamel defects should be restored with an appropriate cast restoration. Placing a cast restoration provides an opportunity for the dentist to change the tooth contours, thus minimizing many of the problems associated with tipped molars.

Clasp assembly designs for significantly tipped molars are often not classical or conventional. Individual ingenuity following the basic principles of RPD design will provide an acceptable clasp design while simultaneously minimizing the need to alter tooth structure. If the degree of the tilt is not great, minor selective grinding procedures will permit conventional clasping arrangements.

RECORDING MOUTH PREPARATIONS
Necessity for recording mouth preparations

RPD therapy is unique in dental practice. The placement of an RPD usually represents the last phase of patient treatment to be accomplished. However, the RPD treatment must be planned in infinite detail before many other phases of treatment begin. Many facets of oral surgery, periodontics, endodontics, restorative dentistry, and orthodontics must be harmonized with the RPD treatment to enhance the success of the total treatment plan. Since these procedures must be accomplished before the impressions are made and the RPD is constructed, there is often a considerable time lapse between the examination, diagnosis, and treatment planning and the actual commencement of the mouth preparations and construction of the RPD. Hence, it is most appropriate and, in fact, necessary to have an accurate record of those mouth preparations that need to be accomplished before and during the RPD phase of therapy. A dentist should never commit these procedures to memory, because of their importance and because of the often considerable delay in the execution of the prosthodontic mouth preparations. For many reasons, it is not unusual to encounter a significant time lapse between the date of treatment planning and the dates of the mouth preparations. Some method of accurately recording the procedures to be done is of paramount importance.

Method of recording, listing, or charting mouth preparations

The method of recording, listing, or charting mouth preparations will depend on the needs and desires of the individual dentist. In the case of dental students, the method will, of course, be that prescribed by the department responsible for teaching the RPD curriculum. In any event, some method should be used to record those procedures needed to prepare the mouth for the RPD (McCracken, 1956). Although most dentists record their mouth preparations on the diagnostic cast, some dentists will, in addition, list the precise mouth preparations on a standard form in the sequence of planned execution. Whatever the technique employed, the purpose is to communicate to the dentist not only the exact mouth preparations that must be executed, but also the proper sequence in which they should be executed for efficiency of performance. This method of recording mouth preparations leaves nothing to memory. An additional advantage of this method is that the record can be placed in the patient's chart and become a permanent part of the patient's record. This can be of enormous value if the treatment becomes the subject of any kind of litigation. Some patient treatments do result in litigation, and an accurate clinical record is mandatory.

Experienced dentists may elect to record mouth preparations directly on the diagnostic cast, relying on their vast experience and clinical judgment to execute the procedures in an efficient sequence. The dental practitioner without this vast experience will do well to use some standard form to chart or record the mouth preparations to be accomplished and the sequence in which they may be accomplished most expeditiously.

Recording on the diagnostic cast

The technique for recording mouth preparations on the diagnostic cast is usually executed using a red pencil to identify the mouth preparations to be accomplished. Teeth to be extracted are marked with an *X*. Some dentists prefer to actually remove the dental stone teeth from the diagnostic cast and identify the extraction site with an *X*. Areas of bony and soft tissue recontouring are outlined with closely spaced parallel lines or shaded with a red pencil. Tooth structures to be altered are outlined or shaded. Included are those procedures necessary to prepare rest seats, guiding planes, modifications of survey lines, occlusal refinements, and removal of interferences. Examples of mouth preparations recorded on the diagnostic cast are shown in Fig. 5-7.

Some dentists prefer to complete all of the mouth preparations on the diagnostic cast ex-

actly as they are to be executed on the patient. These preparations often include tooth preparation and wax-up of surveyed cast restorations. A diagnostic cast so prepared is a useful chairside aid for case presentation and for guiding the dentist through the mouth preparations.

Charting on a prepared form

There are many types of prepared forms used to record mouth preparations. Most have at least two things in common:

1. They indicate a complete listing of all the procedures needed to prepare the patient's mouth to receive the RPD.
2. They indicate the sequence in which the procedures can be executed most expeditiously.

Generally speaking, emergency treatments are not included on the mouth preparation form, since these are usually accomplished before the data gathering process is completed.

Surgical procedures are usually executed first to allow ample time for healing. Other mouth preparations are usually executed in the following general order: endodontic therapy, minor tooth movement, occlusal adjustment, periodontal therapy, restorative dentistry, fixed partial denture prosthodontic therapy, and tooth modifications.

The advantages of listing or charting mouth preparations are that:

1. It ensures completeness.
2. It provides a quick and convenient record of what has to be accomplished to prepare the patient for the reception of the RPD.
3. When the record is properly prepared, it serves as a "road map," guiding the dentist through all of the procedures that must be accomplished in proper sequence and providing sufficient detail to enhance the accuracy of those procedures that are accomplished.
4. It serves as a legal record as to the thoroughness of the mouth preparations and of the treatment plan.
5. It virtually ensures that all procedures will be executed in proper sequence before the impresssion for the master cast is made, since it leaves nothing to memory.

An example of a form appropriate for charting mouth preparations is shown in Fig. 5-8.

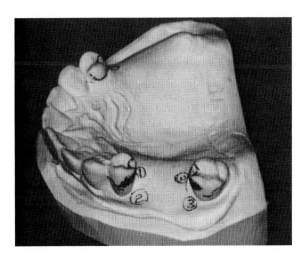

Fig. 5-7. Mouth preparations for preplanned RPD are recorded on diagnostic cast. Areas to be modified have been recorded. Rest seats have been outlined. Tooth surfaces to be reduced to improve survey lines and provide adequate guiding planes are shaded in colored pencil. Circled numbers below shaded areas code amount of tooth structure to be removed.

Many dental schools require students to record all mouth preparations on an appropriate form and to execute them on mounted dental stone casts. The latter practice serves as a "dry run" or preview of the procedures to be accomplished clinically; when completed, the modified cast represents a three-dimensional model of the planned mouth preparations.

Some helpful hints for increasing the accuracy of recording and executing certain types of mouth preparations are discussed next.

Coding selective grinding procedures

Tooth modifications are executed to accomplish specific objectives. When selective grinding (discing) of tooth surfaces is done, the objective is to remove a specific amount of tooth structure from specific areas. Selective grinding so executed provides the tooth modification anticipated. To achieve the degree of accuracy desired during selective grinding procedures,

the dentist must identify and record rather accurately the tooth surfaces to be altered and the amount of tooth surface to be removed. Areas of tooth surfaces to be selectively ground can be identified graphically on the diagnostic cast and in written form on a chart or mouth preparation form.

The amount of tooth structure to be removed should be quantified while mouth preparations are being planned to ensure accuracy in executing the selective grinding procedures, which will be accomplished at a later date. Using a code of 1 to 4, with 1 being a very slight amount and 4 being the maximum amount of enamel that can be removed without penetration, the dentist can chart the amount of selective grinding with relative accuracy. Code 5 can be used for restored tooth surfaces that might logically permit extreme selective grinding. A guide for coding the amount (thickness) of tooth structure to be removed in selective grinding procedures is illustrated below.

Code	Amount of tooth surface to be removed
Code 1	Very little ($^1/_4$ mm)
Code 2	Moderate ($^1/_2$ mm)
Code 3	Large (1 mm)
Code 4	Maximum possible without penetration (1 mm plus)
Code 5	Extreme amount on restored tooth surface

Symbols used in charting mouth preparations

Appropriate symbols or abbreviations should be used to expedite the charting of mouth preparations when they are recorded on a chart or form. A list that might be used for this purpose is suggested below.

Term	Symbol or abbreviation
Survey line	SL
Guiding plane	GP
Interference	Int
Occlusal rest	OR
Incisal rest	IR
Incisal hook rest	IHR
Lingual ledge rest	LLR
Cingulum rest	CR
Facial	F
Lingual	L
Mesial	M
Distal	D
Line angle	LA
Raise survey line	↑ SL or RSL
Lower survey line	↓ SL or LSL
Reduce cusp tip	RCT
Selectively grind	SG

MOUTH PREPARATION CHART

Student _____ Chart No. _____ Student _____

ORAL SURGERY: _____

ENDODONTICS: _____

OCCLUSION: _____

PERIODONTICS: _____

OTHER: _____

		SURVEYED CROWNS					
Tooth	Type of Restoration	Guiding Planes		Rest Seat		Undercut	
		Length	Locat.	Type	Locat.	Amt.	Locat.

	TOOTH ALTERATIONS
Tooth No.	Modifications Required.

Fig. 5-8. Chart used to record mouth preparations for RPD is illustrated. Mouth preparations are recorded in sequence of their execution intraorally.

Other symbols or abbreviations may be used. The goal is accurate communication in the charting procedures.

MODIFYING TOOTH CONTOURS FOR REMOVABLE PARTIAL DENTURES

The contours of natural teeth are usually not suitable to meet the requirements for the proper placement and functioning of an RPD. If the requirements of a sound RPD service are to be met, the existing tooth contours must be changed. If the changes needed can be accomplished within the confines of tooth enamel or of an acceptable existing restoration, the procedures are referred to as tooth modifications or tooth alterations. Thus, when tooth alterations for RPDs are considered, teeth with existing acceptable restorations are treated as sound teeth, and it is assumed that the proposed contour changes can be accomplished without damaging or unduly weakening the existing restorations.

Sometimes the tooth alterations required cannot be accomplished within the confines of sound tooth enamel (or an existing acceptable restoration). In these instances, a restoration must be placed to provide the tooth contours required. (A few exceptions, involving altered forms of tooth structure, will be noted later). When the restoration required is a cast restoration, it is referred to as a surveyed crown. The requirements for surveyed crowns are discussed later in this chapter.

Tooth alterations for removable partial denture frameworks

There are many requirements for RPD frameworks that necessitate some form of tooth alteration. The need for these alterations depends on: (1) the design of the RPD framework and (2) the shape of the tooth or teeth in relation to the chosen path of placement and removal of the prosthesis.

The alterations needed to meet these requirements are listed below in the sequence in which they are generally executed.

1. Selective grinding (enamoplasty) to improve or provide guiding planes
2. Selective grinding to minimize or eliminate interferences between tooth surfaces and various parts of the RPD during insertion and removal
3. Selective grinding to improve survey lines

4. Selective grinding to improve clasp retention
5. Selective grinding to reduce cusp tips or incisal edges of anterior teeth to improve the occlusal plane
6. Alteration of tooth structure to prepare rest seats

It should be routine clinical procedure to smooth and polish all tooth surfaces altered during mouth preparations. Fluoride therapy for altered tooth surfaces is advisable for many patients, depending on their dental caries index.

Preparing guiding planes

Guiding planes are naturally occurring or prepared parallel areas on vertical tooth surfaces that are contacted by certain rigid parts of the RPD framework during the placement and removal of the prosthesis. Guiding planes are generally parallel to each other and to the planned path of placement of the prosthesis (Fig. 5-9). Effective guiding planes, functioning with their metal counterparts on the RPD framework, provide for a single, predictable path of placement and removal (Rudd and O'Leary, 1966; Stern, 1975). The ability of the guiding planes to provide a single, predictable path of placement is illustrated diagrammatically in Fig. 5-10. Functioning guiding planes

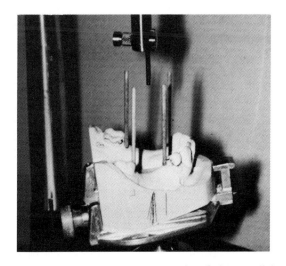

Fig. 5-9. Diagnostic cast is analyzed for parallel guiding planes. Parallel vertical rods (which are parallel to path of placement and removal of prosthesis) are being used to illustrate guiding planes that were identified on either natural or prepared tooth surfaces.

are illustrated in the serial photographs shown in Fig. 5-11. The effectiveness of the guiding planes (preferably two or more) is determined by: (1) their number, (2) their position, (3) their length, (4) their degree of parallelism, and (5) the degree of parallelism of their metal counterparts on the RPD framework. Guiding planes should be prepared on sound enamel or on appropriately restored tooth surfaces. The instrument used to prepare guiding planes is generally a smooth diamond stone with either a cylindric or a tapered point. Keeping the long axis of the diamond instrument parallel with the path of placement when the selective grinding procedures are performed usually creates effective guiding surfaces. Crown ledges on restored teeth provide excellent guiding planes and are discussed later under the heading of surveyed crowns.

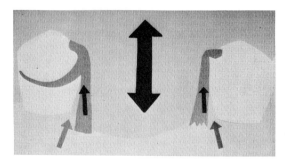

Fig. 5-10. Effectiveness of guiding planes to provide single predictable path of placement and removal is illustrated diagrammatically. Guiding planes are particularly effective when placed on tooth surfaces that oppose each other. Guiding plane contacts tooth surface for several millimeters but does not extend cervically to gingival tissue. Guiding planes may be longer for tooth-supported RPDs than for distal-extension RPDs.

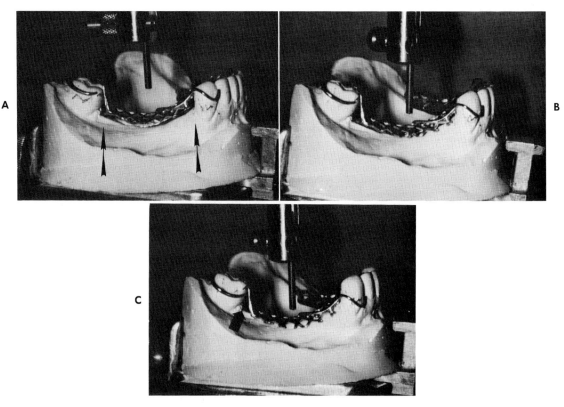

Fig 5-11. A, Guiding planes are illustrated *(arrows)* initially contacting and guiding framework toward its final seating (terminal position). **B,** RPD framework is approximately one-half seated, and guiding planes are directing single, predictable path of placement. **C,** RPD framework is fully seated on master cast. Note severe design compromise forced by interference created by tilted mandibular molar, even though its mesial surface was reduced *(arrow)*. Note that this can be potential area for food impaction. Guiding plane on molar, by necessity, is much shorter than guiding plane on cuspid, which is more parallel to path of placement of prosthesis. Uprighting mandibular molar would have added measurably to treatment effort.

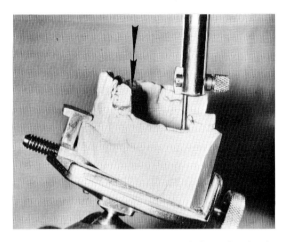

Fig. 5-12. Edentulous space bounded on distal side by mesially tipped mandibular molar. Potential interference has been minimized by choice of path of placement, which uses natural guiding plane *(arrow)* on distal side of mandibular canine. Mesial interference on molar can be further minimized by selectively grinding mesial surface maximally without penetrating enamel (Code 4).

LENGTH. Guiding planes should be longer (occlusogingivally) for tooth-supported than for distal-extension prostheses. Guiding planes on natural tooth surfaces that diverge from the path of placement and removal of the prosthesis will necessarily be shorter than guiding planes on more parallel tooth surfaces (Figs. 5-11, *C,* and 5-12). Proximal guiding planes for all tooth-supported prostheses should be approximately one half to two thirds the length of the occlusogingival dimension of the coronal enamel. The guiding plane should extend from the marginal ridge cervically. Guiding planes on teeth that serve as abutments for distal-extension prostheses should be one third to one half the occlusocervical dimension of the coronal enamel.

From a sagittal view, guiding planes on proximal tooth surfaces appear straight or flat and parallel or nearly parallel to the planned path of placement and removal. They are located on the occlusal portion of the crown, extending from the marginal ridges.

WIDTH. From an occlusal view, guiding planes on proximal tooth surfaces may be straight buccolingually or slightly curved to more or less follow the natural tooth contour. Buccolingually, guiding planes on proximal tooth surfaces should be about two-thirds as wide as the distance between the buccal and lingual cusp tips. This general rule provides guiding planes 3 to 4 mm wide on canines or premolars and 4 to 5 mm wide on molars.

Modifying survey lines

Survey lines can be modified by: (1) changing the tilt of the diagnostic (or master) cast, (2) selectively grinding the tooth (enamoplasty), or (3) placing an appropriate cast restoration (usually a surveyed crown).

TILTING THE DENTAL STONE CAST. When survey lines are modified by tilting the dental stone diagnostic cast, the survey lines on all abutment teeth are affected. The dentist cannot alter the survey line on one abutment tooth by tilting the diagnostic cast without affecting the survey line on all other abutment teeth. Once the final diagnostic cast position has been selected and additional survey line modifications are needed, these can be accomplished by one of the other two procedures.

SELECTIVE GRINDING. Tooth alterations by selective grinding are often necessary to achieve acceptable survey lines for appropriate clasp placement. Practically, survey lines can be lowered but not raised by selective grinding.

It is often desirable to lower survey lines for the correct placement of the shoulder of the clasp assembly (see Fig. 5-7). When survey lines are extremely high and the degree of undercut is severe, teeth are often selectively ground to lower the survey line, thus reducing the degree of undercut so that the retentive arm tip can be placed more gingivally. Survey lines are often lowered so that the nonretentive clasp arm may be appropriately placed at the junction of the middle and gingival thirds of the tooth.

Selective grinding procedures to modify survey lines should be accomplished within the thickness of the enamel. It is reasonable to lower the survey line when it is located in the occlusal third of the tooth: in this area, the enamel is usually of sufficient thickness to permit reasonable selective grinding without penetrating it. It is not reasonable, however, to modify a tooth contour to lower a survey line located in the cervical third of the tooth, because the enamel in this area is very thin and the risk of penetration is very great.

It is not generally possible to raise a survey

line on natural tooth structure by selective grinding. The amount of enamel that would have to be removed to effectively raise a survey line would undoubtedly expose the dentin.

Dentists often ask the question, "How do I know when I have selectively ground the tooth enough to achieve the desired tooth contour?" If the mouth preparations were planned with care and recorded accurately, the dentist should be able to transfer this information to the clinical procedures. Herein lies the value of recording not only the areas to be altered but also the amount. The only sure way of knowing whether the objectives of tooth modification have been met is for the dentist to make an impression, pour it in dental stone, and analyze the dental stone cast for acceptable tooth contours on a dental surveyor before dismissing the patient.

Eliminating interferences with the path of placement and removal of the prosthesis

RPDs are designed to use a specific path of placement and removal. Generally, this is a straight path parallel to the vertical predetermined path as measured by the analyzing rod on the dental surveyor (see Fig. 5-9). Structures that offer interferences or obstructions to the placement and withdrawal of the prosthesis should be carefully evaluated. Interferences or obstructions may be encountered from either the teeth or the associated soft tissues. Interferences from soft tissues undercuts are usually associated with a bony component.

Interferences must be dealt with; otherwise they force compromises in the design, the esthetics, or the fit of the prosthesis that may seriously jeopardize its success. The dentist evaluates interferences with the intent of eliminating them, minimizing them, or designing the RPD around them. Eliminating all interferences is not always practical, and compromises are often necessary.

Minor interferences from tooth surfaces can be eliminated by selective grinding. Moderate interferences can be minimized by selective grinding, by use of block-out (relief) on the master cast, or by a combination of both procedures. The use of a block-out leaves a space, or relief between the area of interference and the prosthesis (see Fig. 5-11, *C*). Severe interferences can be eliminated or minimized by modifying the tooth contours with an appropriate restoration.

Interferences from tooth structure usually result from a tooth whose long axis diverges from the path of placement and removal of the prosthesis. There are usually malposed, tipped, or atypically contoured teeth. Some typical examples of tooth interferences to the path of placement and removal are included in Table 5-2.

The potential for various components of the RPD to interfere with harmonious occlusal relationships is discussed in the section on occlusal considerations in this chapter. Interferences with proper clasp assembly placement are dealt with in this chapter's discussion of survey lines. Impingement on the maxillomandibular space may be the result of enlarged, bulbous tuberosities or extruded teeth. These interferences must be minimized with appropriate therapy (see discussion of extruded teeth in the section on occlusal considerations).

Preparing rest seats

Rest seats are specially prepared tooth surfaces designed to accommodate the metal rest of the RPD framework. Rest seats are also called rest preparations and rest areas. The preparation of rest seats should follow all selective grinding procedures. The rationale for this is simple: if the rest seats were prepared first (particularly proximal occlusal rest seats), the selective grinding to create guiding planes or to lower survey lines would alter the character of the rest preparation. Attempts to redesign the rest seat often result in severe compromises in the rest preparation.

There are many kinds of extracoronal rests employed in an RPD service. Each kind requires a specifically designed rest seat. It should be remembered that it is the rest seat that basically determines the outline, form, size, shape, width, and thickness of the metal rest. If the rest seat is inappropriately prepared, the metal rest cannot possibly accomplish the functions for which it is intended.

FUNCTIONS OF EXTRACORONAL RESTS. To better appreciate the design of extracoronal rests, it is helpful to review their functions. These are to:

1. Serve as vertical stops in the final seating (terminal position) of the prosthesis

TABLE 5-2
Interferences to the path of placement and removal of an RPD

Condition	Interferes with
Crowded, severely overlapped mandibular anterior teeth	Placement of lingual plate major connector
Edentulous space bounded by teeth tipped toward each other	Attachment of minor connectors to rest and clasp assemblies
	Proximal adaption of denture base
	Proximal adaptation of denture teeth
Severe lingual tilt of mandibular posterior teeth	Placement of lingual bar major connector
	Placement of clasp assembly
Terminal abutment tooth of distal-extension base tilted distally naturally or as a result of the chosen path of placement and removal	Attachment of minor connector to rest or clasp assembly
	Attachment of minor connector to proximal plate
	Placement of clasp assembly
	Soft tissue interferences
Labial frenum	Placement of denture base flange (labial bar and swing-lock connectors)
Buccal frenum	Placement of denture base flange
	Attachment of minor connector to bar clasp
Lingual frenum	Placement of lingual bar major connector
Mandibular torus or lingual exostosis	Placement of lingual bar major connector
	Placement of denture base flange
Maxillary torus	Placement of palatal major connector
Bony undercut	
Facial	Placement of denture base flange
	Attachment of minor connector to bar clasp
In mylohyoid ridge	Placement of denture base (lingual flange)

2. Maintain the proper position of the clasp assemblies on the abutment teeth
3. Prevent impingement on the soft tissues adjacent to the abutment teeth by parts of the prosthesis
4. Transmit forces to the abutment teeth
5. Direct occlusal forces along the long axes of the abutment teeth
6. Prevent spreading of the clasp arms when the prosthesis is fully seated
7. Direct food away from tooth contacts and embrasure spaces
8. Assist in resisting lateral forces
9. Prevent extrusion of the abutment teeth
10. Serve as indirect retainers for distal-extension RPDs
11. Determine the proper orientation of the metal framework to the abutment teeth

BASIC TYPES OF REST SEATS. There are two general types of rest preparations (seats), intercoronal and extracoronal. Intercoronal rest preparations are prepared in a restoration such as a crown or inlay. Intercoronal rest prepara-

tions are discussed in the section of this chapter on surveyed crowns. They are never placed in natural tooth structure. Extracoronal rest preparations are placed on natural or restored tooth surfaces.

Rest seats can also be identified according to their location on the tooth surface (that is, occlusal, incisal, cingulum, mesial, distal, facial, or lingual). Most rest seats can further be identified as either proximal rest seats or embrasure rest seats. A proximal rest seat is one located on a proximal surface of a tooth adjacent to an edentulous area (Fig. 5-13, *A*). An embrasure rest seat is one located on a tooth surface adjacent to another tooth (Fig. 5-13, *B*). Some examples of combination terms to describe various rest seats are: (1) proximal occlusal rest, (2) embrasure occlusal rest, (3) embrasure incisal rest, and (4) proximal incisal hook rest.

REQUIREMENTS OF OCCLUSAL REST SEATS. Occlusal rest seats must be prepared so as to accommodate the functions of the metal rests of the RPD framework.

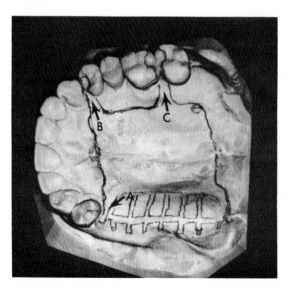

Fig. 5-13. Master cast shows variety of modified basic occlusal rests. *A,* Proximal occlusal rest that is direct component of clasp assembly. *B,* Single embrasure occlusal rest serving as indirect retainer. Note that rest preparation does not cross occlusal surface. *C,* Transocclusal embrasure rest. Note that basic rest preparation flares dramatically toward interproximal embrasure on lingual surface to permit adequate room for minor connector to enter rest area and facially to allow ample room for shoulder of clasp to exit area.

1. Rest seats should be prepared in a manner that will permit the metal rest to direct functional vertical forces along the long axis of the abutment tooth.
2. Rest seats should provide a positive seating of the metal rest in the rest seat on the abutment tooth.
3. A rest seat should have gradual sloping walls; it should be smooth and polished.
4. A rest seat should not have undercuts, sharp angles, or edges.
5. Cavosurface margins should end on self-cleansing surfaces.
6. A rest seat should provide adequate space for sufficient bulk of metal to provide strength in the rest.
7. Rest seats for distal-extension RPDs should allow slight rotation of the metal rest in the rest seat without wedging or torquing of the abutment tooth.

REST SEATS IN NATURAL TOOTH STRUCTURE. When rest seats are placed in natural tooth structure, they are usually placed in sound enamel (Gaston, 1960). There are a few exceptions to this general rule. Teeth that have been severely abraded over a long period of time usually display exposed dentin that is discolored, very dense, and free of dental caries. Experience has shown that it is reasonable to place rest seats in this type of natural tooth structure. Appropriate fluoride therapy should be applied to rest seats prepared in this type of altered dentin. When clinical judgement directs it, these areas of altered dentin should be restored with an appropriate restoration. Another exception are rest seats placed on the incisal edge of mandibular anterior teeth. It is not unusual to penetrate the enamel when placing a rest seat on these surfaces. Clinical practice has shown that slight penetration of the enamel in these areas has not been hazardous to the patient in terms of dental caries susceptibility. This may, in part, be because of the eburnation (making ivorylike) of the underlying dentin or because of the relatively self-cleansing nature of the incisal edge. Generally, however, if the enamel is penetrated during the preparation of rest seats, the area should be restored with an appropriate restoration.

REST SEATS IN EXISTING RESTORATIONS. Rest seats may be prepared in an acceptable existing restoration. It is preferable that the rest seats either completely cover the restoration or be totally contained within it. If it becomes necessary for the cavosurface margin of the rest seat to cross the margin of an existing restoration, the entire area should be made as smooth and self-cleansing as possible. Any deep grooves should be widened, smoothed, and polished. The restoration must be sound and of sufficient bulk to accommodate the rest seat without weakening, and the restorative material must be of sufficient hardness to support occlusal forces without causing excessive wear or breakage of the restoration. Gold and gold substitutes are the most acceptable restorative materials to support rests. Although amalgam alloy is not an ideal restorative material to accommodate rest seats, it is often an acceptable compromise. Rest seats may be prepared in dental porcelain surfaces by using a fine diamond instrument with continuous water spray.

If a cast gold restoration is penetrated during attempts to prepare a rest seat, the restoration can usually be repaired with amalgam alloy or a gold foil restoration. If an existing amalgam alloy restoration is broken during the preparation of a rest seat, it should be replaced with a new one.

Rest seats to be placed in cast restorations that are to be fabricated for the RPD are discussed in the section on surveyed crowns.

OCCLUSAL REST SEATS. There are several variations of occlusal rests and rest seats that accommodate them. They all have similar characteristics to meet the basic principles of design and proper function. They also have specific differences to accommodate specific design requirements or variations in anatomic occlusal form.

There are two general types of occlusal rests; they may be identified according to their relation to either an adjacent tooth or an edentulous space. Proximal occlusal rests are located in a mesial or distal fossa adjacent to an edentulous space (Fig. 5-13, *A*). Embrasure occlusal rests (Fig. 5-13, *B*) are located in a mesial or distal fossa adjacent to another tooth.

Occlusal rests that traverse the occlusal surface between adjacent teeth are identified as transocclusal rests (Fig. 5-13, *C*). Embrasure rests that are not components of clasp assemblies do not generally traverse the occlusal surface. Embrasure rests that are components of circumferential-type clasps (embrasure clasp assemblies) do cross the occlusal surface and are identified as transocclusal rests. The rest seat preparation for each varies slightly.

When two embrasure occlusal rests are immediately adjacent to each other, they may be identified as double occlusal rests or back-to-back rests (Fig. 5-13, *C*). These adjacent occlusal rests have the advantages of:

1. Preventing wedging action between the two adjacent teeth
2. Providing additional support for the RPD
3. Directing food away from the marginal ridges and embrasure spaces
4. Allowing the remaining half of the clasp to serve as a retainer in the event that one of the adjacent teeth is lost.

On occasion, with a nonconventional design, an occlusal rest may approach the occlusal surface from either the midlingual or midfacial surface and be identified as a basic lingual or a facial occlusal rest respectively.

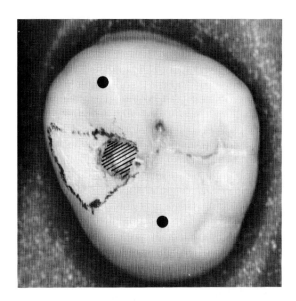

Fig. 5-14. Occlusal view of basic occlusal rest is illustrated. Outline form is basically spoon shaped. Its width at marginal ridge is approximately one half to two thirds of distance between facial and lingual cusp tips. Deepest portion of rest seat is located axially, away from marginal ridge *(large, dark dot)*. Note that outline form of occlusal rest flares slightly toward line angles of tooth as it approaches marginal ridge.

BASIC OCCLUSAL REST SEAT. The difference in the various types of occlusal rest seats can best be appreciated by first considering the preparation required for the basic occlusal rest (a proximal occlusal rest that is not a contiguous component of a clasp assembly). Conventionally, basic occlusal rests are located in the mesial or distal fossa of the occlusal surface of the molars and premolars adjacent to an edentulous space. The outline of the basic occlusal rest, from an occlusal view, is spoon shaped. The occlusal rest's outline also resembles a printed letter U that has been spread apart slightly at its open end. An occlusal view of the basic occlusal rest seat is illustrated in Fig. 5-14.

The occlusal outline of the rest seat for a basic occlusal rest flares only slightly toward the line angles of the tooth as the outline approaches the marginal ridge. The width of the rest seat at the marginal ridge should be one half to two thirds of the distance between the tips of the buccal and lingual cusps (Fig. 5-14).

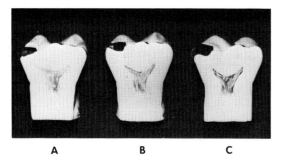

A   B   C

Fig. 5-15. Three examples of basic occlusal rest seat are illustrated in sagittal plane. **A** and **B** illustrate improper rest seat preparation and compromised occlusal rests. **A,** Base of rest seat preparation does not provide positive seat for metal rest. **B,** Marginal ridge is too sharp and has not been adequately reduced. **C,** Acceptable form for basic occlusal rest seat.

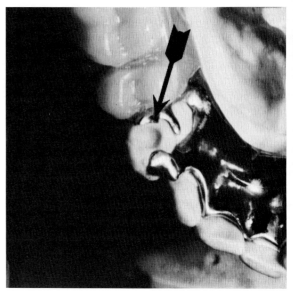

Fig. 5-16. Inadequately prepared rest seat is illustrated. Inadequate reduction of marginal ridge results in weak junction between occlusal rest and minor connector *(arrow)*. Note fractured rest. Usual rest seat resulting from this type of compromise is illustrated.

The deepest portion of the rest seat is located in the fossa area, away from the marginal ridge. This concave area is called the positive seat. It should be 0.5 to 1 mm deeper than the general base of the rest seat. The base of the rest seat should be at right angles to or should make an acute angle with the long axis of the abutment tooth. The positive seat is shown in Fig. 5-14 as a dark dot in the fossa area. The character of the positive seat, in relation to the remainder of the preparation, can best be appreciated in the saggittal view (Fig. 5-15, *C*). Two very common errors in rest seat preparation are also illustrated (Fig. 5-15, *A* and *B*).

The minimum space needed to provide adequate strength and rigidity in the metal occlusal rest is between 1 and 1.5 mm. The rest seats should be prepared with this objective in mind.

Special attention should be given to the marginal ridge segment of the rest seat. The marginal ridge of the abutment tooth must be reduced. This should be done in a manner that will leave a smooth, well-rounded convex surface. Sharp angles on the marginal ridge invite fracture of the rest and the enamel marginal ridge surface (Fig. 5-15, *B*). The reduction of the marginal ridge is necessary to provide space for an adequate bulk of metal as the occlusal rest crosses the marginal ridge to join its associated minor connector. This junction has the potential of being the weakest area of the occlusal rest. Failure to provide adequate bulk in the metal rest at this point often results in fracture of the rest (Fig. 5-16).

The occlusal outline of the basic occlusal rest varies slightly from that of occlusal rests that are components of clasp assemblies, from that of embrasure occlusal rests, and from that of embrasure transocclusal rests. Each of these modifications is discussed later in this chapter.

The proximal outline of the basic occlusal rest seat is generally spoon shaped. The positive seat is definitely concave. The outline over the marginal ridge area follows the general form of the marginal ridge and is usually slightly concave. The marginal ridge must be reduced.

The basic form of the occlusal rest seat, when viewed in the sagittal plane, follows the general contour of the fossa and marginal ridge (Fig. 5-15, *C*). The general outline of the rest seat is spoon shaped. There should be no sharp angles. The rest seat should have gently "flowing," curved surfaces. The positive seat is best envisioned in Fig. 5-15, *C*. The positive seat is the deepest portion of the rest preparation. The base of the rest seat is smooth and concave. From this point toward the marginal

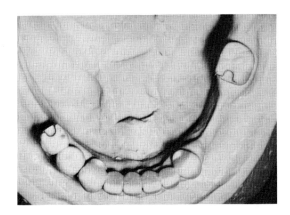

Fig. 5-17. Occlusal view of master cast for RPD. Proximal occlusal rest seats have been outlined in pencil. They illustrate slight modifications desired when occlusal rest seat is to be joined with clasp arm. Note how outline of rest seats flares more dramatically toward line angles of tooth as they approach marginal ridge.

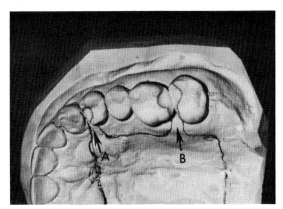

Fig. 5-18. Modifications of basic occlusal rest seat have been accomplished to produce single embrasure rest seat *(A)* and back-to-back transocclusal embrasure rests *(B)*. Note that single embrasure occlusal rest, which is not a component of clasp assembly, does not cross occlusal surface of premolar. Also, note dramatic flare in outline of rest seat as it approaches mesial-lingual line angle. This provides space needed for adequate bulk of metal at junction of embrasure rest and its minor connector. Two adjacent transocclusal embrasure rest seats are illustrated. Rest seats accommodate occlusal rests that are components of clasp assemblies. Note how basic occlusal rest seat has been modified to accommodate greater bulk of metal in interproximal embrasures.

ridge, the concave preparation follows a gentle, smooth-flowing curve. As the preparation approaches and crosses the marginal ridge, the curve changes from concave to convex. The minimum depth of the rest seat should be 1 to 1.5 mm for any portion of the preparation to provide adequate rigidity to the metal rest. The positive seat should be 0.5 to 1 mm deeper than the general base of the preparation.

The preparation for all occlusal rest seats can be made with a number 6 or number 8 round carbide bur or a diamond instrument of a similar size and shape, using either conventional or high-speed instrumentation. The larger instruments are used for preparing rest seats on large teeth and the smaller instruments for small teeth. Following their preparation, all occlusal rest seats should be highly polished.

MODIFICATION OF THE BASIC OCCLUSAL REST SEAT FOR OCCLUSAL RESTS JOINED DIRECTLY TO A CLASP ASSEMBLY. Occlusal rest seat preparations to accommodate occlusal rests that are joined directly to a clasp assembly should be slightly modified to accommodate a portion of the clasp shoulder. From an occlusal view, the rest seat preparation should flare more dramatically buccally and lingually as it approaches the marginal ridge and line angles of the tooth (see Figs. 5-13, *A*, 5-17, and 5-18, *B*).

If the occlusal rest is to attach to a lingual clasp arm only, the modification of the basic

rest seat need flare to the lingual line angle only. If the occlusal rest is to be attached to a clasp having both lingual and buccal arms, the basic rest seat should be modified to flare both to the buccal and lingual line angles (Figs. 5-17 and 5-18). The result is a wider rest seat in the marginal ridge area and a stronger occlusal rest. A basic occlusal rest seat so modified makes provision to accommodate a portion of the clasp shoulder within the natural contour of the tooth, providing strength for the rest and clasp arm while simultaneously minimizing the possibility of occlusal interferences.

MODIFICATION OF THE BASIC OCCLUSAL REST SEAT FOR OCCLUSAL EMBRASURE RESTS. Embrasure rests, which are not components of clasp assemblies, need not completely cross the occlusal surface (Figs. 5-18 and 5-19). Since the minor connector for the embrasure rest approaches the tooth from the embrasure, it is extremely important that there be adequate room for sufficient bulk of metal where the minor connector joins the embrasure rest. To provide the space needed for this juncture, the

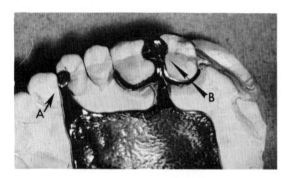

Fig. 5-19. Half of maxillary RPD framework is shown seated on master cast shown in Fig. 5-18. This view provides good example of embrasure occlusal rest *(A)* and transocclusal embrasure rest *(B)*. Note how modification of basic occlusal rest seats shown in Fig. 5-18 has provided strength for metal parts in interproximal embrasures.

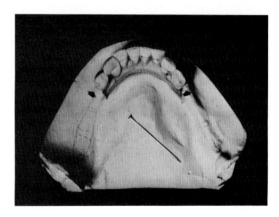

Fig. 5-20. Proximal occlusal rest seats *(arrows)* are shown on distal surface of mandibular first premolars. Their inadequate size is made very obvious when compared with that of head of ordinary straight pin. Occlusal rests that are too small or too thin will not have necessary bulk for strength to resist stresses of function. Rests possessing these characteristics often fracture.

basic occlusal rest must flare even more dramatically toward the lingual line angle than it does for the basic occlusal rest seat that is not a component of a clasp arm. Additionally, it may be necessary to widen the lingual embrasure space to enlarge the interproximal approach for the minor connector.

Embrasure rests are often used "back to back" (Fig. 5-19). When used in this way, they have the advantage of preventing wedging between the abutment teeth, effectively deflecting food away from the marginal ridge, and directing occlusal forces to both abutment teeth. When embrasure rests are used in this manner, both the mesial and distal rest seat must flare dramatically toward the lingual line angles adjacent to the minor connector (most conventionally located in the lingual embrasure).

MODIFICATION OF THE BASIC OCCLUSAL REST SEAT TO ACCOMMODATE TRANSOCCLUSAL, EMBRASURE, AND OCCLUSAL RESTS. Transocclusal and embrasure rests are usually components of clasp assemblies on one or both of the adjacent teeth. In either event, it is important that the basic occlusal rest seat flare toward both the buccal and lingual line angles to provide space for an ample bulk of metal in the interproximal embrasures (Fig. 5-18). The metal thickness in these interproximal flares must provide ample bulk for strength without introducing occlusal interferences. In other words, in addition to adequate bulk for strength, there must be adequate room for the minor connectors to enter

the rest areas and for the clasp shoulders to exit the rest areas (Figs. 5-18 and 5-19).

ASSESSMENT OF THE ADEQUACY OF OCCLUSAL REST SEATS. The adequacy of occlusal rest seats can and should be checked before the impression for the master cast is made. Several techniques may be employed: (1) visual inspection, (2) direct tactile contact, (3) the making of wax imprints or patterns, and (4) the making of a diagnostic cast by the pouring of an impression in dental stone.

Visual inspection should be employed from the moment the preparation is started. The basic outline of the rest seat should be envisioned on the tooth surface mentally as the first amount of tooth structure is removed, and this image should be maintained and intensified until the rest seat evolves. Strangely enough, occlusal rest seats always appear larger in the mouth than they do when they are viewed on the master cast (Fig. 5-20). A soft lead pencil used to outline the base of the (presumably) finished rest seat is of great help in evaluating the outline of the rest seat (Fig. 5-21). The dark contrast of the irregular base vividly demonstrates an obviously inadequate rest seat preparation. An acceptable rest seat for a proximal occlusal rest, which has been shaded with a soft lead pencil, is illustrated in Fig. 5-22. The

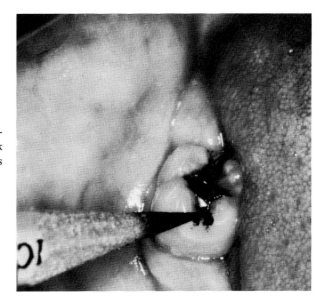

Fig. 5-21. Soft lead pencil is used to check outline form of proximal occlusal rest seat. Dark contrast of small irregular base demonstrates obviously inadequate rest seat preparation.

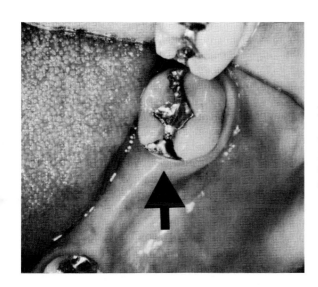

Fig. 5-22. Base of proximal occlusal rest seat *(arrow)* has been shaded with soft lead pencil to assist in assessing its size and outline form. Darker base of rest seat provides excellent contrast with lighter adjacent tooth structure, making assessment easier.

darkened base of the rest seat gives the necessary definition to the outline form to make visual assessment easy.

An explorer or the bur that was used to prepare the rest seat can be helpful in a *direct tactile evaluation* of the rest seat.

Another technique to test the adequacy of the rest seat calls for placing soft wax over the preparation and having the patient bite into tight occlusion. This makes a *wax pattern* of the rest preparation. Its thickness, size, and shape can then be evaluated by the dentist.

Perhaps the best way to assess the adequacy of rest seats and the accuracy of other tooth alterations is to make an irreversible hydrocolloid impression, pour it in dental stone, and obtain a *diagnostic cast* from which the evaluations can be made.

INCISAL REST SEATS. Incisal rest seats, as their name implies, are rest seats located on the incisal edge of anterior teeth. They may be used on any anterior tooth if they can be employed without interfering with the existing occlusion. For this reason, they are more fre-

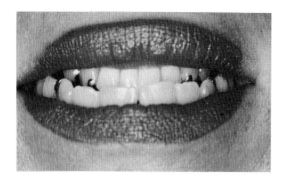

Fig. 5-23. Major disadvantage of incisal hook rest is its lack of esthetic qualities because of display of metal from labial view.

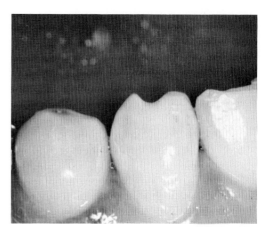

Fig. 5-24. Incisal rest placed centrally on incisal edge of mandibular canine provides best opportunity to direct forces along long axis of tooth. In facial view, incisal rest seat is concave. Depth of preparation should be 1 to 1.5 mm into enamel surface. Outline form should be smooth and should present no sharp angles.

quently used on mandibular anterior teeth. Because of their location on the incisal edge, the incisal rest (particularly the incisal hook rest, with its minor connector), has a greater potential for introducing unfavorable forces on the abutment tooth than do other types of extracoronal rest preparations used on anterior teeth. Yet, clinical practice has shown that incisal rests may be safely employed on anterior teeth that have adequate bony support. This is true even for canines serving as terminal abutments for distal-extension RPDs. The major disadvantage of incisal rests is one of esthetics (Fig. 5-23). They do offer a display of metal not encountered when lingual, cingulum, or lingual ledge rests are employed (Berg and Caputo, 1978). Incisal rests may be employed on any portion of the incisal edge, either mesial, distal, or central. The more centrally placed rest may direct forces more axially along the long axis of the tooth (Fig. 5-24). However, clinical practice has not shown this to be necessary for successful use of incisal rests. Hence, the location of the incisal rest seat might well be determined by the condition of the incisal edge. Marked wear or proximally placed restorations may contraindicate the placement of incisal rests in these general areas.

When the mandibular cuspid is the terminal abutment, incisal and incisal hook rest seats are often placed on the mesial portion of the incisal edge (Fig. 5-25). This location of the metal rest helps resist distal placement of the prosthesis.

The labial and incisal portion of the metal incisal rest should be placed within the normal contour of the tooth. This precludes the possi-

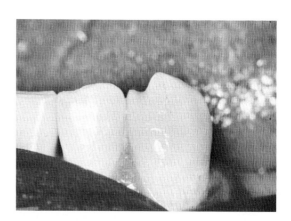

Fig. 5-25. Facial view of incisal hook rest seat preparation on mandibular canine vividly illustrates its size and contour.

bility of occlusal interferences from the metal incisal rest.

Most incisal rest preparations made by dentists are too small, perhaps because of an effort to minimize the display of metal. This is a serious error that all too often results in a fractured rest. If the dentist is committed to placing an incisal rest on an abutment tooth, the rest should be large enough to withstand the stresses of function.

Incisal rest preparations should be minimum of 1.5 mm deep and 2.5 mm wide. Mesiodis-

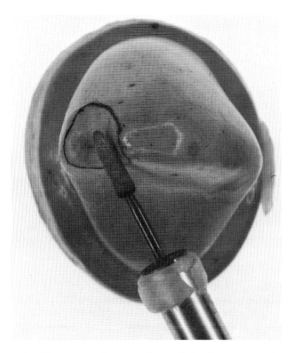

Fig. 5-26. Incisal view of incisal hook rest seat is illustrated on demonstration model. Note angle of carborundum stone in simulated handpiece, which is approximately 40° to the facial-lingual axis of tooth. Reducing a portion of axial wall as outline form approaches lingual surface will provide for ample bulk of material for strength without increasing display of metal from labial view.

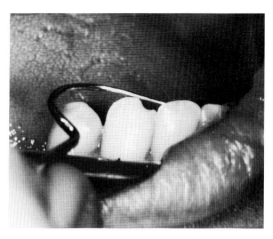

Fig. 5-27. Most incisal rest preparations are made too small, perhaps in an effort to minimize display of metal. This is a serious error that all too often results in a broken rest. If decision has been made to place incisal rest on anterior tooth, rest should be large enough to withstand stresses of function. Explorer is shown being used to check depth of rest preparation in relation to normal tooth contour.

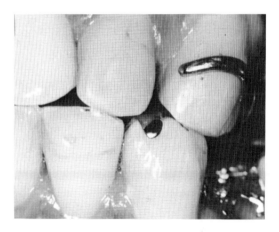

Fig. 5-28. When incisal hook rests are used on anterior teeth, rest seat must be prepared in a way that will permit adequate bulk of metal for strength within normal tooth contour so as not to interfere with tooth contacts in centric or eccentric positions.

tally, the rest seat should be concave (Figs. 5-24 and 5-25). Labiolingually, the rest seat should be slightly convex and carried slightly onto the labial surface. From an incisal view, the axial wall should flare lingually (Fig. 5-26). This will provide an extra bulk of metal for strength without increasing the display of metal from the labial view. The extra strength is significant when the cuspid is the terminal abutment for a distal-extension base RPD.

INCISAL HOOK REST SEATS. Incisal hook rest seats are prepared as a modification of the incisal rest seat. By the preparation's being extended 1.5 to 2 mm onto the labial surface of the tooth as a concave depression, an incisal rest seat is converted to an incisal hook rest seat (Gaston, 1960).

An incisal hook rest has the advantage of providing greater stability than the incisal rest. It has the disadvantage of greater metal display (Fig. 5-23). Incisal hook rests are most often used on mandibular canines. The labial surface

of the mandibular canines is often in tight contact with the lingual surface of the maxillary anterior teeth. It is imperative that a rest seat provide ample room for the "hook" portion of the metal rest so that it can be confined within the normal tooth contour (Fig. 5-27). The metal rest seat must not interfere with tooth contacts in either centric occlusion or in eccentric occlusal positions (Fig. 5-28).

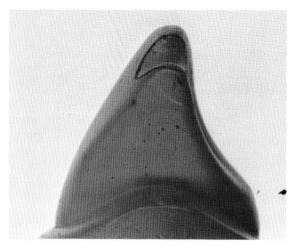

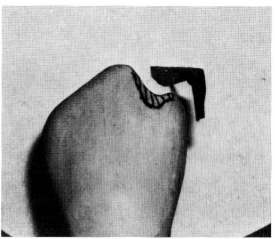

Fig. 5-29. Form of incisal hook rest as viewed from proximal surface of tooth. Note smooth, flowing, convex character of rest seat. Incisal rest seat and incisal hook rest seat are very similar from this view, only difference being that incisal hook rest seat extends onto facial surface for additional 1.5 to 2 mm as concave depression. This extension onto labial surface is vividly illustrated from facial view in Fig. 5-30.

Fig. 5-30. Incisal hook rest preparation is demonstrated on model of mandibular cuspid. Extension of rest seat onto labial surface of tooth is outlined. Note smooth, flowing contour of rest seat with concave positive seat located nearest axial wall and flowing smoothly into convex surface over distal portion of tooth. Simulated metal occlusal rest is shown above incisal hook rest seat. Note similarity between base outline in facial view and base outline of proximal occlusal rest.

The incisal rest seat and the incisal hook rest seat are very similar when viewed from the labial and incisal aspects. The only difference is that the incisal hook rest seat extends onto the labial surface for an additional 1.5 to 2 mm as a concave depression (Figs. 5-29 and 5-30). The general form of the outline of the base, when viewed from the labial aspect, is basically concave and should be approximately 1.5 mm deep and 2.5 mm wide. When the rest seat is located on the mesial or the distal portion of the incisal edge, the base outline should flow smoothly toward the line angle. The similarity between the base outline in the labial view and the base outline of a proximal occlusal rest can be noted in Fig. 5-30. Because of their inherent disadvantages, incisal hook rests should not be used when other types of rests can be employed.

PROXIMAL INCISAL REST SEATS ON MAXILLARY CUSPIDS. Although the proximal incisal rest is perhaps the least esthetically desirable of all rests used on maxillary anterior teeth, it can sometimes be employed to avoid placement of a cast restoration on a tooth in order to obtain a satisfactory positive rest seat. It is usually em-

ployed when the anterior teeth have a deep vertical overlap and the cuspid is located adjacent to an edentulous space (Fig. 5-31). The deep vertical overlap precludes the use of the more conventional rest seat usually placed on maxillary cuspids. The proximal incisal hook rest shown in Fig. 5-27 was employed on a patient whose esthetic values were waived to accommodate his economic status.

"INCISAL-TYPE" REST SEATS FOR MANDIBULAR PREMOLARS. The occlusal anatomy of mandibular first premolars often lacks a definite fossa appropriate for preparation of a satisfactory occlusal rest seat. In these instances, attempts to prepare an occlusal rest seat usually result in either: (1) a totally inadequate rest seat preparation or (2) marked penetration of the enamel surface. The necessity for the dentist to place a restoration to provide a suitable surface for a rest seat can be avoided if the buccal cusp is sound. An "incisal-type" rest seat can be placed on the mesial or distal slope of the buccal cusp to provide a satisfacotry positive seat (Fig. 5-32).

Incisal rests and incisal hook rests can be prepared with a small wheel-shaped or cylin-

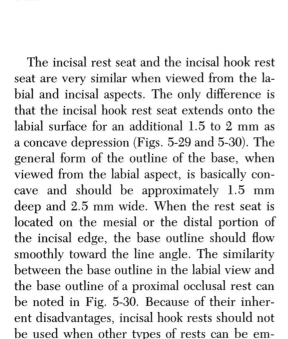

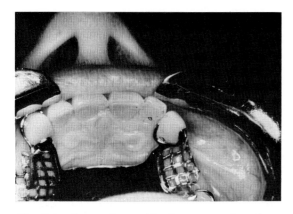

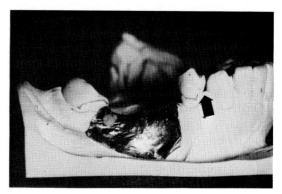

Fig. 5-31. Proximal incisal hook rest is perhaps least desirable of all rests used on maxillary anterior teeth. Its use can sometimes avoid placement of crown on abutment tooth to obtain satisfactory positive rest seat. Deep vertical overlap combined with tight occlusal contacts preclude use of more conventional rest seats usually employed on maxillary cuspids. The tooth contacts on maxillary right cuspid and lateral incisor have been recorded using articulator paper. Note their location close to cervical margin of tooth. Great care has been taken to ensure that lingually placed reciprocal clasp arm does not interfere with normal occlusal contacts.

Fig. 5-32. When occlusal anatomy of mandibular premolar tooth does not provide definite fossa appropriate for preparing satisfactory occlusal rest seat, "incisal type" of rest seat preparation can be placed on mesial or distal slope of buccal cusp to provide satisfactory positive seat *(arrow)*. This eliminates necessity for a metal restoration to provide satisfactory positive seat on abutment tooth.

dric diamond instrument using either conventional or high-speed instrumentation. The outline form of the rest seat should be smooth flowing and void of sharp angles (see Figs. 5-27 and 5-30). All cut tooth surfaces should be smoothed and polished.

CINGULUM REST SEATS. Cingulum rests may be used on the lingual surface of anterior teeth that have a prominent cingulum. They are most often used on maxillary cuspids and incisors (Berg and Caputo, 1978). The nature of tooth contacts in this area makes it imperative that the minor connector reach the cingulum rest preparation without creating occlusal interferences. This requirement can best be met on the basis of information from accurately mounted diagnostic casts. Occasionally, marked wear facets in the cingulum area will alert the dentist to the potential problem of obtaining occlusal clearance in these areas (Fig. 5-33). When there is deep vertical overlap of the anterior teeth, great care must be exercised in evaluating these areas for placing cingulum or lingual ledge rest seats.

A cingulum rest seat should follow the general contour of the cingulum. It can be started

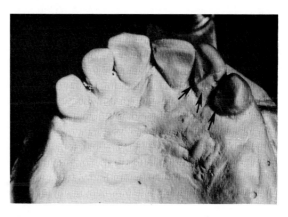

Fig. 5-33. Wear facets *(arrows)* on lingual surface of maxillary anterior teeth near cervical margins should prompt dentist to evaluate these areas with great care when identifying appropriate areas for lingually placed rest seats.

with a number 2 or number 4 round diamond instrument. The base of the rest seat should be placed about 1 mm cervical to the height of the cingulum. The preparation can be finished with a rounded-point cylindric diamond instrument. From the lingual view, the cingulum rest seat should follow the natural contour of the cingulum and slope cervically as the preparation approaches the mesial and distal line angles of the tooth (Fig. 5-34). From the proximal view,

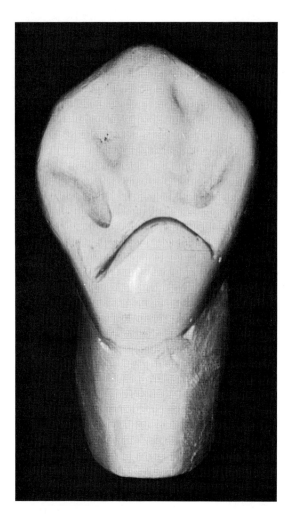

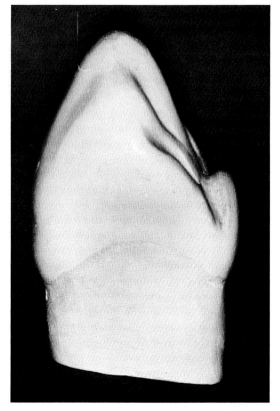

Fig. 5-34. Lingual view of cingulum rest seat preparation is illustrated. Cingulum rest seat should follow natural contour of cingulum and slope cervically as preparation approaches mesial and distal line angles of tooth.

Fig. 5-35. Proximal view of cingulum rest seat preparation is illustrated. Base of rest seat is concave or U shaped. Rest seat should be approximately 1 to 1.5 mm deep. Care must be taken to ensure that lingual axial wall is not undercut.

the base of the rest seat is concave or U shaped (Fig. 5-35). Care must be exercised so that there are no undercuts on the lingual axial wall. The rest seat should be approximately 1 to 1.5 mm deep.

LINGUAL LEDGE REST SEATS. Lingual ledge rests are usually placed on the lingual surface of maxillary anterior teeth. When prepared in natural tooth structure, they are perhaps the least efficient of the anterior rest seats discussed. A lingual ledge rest seat may be placed on any anterior tooth that has lingual enamel of sufficient thickness to accommodate the preparation. Unfortunately, this thickness determi-

nation cannot be made until the preparation of the rest seat is well underway. The lingual ledge rest is usually employed on anterior teeth without a cingulum or on anterior teeth with a cingulum that is not sufficiently prominent to accommodate the cingulum rest preparation. For this reason, the base of the seat (the ledge) must be relatively narrow, which accounts for its relative inefficiency. However, properly prepared, it provides an adequate positive seat (Figs. 5-36 and 5-38). The most satisfactory lingual rest seats are placed on cast restorations, where the ledge can be made wider and the rests can be located more cervi-

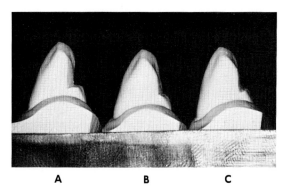

A　　　　**B**　　　　**C**

Fig. 5-36. Some lingual ledge rest seats are illustrated in proximal view. Two of the most common errors made in preparing lingual ledge rest seats are illustrated (**A** and **B**). Acceptable lingual ledge rest seat is illustrated (**C**). In **A**, preparation is too deep and would have penetrated enamel surface. In **B**, rest seat slopes cervically and thus does not provide positive seat.

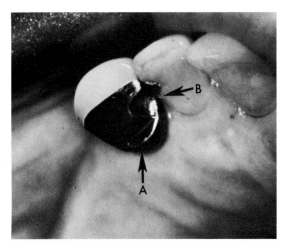

Fig. 5-37. Most satisfactory lingual rest seats are placed on crowns, where ledge can be made wider (*A*) and rest can be located more cervically to avoid occlusal interferences. Note precision-milled recess (*B*) located on mesial surface of tooth. This modification of rest seat, with its metal counterpart, prevents distal displacement of prosthesis. This nonconventional rest preparation is very effective in providing positive tooth support and in preventing distal displacement of prosthesis. It is representative of a combination extracoronal and intercoronal rest seat.

cally to avoid occlusal interferences. The placement of lingual ledge rests and cingulum rests in natural tooth structure is contraindicated when the anterior teeth have an extreme, deep, vertical overlap and tight occlusal contacts. The rest seats would have to be placed so far cervically that the enamel would not be sufficiently thick to accommodate them. Either the cingulum rest or the lingual ledge rest can be placed in a cast restoration; the base of the rest seat can be made sufficiently wide to be efficient, and the rest seat can be placed cervically enough to prevent occlusal interferences (Fig. 5-37). The crown preparation requires sufficient lingual tooth reduction to accommodate the more cervically placed rest seat. Under certain conditions, the need to place a restoration to provide an adequate lingual ledge rest seat or a cingulum rest can be avoided by using a proximal incisal hook rest (Fig. 5-38).

Viewed lingually on teeth without a cingulum, the lingual ledge rest seat should be perpendicular to the long axis of the tooth and located at the junction of the middle and cervical thirds (provided the tooth contacts will permit it), where the enamel is thickest. On teeth with a slight cingulum, the lingual ledge rest seat may curve slightly to follow the curvature of the cingulum if occlusal interferences can be avoided.

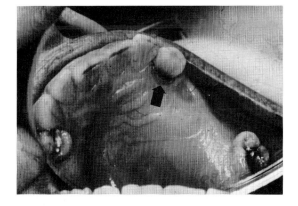

Fig. 5-38. When lingual ledge rest is prepared in natural tooth structure, it is perhaps the least efficient of the anterior rest seats described. However, properly prepared, it provides adequate positive seat. Adequate lingual ledge rest (*arrow*) is shown placed on lingual surface of maxillary canine. Base has been shaded for photographic purposes.

The details of the ledge rest seat can best be visualized from the incisal view (Fig. 5-36). The ledge rest must follow the contour of the lingual surface of the tooth or else the center portion of the ledge will penetrate the enamel. The ledge should be widest (from 1 to 1.5 mm) at the central portion of the lingual surface and gradually tapered to blend in with the mesial and distal line angles of the tooth (Fig. 5-38).

From the proximal view, the base of the rest seat will be flat and perpendicular to the tooth's long axis, or it may have a gentle axial slope. The axial wall should be devoid of any undercuts and should incline slightly toward the labial side. The junction of the ledge with the axial wall should be slightly rounded to be self-cleansing.

Lingual ledge rest seats can be prepared with a cylindric, wheel-shaped, or inverted-cone carborundum stone or diamond instruments. They can also be prepared with carbide fissure burs. The rest seat should be smooth and polished.

ONLAY REST SEATS. Onlay rests are used on the occlusal surface of teeth that are in infraocclusion or on tipped molars. They should cover all or a portion of the occlusal surface of the tooth to restore normal occlusal contacts (see Fig. 5-3, *B*).

The preparation for these rest seats should include widening and smoothing of any deep fissures or grooves to provide a more self-cleansing surface as well as elimination of occlusal or axial undercuts that will prevent seating of the framework.

Creating undercuts

When the final path of insertion and removal of the prosthesis has been chosen, the shape of the tooth may not present acceptable undercuts for clasp retention. Under certain conditions, the tooth surface can be grooved or dimpled to achieve satisfactory retention for clasping. If the tooth surface in question has been restored with an acceptable material and is reasonably parallel to the path of placement and removal, a retentive groove or dimple may be placed. Gold and gold substitutes are ideal materials for these procedures. Amalgam alloy and dental porcelain surfaces are acceptable when wrought wire clasp buccal retentive arms are to be employed.

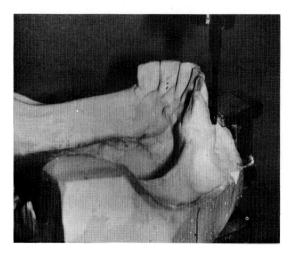

Fig. 5-39. It may be inappropriate to attempt to create undercuts in enamel surfaces by dimpling or grooving under certain conditions. When basic form of tooth is either wedge or cone shaped, tooth surfaces do not even approach paralleling path of placement of prosthesis. Attempts to provide adequate retentive grooves on these surfaces would result in enamel penetration long before adequate groove or undercut could be provided.

Retentive grooves or dimples may be placed in sound enamel in those areas in which the enamel is sufficiently thick to do so (Axinn, 1975). Grooving or dimpling should not be attempted near the cervical margins of teeth, since the enamel is thinnest in this area. The placement of retentive grooves or dimples in sound enamel should be considered only if the tooth surface in question is parallel or nearly parallel to the path of placement and removal. Tooth surfaces that diverge significantly from the path of placement are not suitable for retentive grooves or dimples. Attempts to place such grooves or dimples here would result in enamel penetration long before an adequate groove or undercut could be provided. Although many teeth may pose this problem, canines (particularly mandibular canines) most often do so. When they are wedge shaped, they offer no surface that even approaches paralleling the path of placement (Fig. 5-39). It is best to first restore these areas to an acceptable contour with an appropriate restoration before the retentive area is made.

A dimple or recess in the enamel surface can be made with a number 4 round carbide bur or

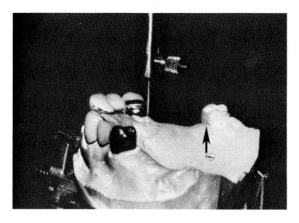

Fig. 5-40. When one or more of abutment teeth are *not* to receive surveyed crowns, path of placement of prosthesis should be keyed on natural tooth surface or surfaces *(arrow)*.

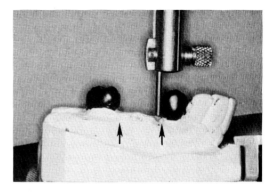

Fig. 5-41. Surveyed crowns should be designed on full arch working casts that are properly oriented to path of insertion and withdrawal of prosthesis. Here, guiding planes *(arrows)* on wax surveyed crowns are being checked to ensure that they are parallel to path of placement and to each other.

with a diamond instrument of similar size and shape. The preparation can be smoothed with a finishing bur and polished with a prophylaxis brush and flour of pumice.

Surveyed crowns

Surveyed crowns are cast restorations that are fabricated for teeth serving as abutments for RPDs (Blatterfein, 1956; Chandler, 1973). The restorations are surveyed while they are being fabricated, using a dental surveyor. The master cast of the abutment tooth preparations is secured to the cast holder and oriented to the planned path of insertion and removal of the prosthesis (Fig. 5-40). The orientation of the master cast is extremely important if the finished surveyed crowns are to provide the design requirements for the RPD (proper guiding planes, survey lines, retentive areas, and occlusal morphologic features) and not introduce interferences to the path of placement.

Full arch impressions should be used to produce the working cast, whether one or all of the abutment teeth are to receive surveyed crowns. The full arch working cast, reproducing the preparation of the abutment teeth, and a dental stone cast of the opposing dental arch should be properly related on a dental articulator. Individual dies should be used to develop the general fit and to perfect the margins of the crowns. The full arch working cast is used to develop the general contours, guiding

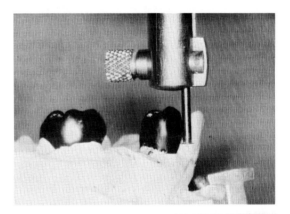

Fig. 5-42. With working cast properly oriented to correct path of placement, undercut gauge is used to check proper amount of retention required in surveyed crown.

planes, survey lines, and occlusal relationships of the surveyed crowns.

When one or more of the remaining natural teeth are not to receive surveyed crowns, the path of placement should be keyed on the natural tooth surfaces, which will provide effective guiding planes (Fig. 5-40). Once the full arch cast is properly oriented to the path of placement, the design requirements for the surveyed crown can be produced in the waxed or partially completed crowns (Figs. 5-41 and 5-42).

When surveyed crowns are being fabricated to support a mandibular RPD that is to be opposed by a maxillary complete denture, the maxillary denture should be carried through the wax try-in stage before the surveyed crowns are completed. This will provide an opportunity to develop an ideal occlusal plane and to incorporate the appropriate compensating curves often needed for complete denture occlusion. These treatment procedures are briefly illustrated (see Fig. 5-4).

When abutment teeth must be restored with surveyed crowns, it provides the dentist with an opportunity to develop ideal survey lines, guiding planes, occlusal rests, and undercuts. For metal surfaces, the form required is developed in the wax patterns of the surveyed crowns (Figs. 5-41 and 5-42). The form for dental porcelain and porcelain-fused-to-metal restorations is developed in the partially completed crowns following the bisque bake (Fig. 5-43). With these opportunities available, there is little excuse for the finished restoration to present sharp marginal ridges (Fig. 5-44), inadequate rest seats (Fig. 5-45), or poorly designed retentive areas.

Conventional crown preparations, however, need to be modified to meet the design requirements of surveyed crown. The previously developed treatment plan will identify the specific design requirements for each surveyed crown. Knowing these in advance of making the crown preparations, the dentist can make appropriate modifications in the abutment

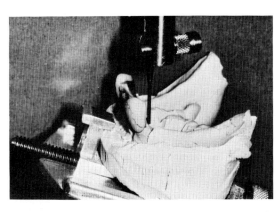

Fig. 5-43. Design for porcelain and porcelain-fused-to-metal restorations is developed in partially completed crowns following bisque bake. Working cast should be oriented to proper path of placement and removal of prosthesis during this procedure.

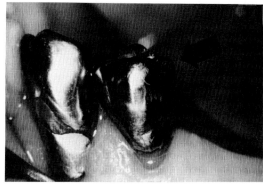

Fig. 5-44. There is little excuse for surveyed crowns not to produce ideal or nearly ideal rest seat preparations. Here, illustration shows inadequately prepared premolar distal occlusal rest seat. Marginal ridge is too high and too sharp *(arrow)*. This results in metal rest that is too thin in marginal ridge area. If such an error is detected before impression for master cast is made, it can be corrected.

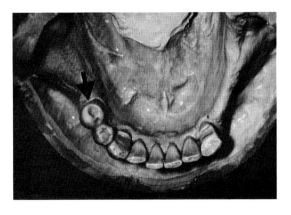

Fig. 5-45. Unacceptable proximal occlusal rest seat is shown from occlusal view. Note that outline of rest seat does not flare toward line angles of tooth. Marginal ridge *(arrow)* is extremely sharp. Usual result of this type of rest seat preparation is shown in Fig. 5-16.

tooth preparation to accommodate the design requirements of the surveyed crown. The reduction of additional tooth surface is usually required in the following instances:

1. To recess rest seats
2. To shorten the clinical crown
3. To reduce severe interferences and undercuts
4. To develop appropriate guiding planes on severely tipped teeth
5. To provide adequate space for the denture teeth in an edentulous space that has been diminished by migration or tilting of the bounding teeth.

Crown ledges

A crown ledge is a form of a lingual ledge rest except that it is placed in the crown of an abutment tooth (Chandler, 1973). Preparations for abutment teeth that are to receive crown ledges require special attention. Additional tooth structure must be removed from the area to receive the crown ledge.

Fig. 5-46 presents diagrammatic illustrations, in the frontal plane, of a surveyed crown with a lingually placed crown ledge. Diagrams B, C, and D show various RPD components (clasp arm and metal component of the lingual ledge recess) as they travel along their path of placement toward their final seating (terminal position). When the RPD is fully seated, the lingual ledge recess is completely filled by its metal counterpart, which serves to reciprocate the labial retentive clasp arm (Fig. 5-46, D). It should be noted that the crown ledge, functioning with its metal counterpart (a component of the RPD framework), serves as a precisionlike guiding plane. The portion of the RPD framework recessed into the crown ledge, when fully seated, completes the contour of the crown and eliminates the projection of the clasp arm on this surface.

When it is mandatory that a surveyed crown be placed on a posterior abutment tooth, the use of a crown ledge is a very desirable treatment modality. It is particularly desirable when additional guiding planes are needed to help direct and control the path of placement and removal of the prosthesis. It is also recommended for patients with overly curious or sensitive tongues.

AVOIDING PROBLEMS

Many dentists have been chagrined during the final phases of RPD construction by problems that would not have arisen if the mouth

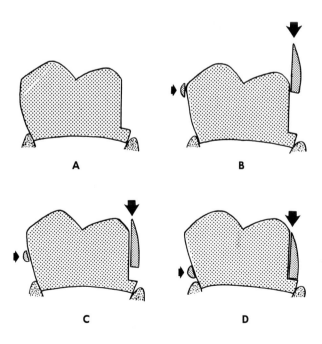

Fig. 5-46. **A,** Cross section of surveyed crown with lingually placed crown ledge is diagrammatically illustrated in the frontal plane. In **B, C,** and **D** various RPD components (clasp arm and metal component of the lingual ledge recess) are shown as they travel along their path of placement toward their final seating. **B,** Metal component of recessed crown ledge has engaged axial wall of crown ledge and is guiding clasp assembly along path of placement. Facial retentive clasp arm has just engaged height of contour. **C,** Metal component of lingual ledge recess is approximately two-thirds seated. Note how axial wall of crown ledge, functioning with its metal counterpart (a component of the partial denture framework), serves as a precision-like guiding plane. **D,** When RPD is fully seated, lingual ledge recess will be completely filled by its metal counterpart and will complete lingual outline of tooth form. Metal counterpart also serves to reciprocate facial retentive clasp arm.

preparations had been properly planned and executed. The following are some examples of these kinds of avoidable problems.

1. The denture base of a mandibular distal-extension RPD must be shortened significantly because of a large, bulbous maxillary tuberosity that should have been reduced previously.
2. The RPD framework has so much retention that it must be dislodged with a rigid instrument.
3. The RPD framework exhibits no retention at all because of improperly planned undercuts on complete cast crowns serving as primary abutments.
4. The patient is unable to close his or her jaws in centric occlusion because the mandibular anterior teeth strike the minor connector leading to a cingulum rest placed too far incisally on a maxillary cuspid.
5. The patient is unable to close his or her jaws in centric occlusion because occlusal rests or the shoulders of clasp arms cause interferences to final closure.
6. The mandibular RPD cannot be seated because the flanges encounter bilaterally opposing bony undercuts in the mylohyoid ridge area.
7. The occlusal rest or a clasp arm fractures just a few weeks after the insertion of the RPD because the amount of tooth structure removed during the mouth preparation was insufficient to permit adequate bulk of metal for these rigid parts of the RPD framework.
8. The patient is unable to incise food after the placement of a maxillary distal-extension base RPD because an extruded mandibular molar produces marked occlusal interferences during protrusive movement.

These are problems that never should occur, since they are readily prevented by exercising reasonable care in making the diagnosis, developing the treatment plan, and executing the previously planned mouth preparations. The previously mentioned problems constitute a distinct disservice to the patient. When these problems are not fully corrected, they pose a significant potential threat to the health of the oral structures and a genuine nuisance to the patient, and they decrease the longevity of the prosthesis. The correction of such defects will often necessitate remaking the RPD after correcting the inadequacies in the mouth preparations that caused the failure.

The dentist may start an RPD health service with an excellent treatment plan, but if the mouth preparations are not executed properly, the results of the treatment effort will be very disappointing.

SUMMARY

Tooth modifications are accomplished to meet the specific needs pertaining to the treatment plan. Each modification is executed to achieve a specific objective. The needs are identified during the examination, diagnosis, and treatment planning, and the objectives and tooth modifications are noted and recorded. The need for specific modifications should be recorded in a manner that will permit the dentist to execute them with as great a degree of accuracy as possible. When this has been accomplished, a significant contribution has been made toward a successful and rewarding RPD experience for both the patient and the dentist.

6 Impressions: Trial fitting of the framework

IMPRESSION PROCEDURES FOR SECURING THE MASTER CAST FOR FABRICATION OF THE REMOVABLE PARTIAL DENTURE FRAMEWORK

Once the remaining teeth in the partially edentulous arch for which a removable partial denture (RPD) treatment has been planned have been properly modified to meet the design specifications of the framework, impressions procedures to secure the master cast must be planned.

The materials of choice to record a partially edentulous dental arch are the elastomeric impression materials. These include the reversible hydrocolloids (agar-agar), the irreversible hydrocolloids (alginate), the mercaptan rubber base impression materials (thiokols), the silicone impression materials, and the polyether impression materials (Henderson and Steffel, 1981). Although any of these materials, when handled correctly and confined in an appropriate tray, will produce consistently good clinical results, the irreversible hydrocolloids are by far the most commonly used in daily dental practice. The reasons for their popularity lie in their ease of handling, convenient availability, relative low cost, and the dependable, accurate dental stone casts that they can produce when properly manipulated (Miller and Grasso, 1981). For these reasons, the irreversible hydrocolloids are the materials of choice for this procedure.

Tray selection for irreversible hydrocolloid impressions

Stock impression trays for partially edentulous arches may be used to make the impression for the RPD framework. These trays are either of a perforated or a rim-lock type (Figs. 6-1 and 6-2). A prime consideration in the selection of a suitable tray is the absolute rigidity that must be afforded by the tray material.

Sturdy, stock metal trays are preferred, since there is little chance they will deform at any time during the impression procedure. However, many dentists do use custom acrylic resin trays that have been constructed on the diagnostic cast.

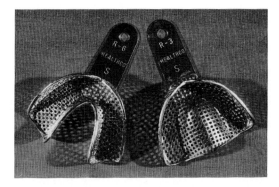

Fig. 6-1. Maxillary and mandibular stock perforated impression trays before modification with modeling compound for irreversible hydrocolloid impressions.

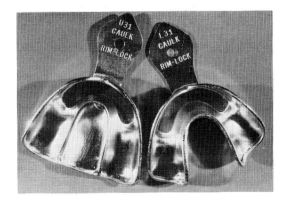

Fig. 6-2. Maxillary and mandibular stock rim-lock impression trays before modification for irreversible hydrocolloid impressions for bilateral distal-extension RPDs.

161

The next technical decision to be made is the selection of the proper size and shape of the tray to take advantage of the dimensional accuracy of the impression material and to include all necessary anatomic landmarks in the impression. An impression tray of the correct size and form for an irreversible hydrocolloid impression material is one that will permit its easy insertion and removal from the mouth with a clearance of one-quarter inch in all regions (Rudd and Dunn, 1967).

When stock metal trays are used, they must be modified to improve the fit of the tray for each individual case. This will ensure an optimal and even amount of bulk of impression material to obtain the desired accuracy from the impression procedure. A uniform thickness of impression material between the surface of the tray and the tissue being recorded will tend to minimize differences in the behavior of the material between a thick section and a very thin one (Miller and Grasso, 1981). A common area in which these differences occur is that of a terminal abutment tooth and the edentulous ridge immediately adjacent to it, which produces an inaccuracy in recording the form of that abutment. The impression tray may also need modification by the addition of extensions to it. This is necessary to secure an impression of strategic anatomic landmarks, such as the mandibular retromolar pads and the maxillary posterior palatal seal area.

The material of choice for these tray modifications is modeling compound because of its rigidity and ease of manipulation. Waxes should not be used, since the impression material will not adhere to them and since, if the wax used is of the soft, pliable variety, it will invariably distort when the impression is removed from the mouth, producing an inaccurate impression. Elastic impression materials will adhere to the modeling compound if the latter is roughened by scraping with a vulcanite scraper and an adhesive, such as Getz's Hold,* is applied to the surface (Fig. 6-3). Alternately, chloroform or rubber cement may be applied to the modeling compound surface and cotton fibers then incorporated onto the tacky surface to ensure adhesion of the impression material to this surface. All excess cotton fibers must be

---

*Teledyne Dental, Elk Grove Village, Ill.

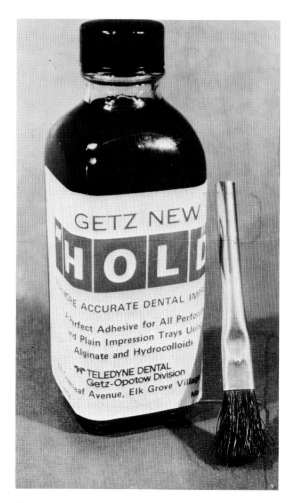

Fig. 6-3. Impression tray adhesive, such as Getz's Hold, is brushed onto modeling compound additions to stock tray to ensure firm union between compound and impression material. When impression is removed from mouth, union between compound and impression material must remain secure to prevent an inaccurate impression.

removed by flaming them slightly and then moistening the remaining fibers before adding the impression material to the impression tray (Rudd and Dunn, 1967).

Modification of the stock maxillary impression tray

After the appropriate stock metal tray for the maxillary arch has been selected, the modeling compound material, which has been softened in a hot water tempering bath, is placed into the hard palate area of the tray and any other areas of the tray corresponding to residual

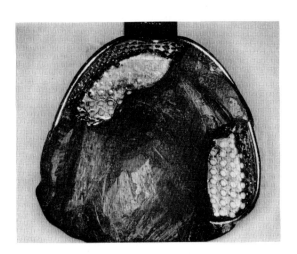

Fig. 6-4. Modeling compound additions have been trimmed away from abutment teeth, and surface area of compound has been roughened to receive adhesive material before impression is made.

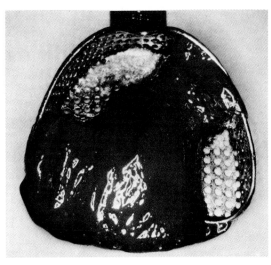

Fig. 6-5. Tray adhesive Hold has been applied to modeling compound surface to achieve firm union between compound and impression material.

ridges. The compound is flamed lightly with an alcohol torch and tempered in the water bath, and the tray is inserted into the mouth, the dentist making sure that the tray is properly centered and that contact is made between the occlusal surfaces of the remaining teeth and the metal of the tray. After the compound has hardened, the tray is removed from the mouth, chilled in ice cold water, and examined for its acceptability. All anatomic landmarks (such as the hard palate, palatal rugae, maxillary tuberosities, and postpalatal seal area) that are desired should be recorded in the compound. If not, additional stick compound can be applied to the deficient areas and the procedure can be repeated until all vital anatomic landmarks have been recorded.

Any contact of the modeling compound with the teeth must be removed by cutting or scraping the compound with a sharp, cutting instrument (sharp knife or Vulcanite scraper). The ultimate goal is to have a uniform layer of the elastic impression material, not the modeling compound, in contact with the teeth and residual ridges. The entire surface of compound is roughened with the scraper to remove any undercut areas in the material (Fig. 6-4). The surface of the modeling compound modification is prepared for the adhesive as outlined above

(Fig. 6-5). The maxillary tray is now prepared to receive the elastic impression material.

Modification of the stock mandibular impression tray

In the same process used for modifying the stock maxillary impression tray, modeling compound that has been softened in a hot water tempering bath is placed into the areas of the selected mandibular tray corresponding to the mandibular edentulous areas, the dentist making sure that there is sufficient material to record vital anatomic landmarks (such as the retromolar pads, the retromylohyoid fossa, the buccal shelf, and the residual ridges). The compound additions are flamed with an alcohol torch and tempered, and the tray is seated to place on the mandibular arch. Care should be exercised to ensure that definite contact has been made between the tray and the occlusal surfaces of the remaining teeth. The tray is removed from the mouth, chilled in iced water, and inspected for accuracy. Stick modeling compound is added to deficient areas until all desired landmarks have been registered. Modeling compound is cut away from around the remaining teeth with a sharp knife. The compound surface is roughened with a knife (Fig. 6-6), and alginate adhesive is painted on the

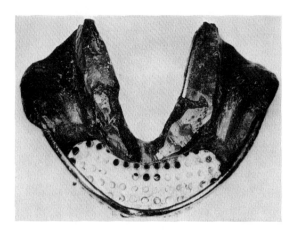

Fig. 6-6. Mandibular impression tray is illustrated. Modeling compound has been trimmed from around abutment teeth, and surface area has been roughened in preparation for application of tray adhesive. Note that all vital anatomic landmarks, such as buccal shelf, retromolar pads, and proper extension into lingual and retromylohyoid fossa areas, have been recorded.

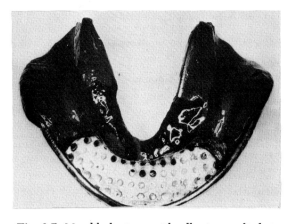

Fig. 6-7. Mandibular tray, with adhesive applied, is now prepared to receive irreversible hydrocolloid impression.

compound as detailed previously. The mandibular tray may now be used to make the mandibular impression (Fig. 6-7).

Use of irreversible hydrocolloid materials in impression making

Irreversible hydrocolloid, or alginate as it is more popularly known, is a powder consisting essentially of sodium alginate and calcium sulfate. When this powder is mixed with water, a latticework of calcium alginate, a gel, is formed (Phillips, 1953). This chemical reaction is irreversible, differentiating this material from the agar-agar type of hydrocolloid impression material, which is classified as reversible because it can be heated repeatedly to become a viscous liquid and then cooled to form a rubberlike gel (Miller and Grasso, 1981).

It was previously stated that the irreversible hydrocolloids, when handled properly, produce consistently good, clinically acceptable impressions from which dental stone master casts can be made for the fabrication of RPD frameworks. However, their relative ease and convenience of use has led dentists to abuse their physical properties. Nevertheless, if these materials are handled meticulously and with strict adherence to basic techniques, dependable results can be anticipated.

Important considerations for handling irreversible hydrocolloid materials

The dentist must standardize all procedures so that variables can be reduced. The manufacturer's directions should be followed implicitly. Although it is best to use individual, single-mix, prepackaged irreversible hydrocolloid to ensure the proper amount by weight of the powder, the bulk-packaged material can be used satisfactorily. Individual measurings of the bulk-packaged material can be dispensed into airtight jars for future use rather than the material's being stored in the original container. The preweighed volume of powder mixed with the manufacturer's recommended volume of room temperature (70° F), deionized water will produce a mix of standard consistency every time. Dispensing bulk-packaged material into individual measurings in airtight jars will prevent contamination of the alginate powder. It will also prevent hydration, especially in humid climates, since the seal of the original container is questionable after once it is opened (Rudd and Dunn, 1967).

The object of spatulation of the powder and water is to thoroughly incorporate all of the powder into the water, producing an homogenous, bubble-free mix. Mixing should be carried out in a flexible, clean, scratch-free rubber bowl with a broad-bladed stainless steel mixing spatula. Mixed material should be pushed against the side of the bowl while the bowl is turned in the opposite direction with the palm of the hand. If available, vacuum mechanical spatulation should be used, because it will ensure a smooth, air-free mix (Rudd and Dunn, 1967).

When the impression material is introduced into the oral cavity at room temperature (approximately 70° F), an immediate increase in viscosity and surface tension of the saliva occurs, resulting in the potential entrapment of air bubbles in strategic locations. To minimize this phenomenon, the dentist should forcibly place the impression material in and on the occlusal surfaces, rest seat preparations, palatal vault, and other critical areas with the index finger before inserting and seating the tray.

Gelation takes place from the tooth and soft tissue surfaces outward to the tray. It is essential that the dentist avoid moving the impression tray intraorally until gelation is complete. Movement of the tray or of the patient during gelation results in internal stress formation that is relieved when the impression is removed from the mouth, resulting in a distorted impression.

All types of hydrocolloids are dimensionally stable only during a brief period after removal from the mouth. The impression should be poured immediately with dental stone, no longer than 10 minutes after removal (Skinner and Hobbit, 1956). The hydrocolloid impression materials dehydrate rapidly, with resultant shrinkage, if they are not poured immediately. If the impression is allowed to stand unpoured, syneresis (water loss) will occur, resulting in the emission of a mucinous exudate that will produce a chalky, inaccurate dental stone cast.

Procedures for making an irreversible hydrocolloid impression

All of the teeth in the dental arch should be given a thorough dental prophylaxis and polishing before the impression procedure, and the polishing agents should be removed by thorough flushing. This will reduce the surface tension of the teeth and facilitate an accurate recording of the dental structures. Excess saliva can be controlled by the use of gauze packs placed in the floor of the mouth or over the ducts of the parotid glands and removed immediately before the introduction of the impression material in the mouth. The teeth are dried gently with the air syringe, with care being taken not to dry them completely. The hydrocolloid materials sometimes adhere tenaciously to a clean, smooth, and dry tooth surface, thereby tearing the impression when the tray is removed from the mouth (Rudd and Dunn, 1967).

The patient is placed in an upright, comfortable position in the dental chair, with the dental arch to receive the impression parallel to the floor.

The water-powder ratio recommended by the manufacturer is used, and the premeasured, room temperature (70° F), distilled water is placed into a clean, dry, flexible rubber mixing bowl. The premeasured powder is carefully added to the water. With a short, stiff spatula, spatulation of the mix is started immediately along the sides of the bowl. A creamy, bubble-free consistency should be attained in no longer than 45 seconds.

The previously modified tray is loaded with the thoroughly spatulated mix, the first portion of impression material being pushed through the holes of the perforated stock tray to ensure that the material is locked securely to the tray. The loading of the tray is completed with the remaining impression material, but a very small amount should be saved for later use. This should not take more than 45 seconds.

The gauze packs are removed from the mouth and the teeth are gently air dried. The previously saved excess impression material is placed on the index finger and forced onto all critical areas, such as rest seats, interproximal embrasure areas, and the hard palate. The loaded impression tray is immediately inserted to place into the mouth.

The position of the impression tray at this time is most important. The dentist should try to center the tray as it was previously positioned when the modeling compound additions were being made. However, caution must be exercised that the tray is not seated completely to tooth contact. The tray should be seated vertically so that a minimum but uninterrupted amount of impression material lies over the occlusal surfaces of the teeth. This will permit an even thickness of impression material to be distributed between the customized stock metal tray and all of the areas that must be recorded

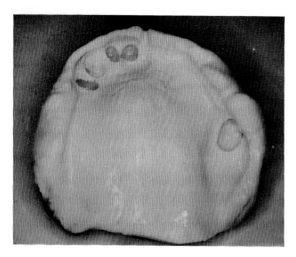

Fig. 6-8. Completed maxillary irreversible hydrocolloid impression. Note thin borders in anterior and thick borders in posterior. Impression material should completely fill cul-de-sac without distending tissue.

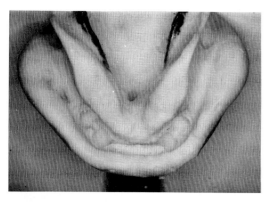

Fig. 6-9. Completed mandibular irreversible hydrocolloid impression. Note in this illustration and in Fig. 6-8 that all vital anatomic landmarks are recorded and that essentially none of modeling compound tray modification areas have perforated through impression material. This offers assurance that even thickness of impression material exists between tray and tissues to be recorded, providing greatest degree of accuracy offered by this material.

in the impression—which was the goal of the tray modification procedures.

The tray must be held immobile intraorally until gelation is complete. When a test sample of the material remaining in the mixing bowl is found to be set, a firm, quick snap of the tray along the long axes of the teeth will deliver the impression from the mouth (Figs. 6-8 and 6-9).

The impression should be rinsed immediately with cold tap water, have the excess moisture shaken off, and then be inspected for anatomic detail and accuracy. If found satisfactory, the impression is sprinkled with a thin coating of dental stone to remove any excess mucous and saliva. The impression is then rinsed again with cold tap water to thoroughly remove all vestiges of dental stone.

The impression is now ready for pouring of the dental stone cast, which should be accomplished immediately. No more than 10 minutes should elapse from the time the impression is removed from the mouth until it is poured. The impression should not be wrapped in a wet towel before the impression is poured in dental stone, since the weight of the towel on the surface of the alginate may cause distortion. While the dental stone is prepared for pouring, the impression should be placed, properly supported through the body and handle of the tray, in a humidor.

Preparation of the dental stone for the master cast

The selection of the dental stone material and its manipulation is most essential in the production of an accurate, strong master cast. Since the master cast must undergo many technical procedures before the final RPD framework is ready for trial fitting into the mouth, an "improved" dental stone material or Class II material should be selected (Phillips, 1973). These improved dental stones have a small degree of setting expansion and an acceptable degree of surface hardness.

Since dental stones are exceedingly susceptible to hydration, these materials should be weighed and stored in tightly sealed glass jars until ready for use (Rudd, Morrow, and Bange, 1969). The manufacturer's recommended ratio is 100 g of dental stone to 24 ml of distilled, precisely measured water.

The premeasured distilled water is poured into a clean, dry, scratch-free rubber or plastic mixing bowl. The dental stone powder is gently sifted into the water and, with a stiff-bladed spatula, manual spatulation is begun. If mechanical or vacuum spatulation is available, either type may be used to distinct advantage. The object of spatulation is to ensure thorough mixing of dental stone powder and water with minimum entrapment of air. Spatulation is accomplished by stirring the mixture vigorously, wiping the material against the sides of the bowl as it is slowly twirled in the hand. The mixing, never to exceed 2 minutes in duration, continues until a smooth, homogenous mass is obtained. Further mixing is not recommended, because gypsum crystals already being formed may be broken, producing a weakened final master cast (Phillips, 1973).

After manual spatulation, the mixing bowl is placed on a mechnical vibrator. The material is kneaded to permit the escape of air that was incorporated into the mixture during the spatulation.

The impression is removed from the humidor, and its surface is very gently air dried. Although excess water should be removed by this process, care should be exercised so that the material is not dehydrated. Essentially, a thin surface film of moisture should be retained without allowing the pooling of water in the deeper crevices of the impression. A properly dried impression will not have a dull appearance but will still retain a shine (Miller and Grasso, 1981).

The dentist places the impression tray on the mechanical vibrator, making sure that the tray itself, not the impression material, contacts the vibrator. This will prevent the possible distortion of the impression. With a small spatula, some prepared dental stone material is added to the distal area of the impression. Using gentle vibration, the dentist moves the material forward so that it pushes the air and moisture ahead of itself. Small increments of material are added continuously at this same distal end. Each new addition of dental stone should push the mass forward (Fig. 6-10). This will ensure that no air bubbles will be trapped in the deeper crevices and that the weight of the material will cause any excess water to be pushed around the dental arch to ultimately be expelled at the opposite end of the impression. This excess water is gently blown out with an air syringe. When the impressions of all of the teeth are filled, dental stone is added in larger quantities until the entire impression is completely filled by vibrating it gently and carefully. Excessive vibration should be avoided when dental stone is poured into an impression of any hydrocolloid material. The flexibility of the material makes it susceptible to distortion (Miller and Grasso, 1981). Harsh vibration of

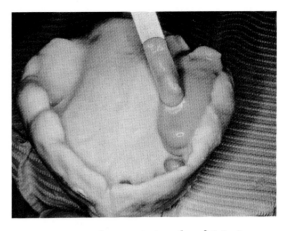

Fig. 6-10. Dental stone is introduced into impression a small amount at a time, starting at distal end, and each additional application pushes stone mass forward.

the impression material can distort it by releasing stresses or by freeing the impression from the tray (Rudd, Morrow, and Bange, 1969).

A two-stage pouring of the master cast, as advocated by Rudd and Dunn (1967), is the technique of choice in this procedure. Recent research results indicate that dental stone should be allowed to set directly against the impression material with the forces of gravity acting vertically against the impression. It was observed that a rougher, more grainy-appearing dental stone cast surface was produced on poured impressions that were inverted before their initial set (Young, 1965). Therefore, after the impression is completely filled with the initial mix of dental stone, it is placed in a humidor at 100% humidity while undergoing its initial set. Again, support should be on the tray and tray handle and not on any part of the impression material while the impression is in the humidor. It is recommended that the top surface of the dental stone be permitted to remain rough and irregular with undercuts to ensure a better bonding when the base of the dental stone cast is ultimately added (Fig. 6-11).

After the heat of crystalization has dissipated, the initially set dental stone cast is removed from the humidor, and the exposed dental stone surface is soaked in slurry water for 3 to 5 minutes as demonstrated by Rudd, Morrow, and Bange (1969). Slurry water is a supersaturated liquid made by allowing dis-

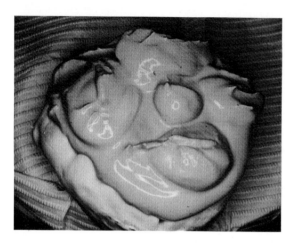

Fig. 6-11. Surface of initial pour of dental stone is left irregular to facilitate better bonding to dental stone base.

carded artifical dental stone casts to sit in a container of water for 48 hours. The resultant liquid is essentially a saturated solution of calcium sulfate and water.

The same dental stone and water-powder ratios are used to make another mix of dental stone for the base of the master cast. This second mix is placed on a glass slab and formed in the shape of a patty. A small quantity of stone is added to the base of the dental stone cast of the impression. The master cast is inverted into this new mix of dental stone. Any excess is carefully trimmed off. The entire assembly— impression, base, and slab—is placed into the humidor.

Between 45 minutes to 1 hour after the initial pour, the dental stone master cast should be separated from the impression material. Once set, the master cast should never be permitted to soak, be wet, or be rinsed in tap water, because dental stone is soluble in plain water (Phillips, 1973). Invariably the surface of the master cast will be etched if it is moistened. In all subsequent procedures in which the master cast will come in contact with water, the water should be slurry water. Therefore, when the impression is removed, it is placed with its master cast in warm slurry water until the modeling compound tray modifications are thoroughly softened. When the impression is gently pried away from the master cast, care should be exercised so that isolated teeth or other important structures are

not inadvertently fractured during this procedure. Any remaining impression material is removed, and the master cast is examined. An acceptable master cast should show a clean, hard, dense surface with anatomic details clearly visible. If the master cast shows a grainy rough surface, it should be discarded immediately and the impression procedures repeated. Then the impression pouring procedures are repeated. If the master cast appears satisfactory, it is ready to be trimmed on a model trimmer.

The master casts should be trimmed only to remove excess dental stone. When the model trimmer is used, reasonable care should be taken to prevent the removal of critical anatomic landmarks. After the trimming is complete, the master cast is washed carefully with slurry water to remove all vestiges of the dental stone sludge produced by the model trimmer. A soft camel's hair brush can be used for this purpose.

The master cast is allowed to thoroughly air dry. It is inspected carefully, and all dental stone nodules that are not located on critical areas are removed. No attempt should be made to "carve out" nodules that exist in critical areas. If such nodules exist, the master cast should be discarded at this time and a new impression planned. If, however, the master cast is deemed acceptable, it is ready to be sent to the dental laboratory. It is accompanied by an appropriately executed dental laboratory prescription (work authorization) and a diagnostic cast with the design of the RPD outlined on it with a number 2 pencil for fabrication of the RPD framework. This cast is now considered the "master cast."

THE WORK AUTHORIZATION (Fig. 6-12)

Almost all dentists delegate many of the various technical phases of RPD service to a commercial dental laboratory, especially fabrication of the RPD framework. The dental laboratory technician must be given specific directions for the laboratory procedures to be performed. The written instructions and diagrams constitute the work authorization (dental laboratory prescription). This is usually augmented with study casts and other materials that have been surveyed and prepared by the dentist. Sometimes it may be necessary to confer with the

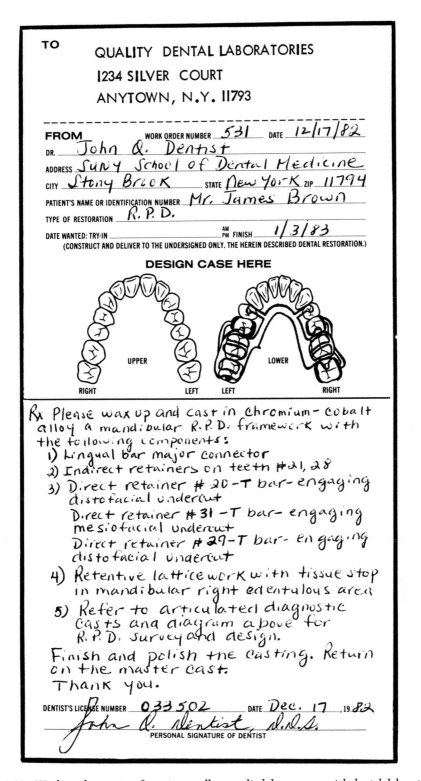

TO

QUALITY DENTAL LABORATORIES

1234 SILVER COURT

ANYTOWN, N.Y. 11793

FROM John Q. Dentist   WORK ORDER NUMBER 531   DATE 12/17/82

DR.

ADDRESS SUNY School of Dental Medicine

CITY Stony Brook   STATE New York   ZIP 11794

PATIENT'S NAME OR IDENTIFICATION NUMBER Mr. James Brown

TYPE OF RESTORATION R. P. D.

DATE WANTED: TRY-IN _____ AM PM FINISH 1/3/83

(CONSTRUCT AND DELIVER TO THE UNDERSIGNED ONLY. THE HEREIN DESCRIBED DENTAL RESTORATION.)

DESIGN CASE HERE

UPPER   LOWER

RIGHT   LEFT   LEFT   RIGHT

Rx Please wax up and cast in chromium-cobalt alloy a mandibular R.P.D. framework with the following components:

1) Lingual bar major connector
2) Indirect retainers on teeth #21, 28
3) Direct retainer # 20 - T bar- engaging distofacial undercut
   Direct retainer #31 - T bar- engaging mesiofacial undercut
   Direct retainer #29 - T bar- engaging distofacial undercut
4) Retentive latticework with tissue stop in mandibular right edentulous area
5) Refer to articulated diagnostic casts and diagram above for R.P.D. survey and design.

Finish and polish the casting. Return on the master cast.

Thank you.

DENTIST'S LICENSE NUMBER 033502   DATE Dec. 17, 1982

John Q. Dentist, D.D.S.

PERSONAL SIGNATURE OF DENTIST

Fig. 6-12. Work authorization form is usually supplied by commercial dental laboratory. However, forms designed by dentists are more likely to meet their needs. Original work authorization is sent to dental laboratory, and carbon copy should be retained by dentist. Above work authorization was used to provide RPD framework shown in Fig. 2-16.

dental laboratory technician over the telephone or in person about various technical aspects of the fabrication of the RPD.

Since the dentist is ultimately responsible for all phases of an RPD, it is incumbent upon him or her to rely upon only a highly competent dental laboratory technician and laboratory. A new dentist in town should learn from competent practitioners the names of the most reliable dental laboratories with which they are familiar. It would behoove the new dentist to evaluate these dental laboratories with a site visit and a discussion with the laboratory owner and dental technicians. The dentist should establish a rapport with the owner and the technicians and respect them as professionals. Mutual respect can be achieved when dentists send the laboratory neat and accurate records, impressions, casts, and detailed instructions.

The work authorization form may be supplemented by written instructions that apply to most cases sent to the laboratory unless otherwise noted. For example, the dentist might request no arbitrary palatal relief, return of all cases for remounting and selective grinding, or return of the prosthesis without trimming the borders. Such instructions can be made into a rubber stamp and printed on the work authorization form. Those instructions that do not apply to that procedure can be crossed off the form. Such information can be included on a form designed by the dentist.

TRIAL FITTING OF THE FRAMEWORK

Whether cast in dental gold alloy or the more popular chromium-cobalt alloys, all RPD frameworks can benefit from careful refinement of their fit. This is especially true of the chromium-cobalt alloys. Since the casting process is not exact, it cannot compensate for the 1.7% shrinkage of these alloys (Crosthwaite, 1979). Also, there are present on the surfaces of both master cast and the refractory cast (a duplicate of the relieved master cast) a multitude of microscopic pores that result in a myriad of microscopic nodules that cannot be completely removed during the metal finishing process. Since these pores are not present on the tooth surfaces, the positive casting nodules must be completely removed from the casting; if they are not, it is possible that the framework will not completely seat in its designed terminal position.

The casting (framework) may appear to, and obviously does, fit the master cast or else the dental laboratory would not have delivered it to the dentist. The apparent fit of the framework may be the result of the casting's having been forced into place on the surface of the master cast. The surface of the master cast should be very carefully scrutinized to locate these abraded areas. Very likely the areas of the casting corresponding to the abraded areas on the cast will have excessive tooth contact in the mouth, preventing the casting from seating completely on insertion.

To prevent the dental laboratory technician from damaging the master cast during laboratory fitting procedures for the framework, the technician can be directed to confine the fitting procedures to a "duplicate fitting" cast, which can be made very easily and conveniently when the refractory cast is being fabricated. This will protect the master cast from the mutilations so often inflicted upon it by many dental laboratories during the fitting procedures.

When the framework is delivered to the dentist, it should be very closely inspected to see that all design features, so scrupulously described in the dental laboratory prescription (work authorization), have actually been produced in the final RPD framework. Using a bright light and high magnification, the dentist should critically evaluate the fit of the casting on the master cast. Major connectors, rests, and clasp assemblies should fit the master cast accurately; otherwise they will not fit the mouth any more accurately. A decision to remake the casting, if it is necessary, should be made at this time.

If the casting appears to fit the master cast satisfactorily, it is ready for the next test. The tissue surface of the casting is examined for nodules and defects in the metal, using bright light and high magnification. These should be removed by the use of high-speed carbide burs or very hard abrasive points and wheels manufactured expressly for this purpose.

The framework is now ready to be inserted into the mouth for the refinement procedures. These procedures can be divided into two steps: (1) fitting of the framework to the abutment teeth and (2) adjustment of the framework to the opposing occlusion (Miller and Grasso, 1981).

Fitting of the framework to the abutment teeth

The casting is positioned over the abutment teeth and, by moderate finger pressure on the occlusal rests, an attempt is made to seat the framework into place. An accurately fitting casting should go into place without any difficulty. If more than a moderate amount of finger pressure is needed to seat the framework, or if it fails to seat fully, measures must be instituted to locate and remove the obstruction or obstructions. Pressure-indicating materials such as Jewelers' rouge in chloroform, Kerr's disclosing wax,* or Detex† aerosol spray are used to disclose the areas of impingement (Fig. 6-13). The disclosing wax or calcium carbonate powder in an aerosol spray is preferred, since either is cleaner and more convenient to use than rouge.

A thin layer of the wax is flowed over all areas of the framework that will contact the hard surfaces of the teeth. The framework is seated firmly into place. It is removed, and the wax is examined for shiny spots where the metal shows through it (Fig. 6-14). Shiny spots produced by guiding planes are disregarded, as are those near the height of contour that occur as the casting seats into place. Shiny spots on rests or other areas occlusal to the height of contour, which indicate that the casting is binding and being prevented from reaching its complete seating, must be relieved. These areas are relieved with abrasive points, and a fresh layer of disclosing wax is reapplied. These procedures are repeated until the casting is completely seated. This will be indicated by the smooth, grayish appearance of the framework showing through a thin layer of wax. To verify the fit in the mouth, the junction of metal and tooth surface should be dried with a gentle stream of air to remove bubbles of saliva that might obscure a discrepancy between tooth and metal. An explorer moved across the margin of the tooth and the metal should reveal a smooth junction with no intervening space. A well-fitting casting will also slide smoothly to place against the abutment teeth. When this state has been reached, the casting can safely be judged to be fitted properly.

---

*Kerr Manufacturing Co., a division of Sybron Corp., Romulus, Mich.

†AeroDent, New Orleans, La.

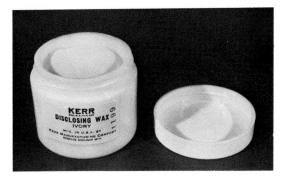

Fig. 6-13. One of the most efficient materials used to reveal areas of impingement on RPD framework is Kerr's disclosing wax. Disclosing wax is applied thinly and evenly to entire tissue side of framework with warm wax spatula.

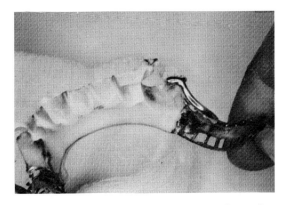

Fig. 6-14. Disclosing wax is used to reveal interference to seating on lingual plate area of mandibular left first premolar in this RPD framework. Contact of guiding plane under distal rest of first premolar should be disregarded, since this is designed contact area.

If these refitting procedures do not successfully remove the obstruction to the final seating of the casting, it unfortunately must be remade. This may occur when the casting extends into an undesirable undercut on a tooth.

Adjustment of the framework to the opposing occlusion

When the framework has been fitted and is completely seated in the mouth, it should then be fitted against the opposing occlusion. In most unilateral and bilateral distal-extension RPDs the remaining dentition has been previously adjusted into the retruded contact posi-

TABLE 6-1

Common problems associated with trial fitting of the removable partial denture

Problem	Possible cause	Solution
RPD framework cannot be fully seated (terminal position)	Inaccurate impression or master cast	Remake the impression or master cast
	Inadequate or faulty RPD survey and design analysis, such as components extended into inadequately blocked (relieved) areas	Resurvey and redesign
	Faulty dental laboratory procedures, such as survey, block-out, duplication, casting, or finishing techniques	Inspect and remake if necessary
	Poorly finished and polished RPD framework, such as nodules on casting in tooth contact or warpage of framework	Relieve, refinish, and repolish
	Excessive clasp retention	Identify and adjust retention of direct retainers
	Careless handling of master cast or framework, causing distortion	Adjust or remake if necessary
	Movement or changes of dentition during interval between impressioning and trial fitting of RPD framework, such as tooth migration, supereruption, or calculus deposition	Localize cause; stabilize, adjust, or remake the RPD framework
RPD framework can be seated (terminal position) but does not have adequate retention	Faulty survey and design analysis	Resurvey, remake, and redesign
	Inadequate mouth preparations	Diagnose and redo mouth preparations
	Inadequate number of abutments	Resurvey and redesign
	Inaccurate impression or master cast; that is distortion of impression or master cast in retentive areas	Redo impression
	Direct retainer (clasp) bent during finishing and polishing	Identify and adjust retention of clasp
RPD framework causes occlusal interferences and inhibits intercuspation	Inadequate mouth preparation	Adjust and correct mouth preparation and redo impression
	Inadequately contoured rests of RPD framework	Recontour rests on RPD framework
	Interference with other RPD components, such as minor connectors or latticework	Adjust interferences and refinish
Wedging effect exists in tooth-bounded edentulous space (felt on weaker abutment)	Guiding plane or inner surface of clasp body located in undesirable undercut	Identify and relieve area
Overretention exists (RPD snaps on and off teeth with a click)	Clasp engages too much of retentive undercut	Polish inside surface of clasp with rubber polishing point or wheel (procedure of choice)
		Shorten end of direct retainer slightly
		Adjust clasp with clasp-bending plier

tion or centric relation occlusion. The mandible should be gently guided to the retruded contact position, and the dentist should visually observe the relationship of the opposing teeth to the RPD framework in this contact position. This occlusal relationship must be identical after the occlusal adjustment of the framework is finished. In other words, the framework must not increase the vertical dimension of occlusion, unless it is specifically intended to do so in an oral rehabilitative program designed to restore a lost occlusal vertical dimension.

The equilibration procedures are designed to eliminate interferences of the framework to a stable occlusal position both in centric and eccentric positions. Adjustments can be made on the metal, on the natural teeth opposing it, or on both. Articulating paper and occlusal indicator wax can be used to reveal the areas of interference. Although the carbon of the articulating paper may not readily transfer to the highly polished metal surfaces of the framework, warming the paper gently over the flame of an alcohol torch will facilitate this marking.

If opposing RPDs are being made, one framework is adjusted by the dentist at a time. Then both frameworks are checked together intraorally. This occlusal equilibration should produce an occlusal relationship that permits the remaining teeth of both the mandible and maxilla to intercuspate harmoniously and simultaneously in the retruded contact position and in all functional movements and that ensures that no part of either framework interferes with normal closure or with any eccentric movement within the patient's functional range (Miller and Grasso, 1981).

When these trial fitting procedures of the framework are complete, all of the areas of metal that have been adjusted must be returned to their original polish and luster by the use of smooth white stones and rubber points impregnated with carborundum. The framework is now ready for the next step in the fabrication of the RPD.

DEVELOPMENT OF THE DENTURE BASE OF THE REMOVABLE PARTIAL DENTURE

If the RPD being fabricated includes only a tooth-borne denture base area, then the master cast secured by the impression technique previously described is a sufficient one on which

to complete the denture base of this type of RPD. Since the support for this denture is provided by the periodontal ligaments of the anterior and posterior abutments bounding the residual ridge, the base of this denture requires only a contact relationship with the residual ridge surface (Applegate, 1965). Therefore, the anatomic accuracy that can be attained by the use of an irreversible hydrocolloid technique as previously described is sufficient to produce a master cast for a tooth-borne RPD.

However, when the design of an RPD includes a unilateral or bilateral distal-extension denture base, a simple impression procedure, one that records only the anatomic form of the residual ridge, is not sufficient to produce the type of RPD service that can preserve all of the remaining oral tissues (tooth, bone, and mucosa) in health (Beresin and Schiesser, 1978; Holmes, 1965). To achieve this often elusive goal requires that the dentist understand both the problems presented by the dual nature of the supporting structures of the partially edentulous ridge and the chronic degenerative processes of residual ridge reduction (Atwood, 1971; Carlsson and associates, 1965; Tallgren, 1972).

Concepts and rationale

The ultimate supporting medium of the RPD is bone (DeVan, 1956). The intermediary attachment medium between the abutment tooth and the alveolar bone is the periodontal ligament; between the denture base and the residual ridge it is the alveolar mucosa or mucoperiosteum. There is an obvious resiliency differential between these attachment media, with the periodontal ligament being essentially nonresilient and the alveolar mucosa exhibiting varying degrees of resiliency (McLean, 1936). As reported by Steiger and Boitel (1959), the resiliency of the tissue-fitting surface of the denture base ranges from 0.4 to 2.0 mm, compared with the resiliency of 0.1 mm for healthy periodontal tissue (see Figs. 1-5 and 6-15). Tissue resiliency is therefore four to twenty times the axial displaceability of the abutment tooth (Steiger and Boitel, 1959). The problem of achieving successful function of an RPD then becomes one of equilibrating this resiliency differential between the relatively nonresilient periodontal ligament of the abutment tooth and

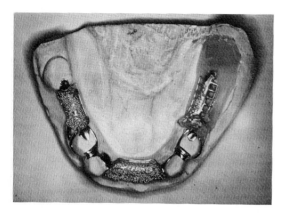

Fig. 6-15. There are differences in displaceability of periodontal ligament versus mucoperiosteum covering residual ridge. Note wax shim on the residual ridge (see also Fig. 1-5).

the more resilient mucosa covering the residual ridge in such a way that, in function, the RPD will generate and dissipate forces equitably between these two media. If this effort is successful and all other factors remain equal, the goal of the RPD service, namely, the preservation of tooth, alveolar bone, and residual ridge, will be enhanced.

If tooth and bone are to be preserved, the dentist must consider not only the equitable distribution of forces to the periodontal ligament and the mucosa but also, and perhaps more important, the direction that these forces take as they impact on these tissues.

The periodontal ligament and the mucoperiosteum are essentially oral connective tissue membranes, and they manifest a greater resistance to axial or vertical loads than to transverse or horizontal loads (DeVan, 1956). Synge's research, using the periodontal membrane of lambs and young calves, revealed a differential of 17.5 to 1 in favor of axial loading. (Gabel, 1934). The results of Synge's experiments led DeVan to conclude, "if we would avoid unduly displacing an oral connective tissue membrane, it would be wise to plan the tooth factors in such a way as to direct the force essentially axial to the natural tooth and essentially perpendicular to the ridge" (DeVan, 1956). This requires that, in effect, the RPD remain stable throughout all functional movements of the mandible, the only positional change permitted is an essentially vertical one.

A stable RPD is one that is able to maintain

its positional relation to supporting bone when functional forces are applied to it (DeVan, 1952a). This obviously is a theorectical ideal. In practical terms, it is a task of monumental proportion, and it is hardly possible to harness all the forces that can be generated on an RPD and its abutments and resolve them into forces that are directed solely axially to the abutments and perpendicularly to the residual ridge. However, that theoretical ideal should be pursued if the goals of RPD service are to be attained.

In considering RPD stability, the denture base, even though properly designed and fabricated, cannot by itself ensure functional stability unless it is complemented by the design of the metal framework and the occlusal scheme of the prosthesis. The framework design should feature rigid major connectors with multiple supporting areas for stress distribution and lateral force attenuation (Steffel, 1951), and the occlusal contacting surfaces should resolve transbolus forces of mastication essentially vertically to the residual ridge and axially to the abutment teeth (Moore, 1962). Only when all three factors—framework, occlusion, and denture base—work in concert, each fulfilling its responsibility to the utmost, can effective RPD stability be developed.

With this in mind, the denture base of the distal-extension RPD should be considered an entity in itself. It should be able to sustain itself by itself, its retention and stability being assured with minimum imposition on the framework. In this regard, principles that apply to impression making for complete dentures must be considered for the distal-extension RPD base (Leupold and Kratochvil, 1965).

There have been many techniques and materials related to impressions for complete dentures that have found their way into the dental literature and clinical practice through the years (Collett, 1965; Starcke, 1975). A general classification can divide these techniques into two categories: tissue placement with pressure techniques, which essentially cause tissue displacement, and nonpressure, or "mucostatic," techniques (Bohannan 1954, Collett 1965). To evaluate the effectiveness of each as it relates to the denture base of the distal-extension RPD requires a review of some basic biologic and physical concepts.

Biologic and physical concepts of impression making

Although the concepts and rationale of the mucostatic school of impression making for complete dentures, espoused by Page, have largely been discredited (DeVan, 1952b), dentists are still indebted to Page and his associates for the explanation of the physical laws of hydrostatics as they pertain to the problem of the denture base (Bohannan, 1954). Essentially, the principles of mucostatics credit interfacial surface tension as being the only retentive means of importance for a denture base (Bohannan, 1954).

Retention, as defined by DeVan (1952b), is that state of a prosthesis wherein functional forces are unable to destroy the attachment existing between the denture and the mucoperiosteum. A stable denture is one that successfully resists the magnitude and direction of functional forces that tend to alter the positional relationship of the denture to its osseous support (DeVan, 1952b). A denture can therefore lose stability but still retain its relationship to the mucoperiosteum; hence, it is still retentive. The thicker the mucoperiosteum, the greater the chance for the loss of stability while retention is maintained. Forces parallel to the mean mucosal plane will always result in displacement of the alveolar mucosa even though the denture is still retentive (DeVan, 1952b). Hence, an RPD base, covering and supported only by a freely movable, resilient alveolar mucosa, can exhibit excellent retention, but it is liable to be very unstable when lateral forces are brought to bear on it. The mucostatic principle disregards completely the retention-enhancing potential of the peripheral seal and the harnessing effect of properly contoured polished surfaces against a functioning musculature (Bohannan, 1954).

Dentist are, however, indebted to Page and his associates for calling attention to the need for registering in an impression the soft tissues of the residual ridge and denture-bearing areas in an unstrained, rest position. Any other position, purposely or inadvertently induced, will compel the tissues, by rebounding, to try to regain their rest position, leading to possible denture base dislodgement and instability (Collett, 1965).

The physical forces affecting the retention of denture bases operate in the film of saliva between the prosthesis and the surrounding tissues. These are the molecular forces of cohesion, adhesion, surface tension, and salivary viscosity. Generally, these forces produce the greatest retentive factors on a denture base when the tissue surface of the base bears a most intimate contact relationship with the mucosal tissues. This produces a film of saliva of minimal thickness that, if the film viscosity is low, produces a retentive potential of the denture base that will successfully resist normal dislodging forces (Brill, 1967).

Brill also points out that there are physiologic forces that are equally as important in denture base retention as the physical forces. These are mainly neuromuscular and are exerted by the cheeks, lips, and tongue. Retention of the denture base is maintained by a constantly changing interplay between the physical and physiologic forces during speech, mastication, and deglutition (Brill, 1967).

Ever since Fish in 1931 and 1933 called attention to the need for fitting the "polished surfaces" of denture bases to the lips, cheeks, and tongue to increase the stability of dentures, much has appeared in the dental literature to support this approach (Brill, 1967; Fish, 1931, 1933; Moore, 1962; Starcke, 1975). The position taken by many (Brill and associates, 1965) is that the critical factor in denture base stability is not the anatomic foundation but rather the muscular function of the lips, cheeks, and tongue and that once residual ridge resorption begins, with a concomitant reduction in the retentive effect of the physical forces, patients acquire a greater ability to retain their dentures by means of the oral musculature (Brill, 1967).

Objectives of development of the distal-extension denture base

With these considerations in mind, three compelling objectives of the development of the distal-extension denture base to secure optimal retention and stability become apparent:

1. The impression procedure and material of choice should permit the reproduction in fingerprint detail of a healthy mucoperiosteum and residual ridge tissue at rest to secure optimal retention by the action of interfacial surface tension (physical forces)

on the distal-extension denture base through the medium of saliva (Brill, 1967).

2. The denture base should be extended to but not encroach on functional muscle attachments, permitting greater distribution of masticatory stresses and a greater area for the development of interfacial surface tension and leading to the production of a peripheral seal (Bohannan, 1954; Kaires, 1956b).

3. The denture base's polished surface contours should be further adapted to the surrounding musculature of the oral cavity to secure active and passive muscular fixation of the denture base, since muscle activity may transcend in importance all other factors responsible for RPD retention (Brill and associates, 1965; Fish, 1933).

Attaining the three objectives above will produce a denture base that will impose minimally on the RPD framework for retention and stability. In fact, such a denture base will enhance the stabilizing potential of the RPD framework. Very often a deficient RPD base, incapable of self-retention and stabilization, will require periodic adjustment of the loose retentive arms of the extracoronal direct retainers, to the detriment of the abutment teeth. On the other hand, distal-extension RPDs with well-developed denture bases will often be found, after years of service, with retainer arms no longer in contact with the abutment teeth, indicating that the denture base is no longer receiving direct retention from the clasping system of the framework, and yet there is no complaint from the patient as to a lack of stability or retention of the RPD (Benson and Spolsky, 1979). This attests to the ability of the denture base to sustain itself by itself, which is of obvious advantage to the abutment tooth. Minimal clasp retention means minimal lateral force potential to the abutment tooth and contributes to its preservation.

Altered cast procedure

The most convenient and effective manner in which to produce an RPD base with the characteristics just described is by the use of the altered (corrected) cast impression technique. A single impression procedure to make an

impression and a subsequent one-piece master cast will not fulfill the prescription for the development of such a denture base (Hindels, 1952; Leupold, 1966).

Essentially, the altered cast technique consists of:

1. Fashioning custom acrylic resin impression trays onto the retention latticework of the RPD framework
2. Developing the denture base impression on these trays
3. Removing the edentulous ridges from the master cast
4. Securing the framework with the developed bases to the master cast
5. Pouring the new impression with dental stone to form a new master cast (altered, or corrected, cast) (Holmes, 1970).

In distal-extension RPDs where the denture bases are relatively small and the residual ridges well formed, or in cases of a unilateral distal extension (Kennedy Class II), complete denture base development may not be required. In these patients, the presence of an adequate number of abutment teeth, permitting relatively large, rigid major connectors and the development of positive cross-arch stabilization by the framework, may permit the omission of the third objective of base development, namely, adaptation of the polished surfaces of the denture base to the functioning oral musculature. A border-molding technique, which ensures positive tissue contact of the residual ridge and the development of borders that will secure a tight peripheral seal, may be all that is necessary to produce a retentive, stable denture base to complement the amply supported framework.

The procedures to produce these denture bases lends themselves very conveniently to the use of modeling compound and free-flowing impression materials such as metal oxide pastes or the elastomeric impression materials.

PROCEDURES FOR BORDER MOLDING THE DENTURE BASE. The following paragraphs present, in step-by step fashion, the procedures used in border molding the denture base.

After the fit of the framework has been refined intraorally, the borders of the residual ridges are outlined in pencil on the master cast.

A small segment of baseplate wax is warmed

over a bunsen burner and adapted to the pencilled outline. The wax will act as a shim, or spacer, between the residual ridge and custom tray.

The retention latticework of the RPD framework is warmed over a flame, and the framework is seated back onto the master cast. The baseplate wax that flowed over the latticework is removed. It should be freed sufficiently in one or two areas so that the autopolymerizing acrylic resin tray material that will be adapted to it will be positively secured (Fig. 6-16).

A separating medium, such as Coe-Sep* is applied to the land areas of the edentulous portions of the master cast. The separating medium should be allowed to dry sufficiently before proceding to the next step.

Autopolymerizing acrylic resin tray material is mixed as directed by the manufacturer. It is adapted to the edentulous areas of the master cast, ensuring positive locking to the framework and complete coverage of the baseplate wax shim.

When the acrylic resin tray material has fully polymerized, the entire assembly is placed in a container of slurry water sufficiently warm to soften the baseplate wax shim material. The framework, with its firmly attached acrylic resin custom trays, is carefully removed from the master cast.

Before the wax shim, which usually adheres to the acrylic resin, is removed, the excess tray material is reduced to the borders of the shim by use of acrylic resin trimming burs mounted on a low-speed handpiece.

The casting is reseated back onto the master cast after the wax shim has been completely removed to ensure that the acrylic resin custom trays meet the specifications of the pencilled outline (Fig. 6-17).

The framework, with attached acrylic resin impression trays, is seated in the mouth. The functioning border tissues bounding the edentulous areas of the mouth are manipulated by the dentist to determine how much the borders of the acrylic resin tray must be reduced to permit these tissues to move without impingement from the tray borders. Usually 2 mm or more should be removed to permit free move-

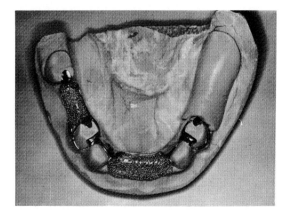

Fig. 6-16. Framework of this unilateral distal-extension RPD has been applied to wax shim over residual ridge of master cast. Portion of latticework of framework has been cleared of wax to permit firm union between autopolymerizing acrylic resin tray and framework.

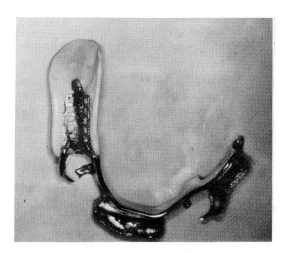

Fig. 6-17. Tissue-fitting surface of custom impression tray.

ment of these tissues and to provide adequate clearance for frena and muscle attachments. When the acrylic resin trays are properly contoured, the mandibular trays should cover the retromolar pads, extend onto the buccal shelf, and have their lingual borders placed between the resting and active phases of the lingual vestibular areas, as described by Smutko (1979). The maxillary trays should have a form resembling a custom tray ready to be border molded for a complete denture.

---

*Coe Laboratories, Inc., Chicago, Ill.

The custom acrylic resin trays are now ready for border molding. Low-fusing modeling compound, tempered in a heat-controlled water bath, is placed on the trimmed borders of the acrylic resin trays and, section by section, molded by the physiologic action of the tongue, cheeks, and lips. Through a combination of sucking and swallowing movements performed by the patient and finger manipulation performed by the dentist, denture borders are created around which resilient, movable tissue can function without discomfort to the patient or dislodgement of the denture base. Care must be exercised to ensure that the dentist's fingers stabilize the framework on the abutment teeth as the patient performs these functional movements. Digital pressure on the trays could unseat the framework anteriorly and should therefore be avoided.

When the border molding is complete, the framework is removed from the mouth and inspected (Fig. 6-18). Any excess modeling compound that has flowed inside the tray is trimmed away with a sharp scalpel without reducing the length of the border (Fig. 6-19).

Since one of the objectives of the impression procedure is to secure an impression of the alveolar mucosa in an undistorted condition, vent holes may be drilled in the acrylic resin tray to permit escape of the impression material in making the corrected impression, minimizing any effects of a hydraulic system that would be set up between tray, impression material, and resilient alveolar mucosa, which would tend to displace the resilient mucoperiosteum.

To secure the corrected impression, the impression material (either a metallic oxide paste or mercaptan rubber base) is prepared as directed by the manufacturer. The choice of impression material for this procedure is based in part on the displaceability of the mucoperiosteum and the severity of tissue undercuts (usually located in the retromylohyoid area). The internal portion of the tray is loaded with the impression material, but not overloaded. A thin layer of material is carried over the border-molded areas. When the impression material is ready to be placed in the mouth, the framework is seated onto its abutment teeth and digital pressure is applied to the casting and the teeth only, to ensure their proper ap-

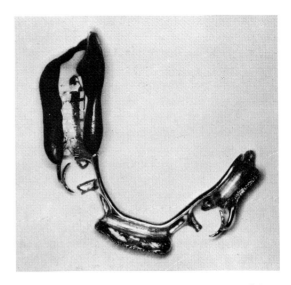

Fig. 6-18. Tissue-fitting surface of untrimmed border-molded custom impression tray.

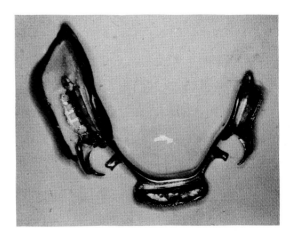

Fig. 6-19. Completed border-molded and trimmed impression tray. Modeling compound that has been laminated inside impression tray has been trimmed away. Note that border length and width have not been reduced. Impression tray is now ready to receive final impression material.

position. Under no circumstances should finger pressure be placed on the acrylic resin trays. This might cause not only an unseating of the framework anteriorly but also an undesirable displacement of the underlying alveolar mucosa. When the impression material reaches its initial set, the border tissues are activated, the

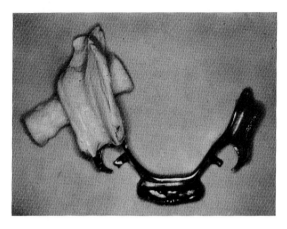

Fig. 6-20. Final impression made in metallic oxide paste.

mandible is closed just short of occlusal contact, and the impression material is permitted to set against the tissues that are now in their normal unstretched position. Positive finger pressure on the RPD framework is maintained throughout the entire setting of the material.

The framework, with the impression, is now removed from the mouth. All excess impression material is trimmed to expose the finishing lines of the framework. The framework should be carefully inspected to see that none of the impression material has penetrated under the occlusal rests. If this has occurred, an improper relationship has been recorded between the residual ridge and the framework, necessitating the remaking of the corrected impression. Ideally, the impression should be free of air bubbles and pressure spots from the tray, compound, or framework (with the exception of the tissue stop of the framework) and should exhibit an accurate, minutely detailed negative of the tissues of the residual ridge and denture-bearing areas and the mucobuccal reflection (Fig. 6-20). An impression with these favorable characteristics can be expected to produce an RPD base whose retention is assured by interfacial surface tension created by a close adaptation of the denture base to the tissues of the residual ridge and denture-bearing areas and a tight peripheral adapation that maintains the border seal throughout normal function. If the impression is defective in regard to any of these criteria, it should be rejected and remade. If, however, the impression is deemed

acceptable, the next step is to alter the master cast to receive the corrected impression.

The edentulous portions of the master cast are cut away with a jeweler's saw. A series of bur cuts to create mechanical locks is then introduced into the cut portions of the remaining master cast to effect a stronger union between the old and new master cast. A separating medium such as Coe-Sep is applied to the remaining dental areas of the master cast and allowed to dry. This will permit the removal of any new dental stone material that may seep out from under the boxed and rimmed impression during the pouring of the new master cast.

The framework with the corrected impression is seated on the abutment teeth. The framework is secured to the cast with sticky wax, all surfaces being sealed carefully.

Rimming wax is sealed to the borders of the impression, and then the entire assembly is boxed.

The assembly is placed in slurry water, and the master cast is soaked thoroughly.

A uniform mix of Class I dental stone (Phillips, 1973) is prepared as directed by the manufacturer. Dental stone material is poured into the boxed and rimmed impression, and the impression is placed aside to set. A Class I dental stone rather than a Class II dental stone is desired in order to facilitate recovery of the completed RPD base after the RPD is processed in heat-cured acrylic resin.

After the new dental stone cast has set, the rimming and boxing wax is removed. The new master cast is placed in warm slurry water to soften the modeling compound. When the compound has softened sufficiently, the framework is carefully removed from the new master cast. The master cast is set aside. (These steps are illustrated in Figs. 6-49 to 6-55 for a maxillary RPD).

The impression material and custom acrylic resin trays are removed from the retention latticework of the framework by heating the acrylic resin carefully with an alcohol torch. The acrylic resin is gently heated to soften it until it can be detached from the framework. The framework is then carefully inspected. All residual material—baseplate wax, acrylic resin, and impression material—must be removed from the framework. Any scratches produced on the framework during the technique must

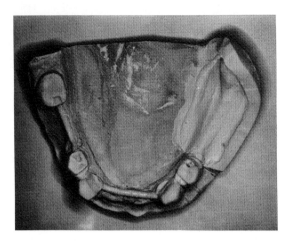

Fig. 6-21. Altered cast ready for mounting procedures.

be repolished. After the altered cast has been trimmed on a model trimmer, the framework is placed on the new master cast to ensure that the casting now fits as precisely as it did before the cast-altering procedures.

All remaining wax and residual impression material is removed from the new altered cast. Any new dental stone that may have inadvertently seeped into the original master cast may be removed easily at this time. The separating medium applied to this area before pouring the new master cast makes this possible. The master cast (altered cast) is trimmed neatly on a model trimmer. It is now ready for the mounting procedures necessary for the final phase of the fabrication of the RPD (Fig. 6-21).

Denture base development for removable partial dentures with extensive edentulous areas

The border-molding technique just described is not considered sufficiently effective in producing a retentive and stable denture base for an extensive RPD in a patient with only six or fewer anterior teeth remaining or for a bilateral distal-extension RPD in a patient with excessively resorbed residual ridges (Beresin and Schiesser, 1978; Moore, 1962). The harnessing effect of muscular fixation acting on the polished surfaces in the denture base will provide the necessary denture base stability and retention to effectively reduce the load placed on the few remaining teeth for this func-

tion (Brill, 1967; Fish 1931). This should be expected to produce an RPD that can noticeably lengthen the life expectancy of the remaining teeth and, as a result of the inherently stable nature of such denture bases, contribute to the preservation of the remaining residual ridges (that is, not increase the rate of residual ridge reduction).

The technique used in these situations is essentially an altered cast technique, as previously described, but it is characterized by an intermediate step designed to secure active and passive muscular fixation of the denture base by using the musculature of the oral cavity to ensure and increase the retentive potential of the denture base.

The most important muscles in this regard are the buccinator, the orbicularis oris muscles, and the intrinsic and extrinsic muscles of the tongue. By capturing the action of these structures on the polished surfaces of the denture base, both active and passive muscular fixation can be developed. Active fixation occurs when the tongue is pressed against the cheek and the buccinator is simultaneously pressed inward toward the oral cavity. This simultaneous pressure will stabilize a denture against its foundation. Passive muscular fixation can be developed to stabilize a mandibular denture base by using the mass and weight of the musculature acting on appropriately developed inclines of the polished surfaces of the denture base. In essence the denture base is wedged down onto its foundation by the tongue and cheeks (Brill, 1967).

Several techniques have been reported to secure this type of base development both in complete and removable partial dentures (Beresin and Schiesser, 1978; Fish, 1933; Lott and Levin, 1966). The procedure described here uses a "mouth temperature" wax, Kerr's Iowa wax,* to develop as much of the polished surface of the denture base as is deemed necessary to impart the desired retentive characteristics (Henderson and Steffel, 1981). The wax is placed in a storage container, which is then placed in a heating bath to render the wax fluid. When fluid, the wax is applied with a sa-

---

*Kerr Manufacturing Co., a division of Sybron Corp., Romulus, Mich.

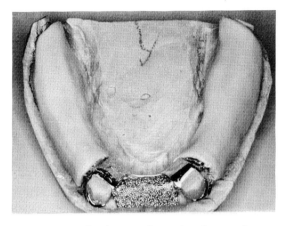

Fig. 6-22. Occlusal view of completed autopolymerizing acrylic resin impression tray for bilateral distal-extension base RPD before border reductions for wax base development.

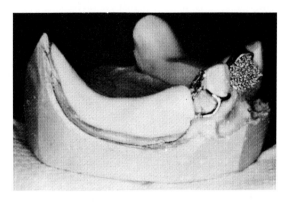

Fig. 6-23. Impression tray seated back on master cast after border reduction to prevent muscle impingement.

ble brush to appropriately fashioned impression trays that are secured to the RPD framework in the manner previously described for the border-molded technique. At mouth temperature, the wax has a consistency that lends itself most effectively to capturing the form of the functioning musculature as it relates to the border and sides of the custom acrylic resin impression trays.

Once the wax development is completed, a laboratory plaster cast is made in this impression; from this, another acrylic resin tray, again secured to the framework, is fashioned to make the final, or corrected, impression. This final impression is made not only of the residual ridge and peripheral seal area but also (and perhaps most important) of the functioning oral musculature as it is related to the so-called polished areas of the denture base.

PROCEDURES FOR DEVELOPING THE DENTURE BASE USING MOUTH TEMPERATURE WAX. The following paragraphs present, in step-by-step fashion, the procedures used for developing the denture base using mouth temperature wax.

Impression trays are fabricated on the RPD framework in essentially the same manner as that previously described for border-molding procedures (Fig. 6-22).

After the borders of the tray have been reduced to avoid muscle impingement (Fig. 6-23), the assembly is removed from the mouth and replaced on the master cast. Blocks of

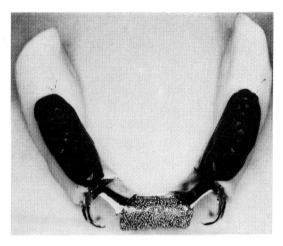

Fig. 6-24. Modeling compound occluding contact segments have been attached to occlusal surface of impression tray. Note shallow indentation in surface of compound segments of opposing occlusal surfaces. This will permit opposing cusp tips easy access into and out of fossae of contacting segments without torquing and dislodging impression tray while base development procedures are being performed by patient.

modeling compound or hard baseplate wax are made and attached to the occlusal surface of the acrylic resin custom trays to act as occluding contact segments for the opposing dentition (Fig. 6-24).

The occlusal contacting segments are warmed with an alcohol torch and tempered in

Fig. 6-25. Iowa wax is placed in small metal container that is placed in hot-water bath as illustrated. Hot-water bath softens wax and prepares it for use.

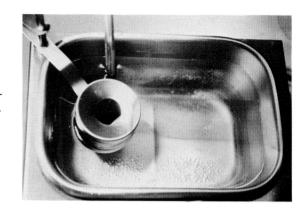

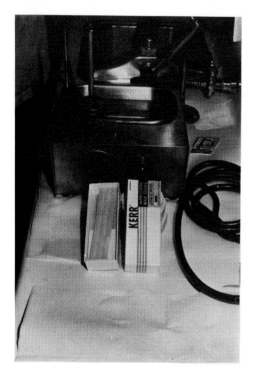

Fig. 6-26. Equipment and materials necessary to develop wax base are illustrated. They include thermostatically controlled hot-water bath, metal container holding impression wax material, thermometer, $1/4$-inch wide sable brush to apply softened wax, and wax (supplied in stick form).

warm water, and the framework is placed into the mouth. The patient is instructed to close the jaws in centric relation occlusion. The modeling compound is trimmed so that the occlusal surface presents a flat plane with only the tips of the opposing dentition making contact with the compound or wax.

The Iowa wax is prepared for use by being placed in a storage container (Fig. 6-25) that is suspended in a hot-water bath and heated until the wax becomes liquid. The wax should never be softened in a flame, because this will vaporize important constituents of the wax and alter its physical properties (Fig. 6-26).

A soft sable brush, approximately a quarter of an inch wide, is used to paint the fluid wax into the internal aspect of the acrylic resin trays. When sufficient wax has been brushed into the trays, the assembly is carried to the mouth and seated gently into place. The patient is requested to close the jaws to occlusal contact. The material is left in the mouth for 1 to 2 minutes.

The impression is removed from the mouth, and the surface of the wax that had been in contact with the residual ridge is examined. The objective at this time is to ensure even contact of the mouth temperature wax with the tissues covering the residual ridge. Firm contact of the wax with tissue will produce a glossy

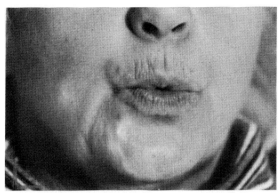

Fig. 6-27. Patient's masculature develops buccal flanges of wax impression by appropriate functional movements of tongue, lips, and cheeks. Marked protrusion is effected by patient's enunciating sound *proo,* as is illustrated here.

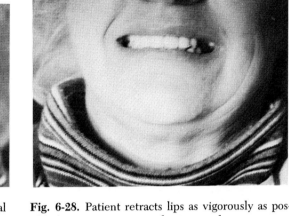

Fig. 6-28. Patient retracts lips as vigorously as possible by enunciating sound *wiss* or *whee.*

surface, indicating adequate condensation of the surface of the wax. Voids in the wax or lack of tissue contact will be evidenced by a dull surface appearance to the wax. Additional wax is brushed onto the dull areas, and the impression reseated into the mouth. Occlusal contact is again made. This procedure is repeated until firm contact is made between wax and tissue, as evidenced by the production of a shiny wax surface throughout the entire residual ridge and denture-bearing areas.

When complete tissue contact is made, wax can be applied to the peripheral areas, with the expectation that the new layer of wax will adapt itself to the functioning musculature and begin the development of this most important surface of the ultimate denture base.

The essential muscle action used to develop the buccal flanges are lip and cheek movements consisting of a marked protrusion and retrusion of the lips as in sounding *proo-wiss* (Figs. 6-27 and 6-28). The *wiss* movements should be made to retract the corners of the mouth as far as possible (Merkeley, 1959b). When a maxillary denture base is developed, the coronoid process of the mandible should be made to function against the wax on the disto-buccal border of the maxillary tray by the alternate movement of the mandible in a side-to-side and protrusive manner (Smutko, 1979) (Fig. 6-29).

The muscle activity necessary to produce properly developed lingual and retromylohyoid

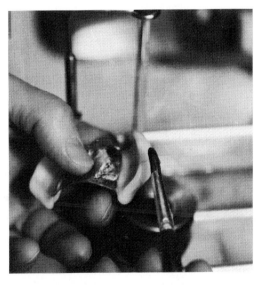

Fig. 6-29. Additional wax is brushed onto buccal surface of tray of this maxillary bilateral distal-extension RPD during base development. Good contact between wax and mucosa will result in well-condensed, shiny, and smooth wax surface. Irregular, dull wax surface is indicative of lack of good tissue contact.

denture flanges is accomplished by the patient's alternately placing the tongue into the right cheek and then into the left cheek, followed by a wiping the lips with the tongue. The patient should constantly be reminded to suck and swallow; these physiologic activities of the musculature, being normal, will help pro-

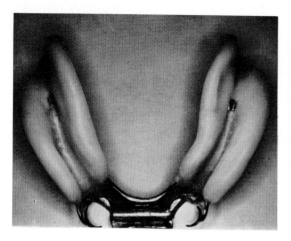

Fig. 6-30. Completed wax developed base illustrating amount of buccal and lingual development that can be attained.

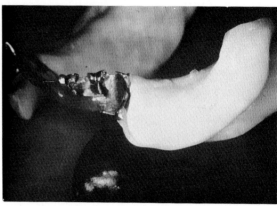

Fig. 6-31. In this developed base, occlusal contacting segments have been omitted, because ample number of stabilizing and retaining abutment teeth ensured positional relationship of impression tray while base-developing procedures were being performed.

duce denture base surfaces well disposed to retention and stability during function.

Additional mouth temperature wax is added incrementally to the buccal and lingual surfaces of the impression trays until all of the areas show well-condensed wax surfaces, indicating optimal contact of wax surfaces to the functioning musculature.

Once this state of denture base development has occurred, the entire assembly is replaced in the mouth and allowed to remain for 8 to 12 minutes to permit as close an adaptation of the wax to all areas as possible. Periodically during this final insertion the prescribed muscular movements are performed to continue the adaptation of the wax to the functioning musculature (Fig. 6-30).

When this phase is completed, ice-cold water is poured into the mouth to chill the wax thoroughly. An aspirator is used to suction off the water. When thoroughly chilled, the wax impression may be removed, with care being exercised so that the wax is not distorted during removal of the framework (Figs. 6-31 and 6-32).

A sharp line is scribed on the buccal and lingual aspects of the wax development to indicate the extent of the muscle-adapted area of the base to be recorded in the final impression.

At this time, the wax impression can be rimmed and boxed, and a model plaster cast can be poured into this impression. This is rather difficult to perform without distorting the carefully created flanges. A more convenient procedure is to make a cast in the manner described in the next paragraph.

A piece of carding wax is placed over the inner surfaces of all of the retentive clasp arms of the framework. A uniform mix of laboratory plaster is made. The tissue surface of the wax trays is filled with the laboratory plaster. The remainder of the laboratory plaster mix is placed on a glass slab. From this, a patty approximately 4 inches square and 1 inch thick is made. After the tissue surface of the tray is filled with laboratory plaster, the impression is inverted onto the patty, forcing the impression into the surface of the laboratory plaster up to the scribed line on the side of the wax impression until the scribed line is visible in its entirety. All areas of the framework are freed of excess laboratory plaster except the occlusal rest areas and the inferior border of the lingual bar.

When the laboratory plaster is set, the cast is trimmed on the model trimmer to produce a land area of approximately one-quarter inch around the entire assembly (Fig. 6-33). The cast is then submerged in hot water to soften the wax for removal of the impression tray and the recovery of the plaster cast (Figs. 6-34 and 6-35).

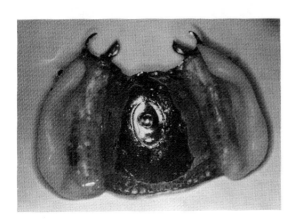

Fig. 6-32. Base of maxillary bilateral distal-extension RPD. Note very thick lamination of wax that has extruded onto palatal aspects of major connector. This is unavoidable and clinically insignificant. Lamination should be removed before laboratory plaster cast is made.

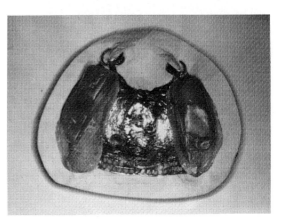

Fig. 6-33. Maxillary wax base in its laboratory plaster cast before recovery of the cast. Note that in this instance, hard, pink baseplate wax serves as occluding contact segments instead of modeling compound.

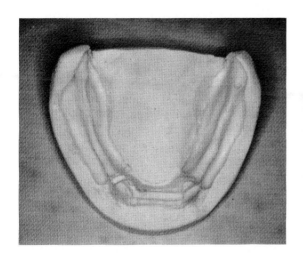

Fig. 6-34. Finished mandibular laboratory plaster cast after recovery from wax impression. Note how tissue bar between abutments, canine cingulum rests, and inferior surface of major connector act as positive seats for RPD framework.

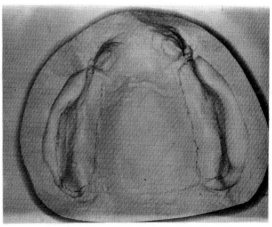

Fig. 6-35. Finished maxillary laboratory plaster cast. Note positive seating for framework on cingulum rests and palatal major connector.

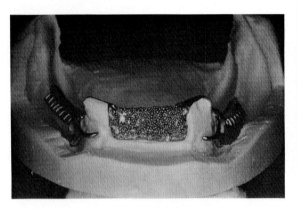

Fig. 6-36. Mandibular RPD framework seated on laboratory plaster cast after removal of impression trays from framework. Note that retentive arms of framework do not engage laboratory plaster cast. This was facilitated by addition of carding wax to clasp arms before impression was poured.

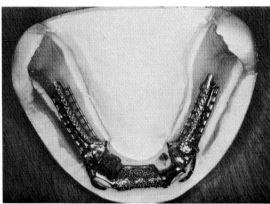

Fig. 6-37. Wax shim has been placed over residual ridge, framework has been adapted to shim, and soft acrylic resin liner has been applied to concave buccal areas of laboratory plaster cast.

Once the impression tray is removed from the cast, the acrylic resin custom tray is carefully heated and removed from the framework, as described previously.

The framework is now replaced onto the laboratory plaster cast. If the procedure has been performed correctly, the framework should have a very positive seat on the cast (Fig. 6-36). The occlusal rest areas and the inferior border of the lingual bar of the mandibular framework and the palatal area of the maxillary framework will ensure this positive seat.

The next step is the fabrication of the acrylic resin trays for the final, or corrected, impression. A single thickness of baseplate wax is adapted to the crest of the residual ridge on the laboratory plaster cast. Coe-Sep separating medium is applied to all of the surfaces of the cast included in the developed areas.

The retention latticework of the framework is warmed over a flame and seated onto the plaster cast through the wax shim. The excess wax that has flowed over the latticework is removed, freeing the latticework sufficiently for adequate retention to the acrylic resin tray material that will be adapted to it.

The contacting musculature usually produces concave surfaces in the laboratory plaster cast, primarily on the buccal aspects. If hard-tray acrylic resin were placed in these cast convexi-

ties, the final impression would be very difficult to separate from the ultimate altered cast without destroying these muscle adapted surfaces. Hence, precautions must be taken to avoid this eventuality.

After the separating medium has dried, an autopolymerizing soft acrylic resin liner, such as Coe-Soft,* is mixed according to the manufacturer's directions and adapted to the convexities of the laboratory plaster cast produced by the functioning musculature at the borders of the tray. Care should be exercised that the soft liner is limited to the concave areas only. The soft liner should not extend to the wax shim or in any way contact the metal framework (Fig. 6-37).

Once the soft liner has fully polymerized, a portion of regular, hard, autopolymerizing acrylic resin tray material is mixed and adapted to the soft liner, the framework, and the remaining portions of the laboratory plaster cast of the edentulous areas (Fig. 6-38). This completes the fabrication of the tray for the final impression (Fig. 6-39).

When the acrylic resin has fully polymerized, the base side of the laboratory plaster cast is placed onto the model trimmer and reduced to just short of contact with the tray material.

---

*Coe Laboratories, Inc., Chicago, Ill.

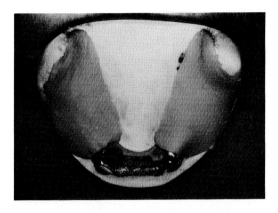

Fig. 6-38. Hard, autopolymerizing acrylic resin has been adapted to master cast to complete fabrication of final impression tray.

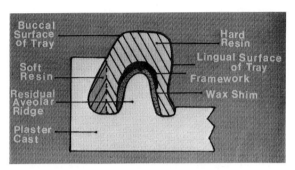

Fig. 6-39. Cross-sectional view through final impression tray, showing relationship between hard and soft acrylic resin materials of tray. Use of soft acrylic resin material in buccal concavities of laboratory plaster cast will facilitate removal of tray and recovery of final altered cast without damage to cast or framework.

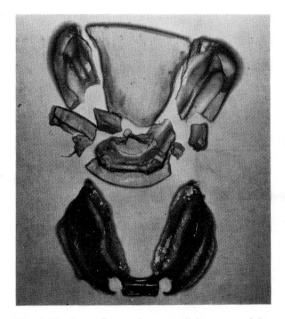

Fig. 6-40. Several taps from small hammer, delivered at base of plaster cast, have fractured cast into several pieces, permitting recovery of final impression tray. Use of laboratory plaster instead of dental stone simplifies fracturing of cast and recovery of final tray without damage to either tray or framework.

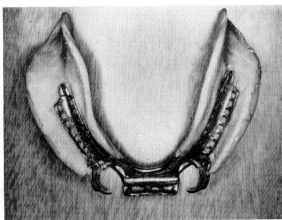

Fig. 6-41. Mandibular final impression tray. Note soft acrylic resin applied to buccal periphery of tray.

The cast with the assembled tray is placed in hot water for a few moments to soften the wax shim. Then, with several taps of a small hammer applied to the base of the plaster cast, the cast is fractured in several areas to permit recovery of the custom acrylic resin trays (with their developed areas) without injury to either the framework or the trays (Fig. 6-40).

The trays are trimmed of any excess acrylic resin, and the wax shim is removed. The impression tray is now ready for the final impression (Fig. 6-41). (See Figs. 6-42 through 6-48 for an alternate procedure for fabricating final impression trays for the maxillary arch.)

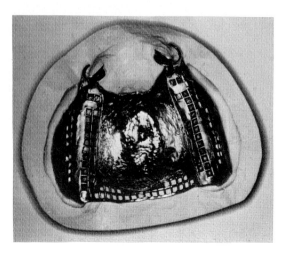

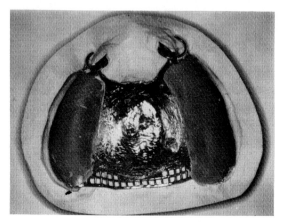

Fig. 6-42. Adaptation of maxillary RPD framework to wax shims.

Fig. 6-43. Adaptation of hard-tray acrylic resin to framework and shims before application of soft acrylic resin to buccal convexities.

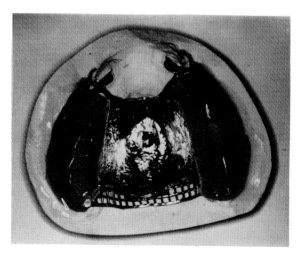

Fig. 6-44. Application of soft acrylic resin to buccal convexities and to previously polymerized hard acrylic resin tray material. Monomer and polymer of soft acrylic resin must be accurately proportioned to yield thick, fluid mixture that wll readily flow into buccal space between cast and hard acrylic resin.

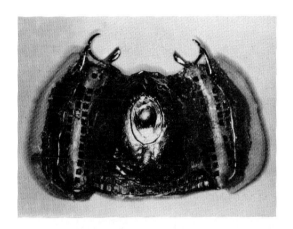

Fig. 6-45. Finished final maxillary impression tray. Note soft acrylic resin applied to buccal areas of impression tray. This alternate tray preparation technique will also produce a serviceable tray for final impression.

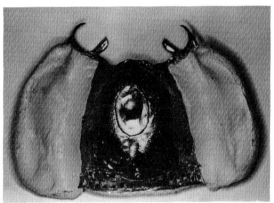

Fig. 6-46. Metallic oxide final maxillary impression.

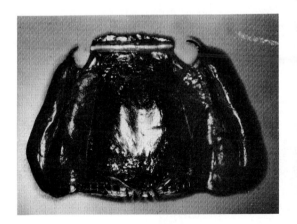

Fig. 6-47. Thiokol rubber base final maxillary impression.

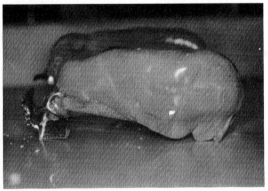

Fig. 6-48. Extent of impression of buccal musculature that was recorded in impression shown in Fig. 6-47.

A free-flowing metallic oxide paste or an elastomeric impression material is mixed according to the manufacturer's direction and loaded into the tray. Impression material is wiped along all flanges of the impression tray in contact with functioning musculature. The impression tray with the framework is introduced into the mouth and gently seated to place. Care must be exercised to assure that the framework is positioned accurately on its abutment teeth. No digital pressure is ever exerted on the trays over the edentulous areas. The patient is instructed to perform the previously described muscular movements while the impression material is setting. Just before it sets, the patient is advised to relax the musculature and bring the tongue up and out to the lower lip when the final mandibular impression is made.

When the impression material has set, the entire assembly is removed from the mouth and inspected for accuracy (Figs. 6-46 through 6-48). If found acceptable, the final altered cast is fashioned in the manner described for procedures for border-molding the denture base and illustrated in Figs. 6-49 through 6-55, with

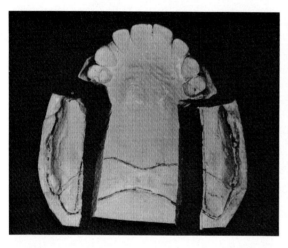

Fig. 6-49. Residual ridges of laboratory cast that is to be altered on this maxillary RPD have been sectioned and removed by use of thin, sharp saw such as jeweler's saw.

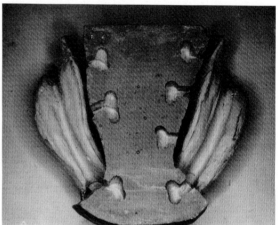

Fig. 6-50. Mandibular final impression has been secured with sticky wax to master cast after anatomic residual ridges have been removed by use of jeweler's saw. Note dovetails in base of laboratory cast to mechanically lock new additional dental stone.

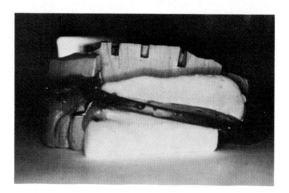

Fig. 6-51. Rimming wax has been applied to buccal surface of maxillary final impression, illustrating extent of this surface that will be incorporated into final denture base.

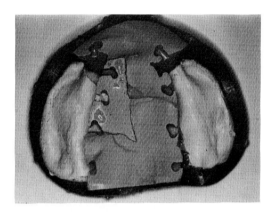

Fig. 6-52. Rimming wax is applied completely around final impression and master cast.

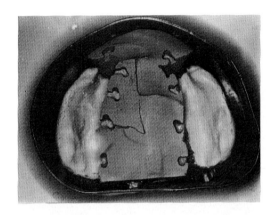

Fig. 6-53. Maxillary final impression is boxed in preparation for pouring it with dental stone.

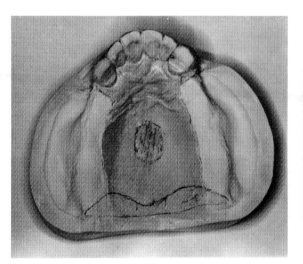

Fig. 6-54. Final maxillary altered master cast.

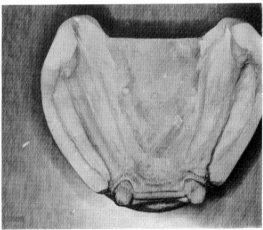

Fig. 6-55. Final mandibular altered master cast.

the exception that when the final impression is rimmed, the entire muscularly developed surface of the impression is preserved, not just the border area (Figs. 6-56 through 6-58). This will permit the harnessing and stabilizing effects of an active musculature to operate on the ultimate denture base, whether maxillary or mandibular, and impart to that denture base properties of retention and stability that will tend to provide the greatest longevity for the abutment teeth and residual ridges.

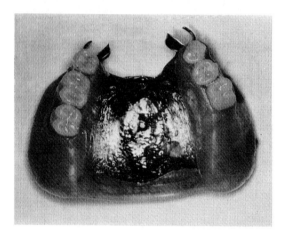

Fig. 6-56. Occlusal view of completed maxillary RPD.

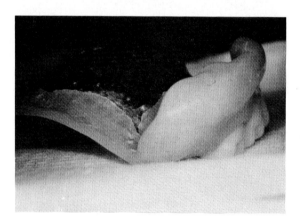

Fig. 6-57. Right posterior aspect of maxillary RPD showing buccal convexities developed by functioning musculature. Distobuccal area of denture base has been fashioned by action of coronoid process of mandible and buccinator muscle.

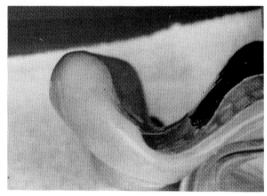

Fig. 6-58. Same features illustrated in Fig. 6-57 as they appear on left side of RPD.

7 Maxillomandibular relations

PURPOSE AND FUNCTION OF DENTITION

Teeth come together (occlude) primarily to tear and grind food in preparation for swallowing and digestion. Maximum chewing efficiency may be achieved when all natural teeth are present. But, as teeth are lost because of disease or trauma, masticatory efficiency decreases (Bates, 1975). Adaptation generally occurs, and few young people suffer, at least nutritionally, from the partially edentulous state. However, human beings age biologically and, as a rule, do not retain their youthful resiliency in late or even early middle age. Physiologic adaptation to the partially edentulous state that is satisfactory during an individual's early decades may not be adequate in later years. Some type of prosthesis, whether fixed or removable, is usually necessary to complement the function of the remaining natural teeth. The general pattern of tooth loss in humans proceeds in a predictable fashion: (1) loss of maxillary posterior teeth, (2) loss of remaining maxillary anterior teeth, (3) loss of mandibular posterior teeth, and finally (4) loss of mandibular anterior teeth, all with intervening prosthodontic replacements (Brewer and Morrow, 1980). Aiding digestion is not the only reason for the replacement of natural teeth. Maintenance of proper support for the orofacial musculature, esthetic appearance, proper speech production, prevention of tooth movement, maintenance of the morphologic face height, prevention of the temporomandibular joint (TMJ) dysfunction syndrome, and maintenance of the patient's psychologic well-being all depend, to some extent, on support from the natural teeth or a prosthesis.

SUCCESSFUL PROGNOSIS FOR A REMOVABLE PARTIAL DENTURE

Intelligent coordination of many biologic and technical factors by the dentist has much to do with the patient's successful use of a prosthesis. However, the patient's attitude and expectations of treatment are the other major component to success (Zarb and associates, 1978). For a removable partial denture (RPD) to function well, the framework design, the denture base contours, and the patient's care and use of the prosthesis must all be meticulously planned. Of equal importance to a long-term successful prognosis for an RPD is how the prosthetic teeth on the prosthesis function with the dentition in the opposing dental arch. The contact of opposing teeth in the dental arches is referred to as occlusion. The proper development of RPD occlusion depends on the meticulous completion of several procedures. When the dentist performs these procedures adequately, an RPD will aid in accomplishing a fundamental prosthodontic principle: to preserve what remains.

The adaptive capacity of an individual is greatest in the second and third decades, bearing in mind differences between biologic and chronologic age. Therefore, the patient's ability to adapt to a new occlusal environment in the fourth decade and beyond is more difficult. When developing an occlusal scheme on an RPD, the dentist must carefully create an occlusion that taxes the adaptive capacity of the patient to the least extent possible. To achieve this, the occlusion is developed with an effort to maintain the stomatognathic system as it presently exists rather than to restore total function or dramatically alter esthetics. Certain generally accepted prosthodontic procedures and practices can be used by the dentist to guide the development of an occlusion. The first of these procedures, diagnosis, catalogues the patient's present oral conditions. After this knowledge is established, a treatment plan can be formulated that will maintain a healthy occlusal system.

For the dentist, treating a patient with an

RPD can be likened to taking a trip. There is a starting point, the diagnosis; an itinerary, the treatment plan; a journey, the actual treatment; a destination, the completed treatment; and a return, recall and maintenance. When the dentist fails to complete any of the steps during the course of treatment, the result will be delay, frustration, and perhaps an inability to satisfactorily complete the journey.

DIAGNOSIS

A diagnosis made by the dentist is necessary to determine the basis for patient treatment. The length and destination of the trip will be unknown if the starting point is a mystery. Part of the diagnostic effort involves the gathering of data related to the patient's occlusion. Information about the patient's existing occlusal scheme can be derived from three sources: (1) a roentgenographic survey, (2) intraoral examination, and (3) evaluation of mounted diagnostic casts. The information obtained from these sources must be cross-correlated to arrive at a complete and accurate diagnosis. To make an accurate diagnosis, the dentist must first know what to look for from these three sources of information.

Roentgenographic survey

A radiograph is a two-dimensional representation of a three-dimensional object. Even a complete roentgenographic survey cannot be relied on exlusively to provide the dentist with all of the necessary diagnostic information. Yet, certain radiographic signs are suggestive of pathologic changes that may have been caused by the occlusion (Fig. 7-1). Radiographic signs of occlusal pathosis that the dentist must look for are: (1) widening of the periodontal ligament space, (2) angular bony defects, and (3) changes (either thickening or thinning) of the lamina dura. These radiographic signs should be correlated with clinical evidence found during the time of patient examination to determine any emerging pattern indicative of occlusal pathosis.

Intraoral examination

A "chairside" occlusal analysis during the patient's diagnostic visit should be structured to reveal signs and symptoms of occlusal pathosis. The structure of this clinical examination must

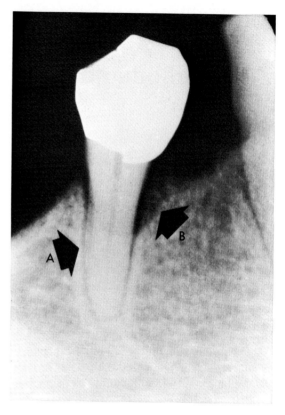

Fig. 7-1. Radiographic suggestion of trauma from occlusion. There appears to be widened lamina dura on distal side *(A)* and infra-bony defect on mesial side *(B)*. Balancing protrusive and lateral contacts were apparent clinically.

also permit the determination of normal physiologic occlusion.

If occlusal pathosis is present, its signs are likely to be found during: (1) testing of the teeth for the presence or absence of mobility patterns, (2) charting of periodontal pockets, (3) examination for severe dental attrition, and (4) determination of deflective occlusal contacts from centric relation to centric occlusion. Normal physiologic occlusal contacts in centric occlusion and eccentric positions are also found and may include:

1. *Canine guidance,* in which the only natural teeth that contact in lateral eccentric movements are the canines (Fig. 7-2)
2. *Posterior group function,* in which two or more posterior teeth in each dental arch contact in a working-side lateral eccentric movement; the canines may or may not be included in this movement (Fig. 7-3)

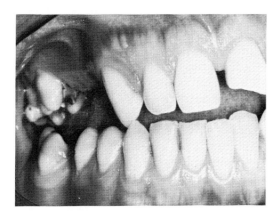

Fig. 7-2. Canine guidance. During right lateral eccentric movement canine tooth discludes posterior dentition.

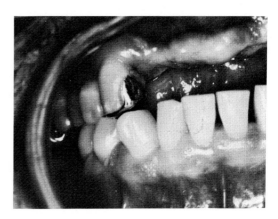

Fig. 7-3. Posterior group function. Maxillary right canine and premolar teeth are in group function contact with mandibular right canine and premolar teeth, with mandible in right lateral eccentric position.

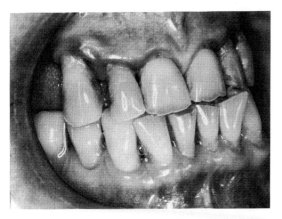

Fig. 7-4. Anterior group function. During right lateral eccentric movement maxillary central, lateral, and canine teeth are in group function contact with mandibular right central, lateral, canine, and first premolar teeth.

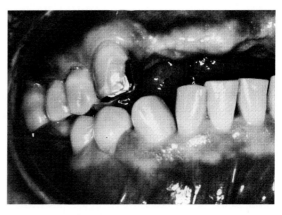

Fig. 7-5. Posterior cross arch balance. This is same patient as in Fig. 7-3, but with mandible in left lateral position. Maxillary right premolar teeth are in balancing contact with mandibular premolar teeth.

3. *Anterior group function,* in which two or more incisors in each dental arch contact in a working-side lateral eccentric movement; the canines may or may not be included in this movement (Fig. 7-4)
4. *Cross arch balance,* in which one or more teeth contact on the nonworking side during a lateral eccentric movement (Fig. 7-5)
5. *Incisal protrusive guidance,* in which the maxillary and mandibular anterior teeth disclude the posterior teeth in a straight protrusive movement (Fig. 7-6)

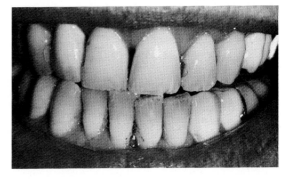

Fig. 7-6. Incisal protrusive guidance. During protrusive movement of mandible anterior teeth disclude posterior teeth.

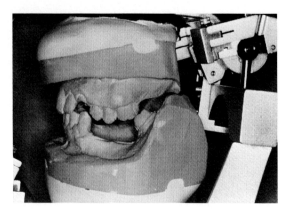

Fig. 7-7. Posterior protrusive guidance. During protrusive movement maxillary left first molar is in contact with mandibular left third molar.

6. *Posterior protrusive guidance,* in which any posterior teeth contact in a protrusive movement (Fig. 7-7).

Naturally, in the absence of signs and symptoms, any of these occlusal contacts may be functional and physiologic for any particular patient. However, any of these occlusal contacts may be pathologic when certain signs and symptoms are present. For instance, a retrusive contact from centric relation between the mesial incline of the distolingual cusp of a maxillary first molar and the distal incline of the distobuccal cusp of a mandibular first molar may cause an angular bony defect on either natural tooth, with furcation involvement, severe occlusal wear, or excessive tooth mobility. On the other hand, when this situation occurs, there may be no pathologic signs of occlusal trauma evident at all. Whether occlusal pathosis is manifest depends in part on both the intraoral environment and the patient's capacity to adjust to these occlusal contacts.

The first step in the diagnostic process is for the dentist to gather the evidence. The second step is to correlate this evidence and determine if the patient's existing occlusion is physiologic or contributing to pathosis.

Examination of the mounted diagnostic casts

As important as both the roentgenographic survey and intraoral examinations are, a thorough occlusal analysis can only be obtained after examination of the mounted diagnostic casts. It is imperative that all diagnostic casts

be mounted on a suitable dental articulator in the correct maxillomandibular relation to complete the diagnosis of the occlusion.

The relationships between the jaws and teeth that can be visualized from the mounted diagnostic casts must be identified before treatment planning can begin. This knowledge is necessary for three reasons:

1. The existing initial tooth contacts must be identified and analyzed for factors that may contribute to existing pathosis or act as potential causes of damage to a future planned occlusion.
2. The design of the occlusal scheme of the RPD must reflect decisions made about the occlusal plane and the type and distribution of occlusal contacts between the RPD and remaining natural dentition. The occlusal plane and occlusal contacts can best be visualized and identified when studied outside the mouth on mounted diagnostic casts.
3. The framework design and denture base extension may be influenced by the patient's existing occlusion and maxillomandibular relations.

Planning an occlusal scheme, whether for a balanced or nonbalanced occlusion, requires the dentist to decide whether changes must be made in one or more of five areas: (1) the character of the opposing dentition (whether it is a prosthetic or natural dentition), (2) the location and amount of the initial tooth contact, (3) the plane of occlusion, (4) the position in which the occlusion will be established (such as centric relation or centric occlusion), and (5) the type and number of lateral tooth contacts that occur during eccentric mandibular movements.

For the dentist to make these decisions rationally, diagnostic casts should be mounted on a dental articulator, using a face-bow transfer procedure and a centric relation record at an acceptable occlusal vertical dimension.

Hinge axis location and face-bow transfer procedure

When the mandible opens and closes, it moves in one of two basic ways. The first opening movement of the mandible from centric occlusion is rotation around an imaginary axis that passes approximately through the center of the mandibular condyle bilaterally (Fig. 7-8). The

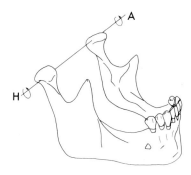

Fig. 7-8. Mandible rotates around line *HA* through condyles in simple hinge axis movement.

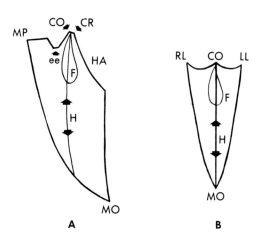

Fig. 7-10. Border movement of jaws. **A,** Envelope of mandibular movement as seen from side. *MP,* Maximal protrusive position of mandible; *ee,* edge-to-edge relationship of maxillary and mandibular anterior teeth; *CO,* centric occlusion; *CR,* centric relation; *HA,* hinge axis opening; *MO,* maximum opening; *H,* habitual closure; *F,* general area in which function occurs. **B,** Envelope of mandibular movement as seen from anterior view. *RL,* Right lateral position; *CO,* centric occlusion; *LL,* left lateral position; *MO,* maximum opening; *H,* habitual closure; *F,* general area in which function occurs. (Modified from Posselt, U.: Acta. Odontol. Scand. [Suppl.] **10**:3, 1952.)

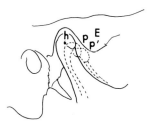

Fig. 7-9. Ginglymoarthrodial movement of jaw. Condyle may have pure rotatory movement around point *h* or may move anteriorly along articular eminence *(E)* to points *p* and *p'* for protrusive movement of jaw, or both movements may be combined.

mandible can rotate around this imaginary axis until its motion is limited by the maximum length of the masticatory muscles, ligaments, and fascia. This is known as a hinge axis movement or the posterior border movement of the mandible. The maximum opening of the mandible, as measured vertically between the anterior teeth, varies from 15 to 30 mm in the average adult. The second basic movement, called translation, is the forward and downward sliding of the mandibular condyles and articular disc along the anterior superior wall of the glenoid fossa (Fig. 7-9). A combination of these two movements can produce a very large mandibular opening. Humans do not usually open their mandible maximally, whether by a pure hinge axis movement alone or in combination with a translatory movement. Yawning might be considered a maximal opening movement. These maximal openings are referred to as border movements. The cyclical jaw movements of

mastication usually occur within these extreme border movements (Fig. 7-10). However, when a dental articulator is used to study the occlusion or to construct an RPD, locating and recording the hinge axis border movement of the mandible is necessary. A hinge axis recording (positional record) is necessary because the mandible will only open and close in this position when the mandibular condyles are in centric relation.

The maxillomandibular relation called centric relation is by definition the most posterior superior unstrained position of the mandibular condyles in the glenoid fossa from which eccentric movements can be made. This is an anatomic (bone-to-bone) position, in contrast to the neuromuscular (tooth-to-tooth) position, and can be repeated by the dentist to within very small tolerances. Since this anatomic position is free from the dictates of the teeth, periodontal ligament, and neuromuscular system

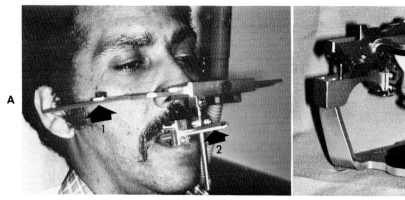
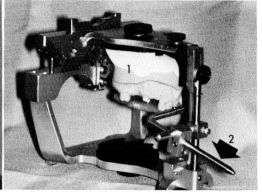

Fig. 7-11. A, Face-bow in place. *1,* Face-bow; *2,* face-bow fork. **B,** Cast mounted on artic- ulator. *1,* Face-bow fork in place; *2,* face-bow fork.

yet intimately related to occlusal function through the border movements of the mandi- ble, it is the ideal starting place from which to mount diagnostic casts to study the patient's occlusion. Mounting diagnostic casts on any dental articulator demands that their occlusal surfaces be related to the dental articulator in the same manner as they are to the patient's hinge axis.

Practically, the position of the maxilla is eas- iest to relate to the hinge axis of the mandible because it is fixed to the skull. The mandible, however, because of its muscular and soft tis- sue suspension beneath the skull, moves quite easily from side to side and up and down and makes the location of a hinge axis more diffi- cult. The occlusal surfaces of the maxillary teeth can be related to external facial land- marks over the location of the hinge axis quite easily. To record this positional relation, an in- strument known as a face-bow is commonly employed by the dentist (Fig. 7-11, *A*). It is called a bow because it has a bow shape. The imaginary line connecting the hinge axis points of the mandibular condyles is analogous to the bow string. To complete the analogy an arrow- shaped instrument called a face-bow fork is used to record the position of the maxillary teeth in relation to the hinge axis. The face- bow fork consists of a rod with U-shaped prongs on one end. Hard wax or stick com- pound is attached to the prongs, and a registra- tion of the cusp tips of the maxillary teeth is made. The face-bow fork is attached to the cen- ter of the face-bow, which has been positioned

over the hinge axis location by a lock nut or screw arrangement. Each type of face-bow has hinge axis location and mounting procedures that must be followed implicitly when the max- illary cast is mounted on the dental articulator (Fig. 7-11, *B*).

After the maxillary cast has been mounted on the dental articulator, the mandibular cast is mounted in centric relation to the maxilla by means of a centric relation record.

As previously noted, centric relation is an anatomic position (bone to bone), not a tooth- determined position (neuromuscular). When recording centric relation, the dentist must not allow the teeth to touch, because any tooth contact, however slight, might cause a reflex deflection of the mandible away from centric relation. The patient is guided along the hinge axis closure by the dentist until a position is reached that is just short of the first tooth con- tact. The centric relation record may be made by using any one of several recording materi- als, such as elastomeric impression materials (polyether or silicone), impression plaster, compound, or wax.

When this recording method is used, the di- agnostic casts mounted on the dental articula- tor must close through a distance that is the same as the thickness of the recording me- dium. It is apparent that the teeth and the di- agnostic casts must be on the same arc of clo- sure to permit the teeth to contact on the den- tal articulator as they do intraorally.

If the diagnostic casts are mounted arbitrar- ily on a dental articulator too far anteriorly

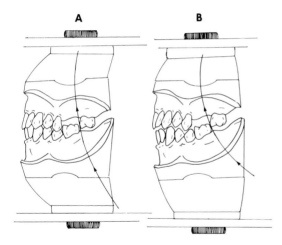

Fig. 7-12. Difference in arcs of closure with and without face-bow transfer. **A,** With face-bow transfer radius of arc of closure is same as hinge axis closure, so initial tooth contacts are same on articulator as in mouth. **B,** Without face-bow transfer arbitrary mounting of casts results in posterior closure to condyles. Radius of arc of closure is shorter than hinge axis radius. Smaller arc results in false "premature" centric relation contact.

without using a face-bow transfer procedure, the distance from the hinge axis to the teeth (the radius of the arc of closure) will be greater than that which exists in the patient. Thus, when the diagnostic casts are closed to first tooth contact, the anterior teeth will meet before the posterior teeth. Conversely, when the diagnostic casts are mounted too far posteriorly between the members of the dental articulator, the radius of the arc of closure will be shorter than in the patient and the posterior teeth will contact before the anterior teeth (Fig. 7-12).

With the diagnostic casts mounted too far anteriorly, an existing premature (deflective) tooth contact in centric relation between a maxillary mesial incline and a mandibular distal incline might not be apparent when the diagnostic casts are examined. The greater arc of closure would allow the casts to occlude in a more vertical manner, thus avoiding or diminishing the prematurity. Thus, a deflective tooth contact might not be found when one actually exists. In the second example, where the diagnostic casts are mounted too far posteriorly on the dental articulator, a premature contact could be thought to occur, because the shorter arc of closure might bring closely approximated

tooth inclined planes into premature contact, when none exists intraorally. In either case, the mountings would be an inaccurate representation of the actual clinical situation and would lead to an inappropriate diagnosis.

Factors to be studied on the mounted diagnostic casts

CENTRIC RELATION, CENTRIC OCCLUSION, AND INITIAL TOOTH CONTACTS. Centric relation is an anatomic position and, more specifically, a neuromuscular position. It is a position dictated by the muscles attached to the mandible and articular disc and ligaments and not dictated by tooth position. The established definition of centric relation, as defined in the *Glossary of Prosthodontic Terms* (1977), is given in terms of jaw movement, not tooth position. As defined, it is the most posterior position of the mandibular condyle in the glenoid fossa from which unstrained lateral movements can be made at a given vertical dimension. Centric relation is not a point position. Because it is a position controlled by the neuromuscular system, it can vary (but only slightly) from day to day and hour to hour (Shafagh and associates, 1975).

Centric occlusion, on the other hand, is a tooth position. This maxillomandibular relation is the position of the maxilla in relation to the mandible when the teeth are in maximal intercuspation. Centric occlusion can change through attrition, tooth migration, and tooth loss, but it will do so very slowly. Teeth can and do move with time, but over a short period of time, centric occlusion will change imperceptibly. Over a long period of time, the change can be considerable. A majority of adult patients demonstrate two separate maxillomandibular positions: a neuromuscular position, centric relation, and a tooth-contacting position, centric occlusion (Ramfjord and Ash, 1971).

One position is anatomic, and the other intercuspal, but both require a functional neuromuscular system to achieve their respective posture. The entire neuromuscular system constantly adapts to many stimuli. As a bolus of food is chewed, the muscles of mastication automatically regulate their contractive force on the basis of the consistency and size of the food bolus. The exact mediation of the automatic regulation is not precisely known. However, a neuromuscular reflex arc is involved that sends sensory afferent signals from the receptors found in the periodontal ligament, mucoperiosteum, and tongue and cheek to the central nervous system. These afferent signals are received and computed, and an efferent motor signal is sent to the muscles of mastication to regulate the speed and force of contraction. Given this reflex mechanism, if excessive pressure were placed on a tooth or several teeth, whole muscles or certain muscle bundles might contract prematurely to reposition the mandible when an afferent signal indicating an excessive or premature contact was delivered to the central nervous system. When initial tooth contact occurs on an inclined plane, the mandible cannot find a stable position. Therefore, the muscles of mastication will selectively contract to shift the mandible away from this unstable position until a positive occlusal and stable mandibular position is reached. This neuromuscular self-protective mechanism has its limitations, which vary with the individual. The amount of adaptation to deflective tooth contacts or to missing or malposed teeth that can occur for each individual without causing pathosis is of primary concern to the dentist.

Only when diagnostic casts are mounted in centric relation can the occlusal information of the patient, portrayed in three dimensions, be understood. This information demonstrates initial tooth contacts and subsequent tooth positions. It must then be correlated with that from the radiographic and intraoral examination so that the dentist can determine the individual's adaptive ability.

When the mounted diagnostic casts are examined in centric relation by the dentist, specific areas to be observed initially are: (1) interferences from centric relation to centric occlusion caused by deflective tooth contacts and (2) the magnitude and direction of the interferences from centric relation to centric occlusion. These are important considerations in planning the prosthesis. Knowing what differences exist between centric relation and centric occlusion position will permit future planning for any occlusal adjustments necessary to achieve harmonious and simultaneous contact during function.

PLANE OF OCCLUSION. The second factor to be studied on the mounted diagnostic casts is the plane of occlusion. The plane of occlusion of the natural dentition can be visualized as an imaginary curved plane that connects the incisal edges of the anterior teeth with the cusp tips of the posterior teeth. This anteroposteriorly and mediolaterally curved plane is important functionally, because it allows the mandibular teeth to be cradled within the confines of the maxillary dental arch. This effect aids both in protecting the soft tissues from injury and in stabilizing the mandible during final closure to centric occlusion. It neatly bisects the oral cavity into a superior, or maxillary, half and an inferior, or mandibular, half. Any dramatic changes in the symmetry of the occlusal plane from tooth loss or migration may cause a problem.

A disruption of this imaginary curved plane will occur when an unopposed maxillary or mandibular tooth continues to erupt passively into the opposing edentulous space. This extrusion would cause a corresponding indentation in the opposing occlusal plane. During a protrusive (translatory) movement of the mandible, this extruded tooth might contact the proximal surface of the tooth bounding the indentation. This action would deflect the mandible downward as it tried to continue on its anterior-inferior path (Fig. 7-13). This situation frequently causes considerable stress in the adaptive capacity of the teeth, bone, and musculature. When the patient's adaptive processes cannot contend with this increased stress, TMJ dysfunction, increased tooth mobility, changes in the lamina dura, and severe tooth wear can result.

Often it is not just a single tooth but a whole dental arch segment that extrudes and invades the opposite dental arch when there are no opposing teeth (Fig. 7-14). The plane of occlusion, in this instance, rather than being more or less gently curved becomes warped as one side (or a portion of one side) of the dental arch extrudes. Obviously, an occlusal scheme developed on a prosthesis constructed to replace these missing teeth must address itself to this skewed occlusal plane.

ANTERIOR AND POSTERIOR DETERMINANTS OF OCCLUSION. Alone, an extrusion from or into the occlusal plane or a twisting of that plane will not be the sole factor governing the

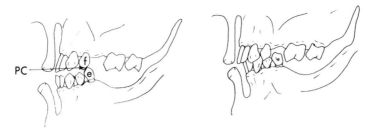

Fig. 7-13. Protrusive interference from extruded tooth. Mandibular second premolar tooth (*e*), because it is extruded, makes protrusive contact at *PC* with maxillary first premolar tooth (*f*).

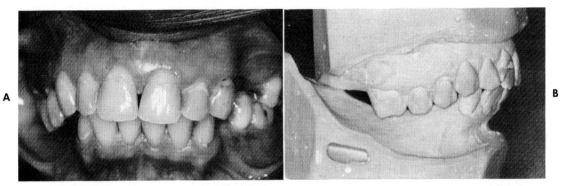

Fig. 7-14. A, Right side of maxillary arch has extruded and is touching mandibular residual ridge. Mandibular right second premolar has invaded edentulous space on maxillary left side. **B,** Mounted study cast of patient illustrated in **A** shows extruded maxillary segment contacting mandibular edentulous ridge.

function of eccentric mandibular movements. There are two other determinants that affect the magnitude of the impact of an altered occlusal plane on any prosthodontically developed occlusion: anterior and posterior guidance. The more influential of these is anterior, or incisal, guidance.

INCISAL GUIDANCE (ANTERIOR DETERMINANT). Incisal guidance is the term used to describe the influence of the maxillary and mandibular anterior teeth on the eccentric movements of the mandible. As the muscles contract to protrude the mandible, the incisal edges of the mandibular anterior teeth may meet the inclined planes of the lingual surfaces of the maxillary anterior teeth, and guide the protrusive movement of the mandible. The result of this anterior force on inclined planes is the opening movement of the mandible. Depending on the length and inclination of the maxillary anterior teeth, the mandible can be opened quickly or

slowly, through either a long or a short distance. A steep incisal guidance is the result of long (increased vertical overlap), vertically inclined maxillary anterior teeth. A shallow incisal guidance, in contrast, is the result of labially inclined or short (decreased vertical overlap) maxillary anterior teeth (Fig. 7-15). If the incisal guidance is steep, a single tooth or segmental extrusion from the plane of occlusion may not create a posterior interference when the mandible is protruded. However, if the incisal guidance is shallow, even a small extrusion from the plane of occlusion probably will create a posterior protrusive interference.

CONDYLAR GUIDANCE (POSTERIOR DETERMINANT). The posterior determinant of occlusion is the structure of the TMJ bilaterally. The movement of the mandibular condyle in its glenoid fossa is a guided movement. The movement of the mandibular condyles and articular disk away from centric relation is guided pri-

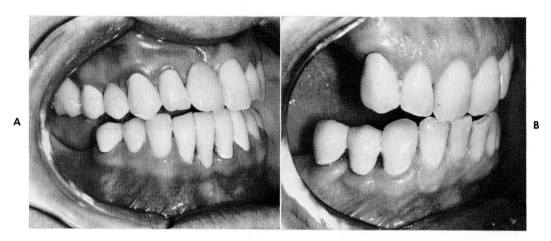

Fig. 7-15. A, Shallow incisal guidance. **B,** Steep incisal guidance. Space between maxillary canines in **A,** where guidance is shallow, appears nonexistent even though it does exist, whereas space is considerably greater in **B,** where incisal guidance is much steeper.

marily by the superior and the lateral walls of the glenoid fossa. There are two directions of movement to consider: anterior and medial.

The superior wall (roof) of the glenoid fossa has an anterior inferior inclination, so in a straight anterior pull of the mandible caused by an even contraction of the lateral pterygoid muscles (and suprahyoid muscles), the mandibular condyles will be guided inferiorly as well as anteriorly (see Fig. 7-9). When only one of the lateral pterygoid muscles contracts, it pulls the mandibular condyle and articular disk medially and inferiorly from its resting position. The insertion of this muscle is anterior, inferior, and medial to the head of the mandibular condyle, so the condyle is pulled forward, downward, and inward when it contracts (Fig. 7-16). It is guided in this direction by the slope of the superior wall and the inward or medial slope of the medial wall of the glenoid fossa (Fig. 7-17).

When tooth structure is used to guide the opening of the mandible, the simple anterior and inferior protrusive movement of the mandible is controlled or determined by: (1) the length and inclination of the maxillary incisors (referred to as incisal guidance) and (2) the inclination of the superior wall of the glenoid fossa (referred to as condylar guidance). The primary anterior lateral eccentric movement of the mandible is controlled predominantly by the length and inclination of the canines and buccal cusps of the posterior teeth (group function) or by these features of the canines alone

(canine guidance). The secondary posterior lateral eccentric movement of the mandible is controlled by the structure of the medial and superior walls of the glenoid fossa.

In general, incisal guidance is the dominant influence in programming mandibular movements; however, condylar guidance becomes increasingly more important when incisal guidance is shallow. Therefore, an extrusion from the plane of occlusion may or may not be a potential interference in either protrusive or lateral eccentric movements of the mandible, depending on the inclination of the superior and medial walls of the glenoid fossa and the length and inclination of the maxillary anterior teeth. If the mandible is guided open posteriorly by a steeply inclined superior wall, an extrusion from the occlusal plane may not be an interference; however, if the inclination of the superior wall is shallow, an extrusion from the occlusal plane presents an interference. However, because condylar guidance has greater influence during eccentric mandibular movements in the posterior plane of occlusion than anterior guidance, the position of the extrusion in the dental arch in relation to the occlusal plane is important in determining whether an interference in a protrusive movement will be manifested (Fig. 7-18).

COMPENSATING CURVES IN A PROSTHESIS VERSUS THE CURVES OF SPEE AND WILSON IN NATURAL TEETH. The morphologic features of the anterior and posterior determinants have a direct bearing on the type and amount of com-

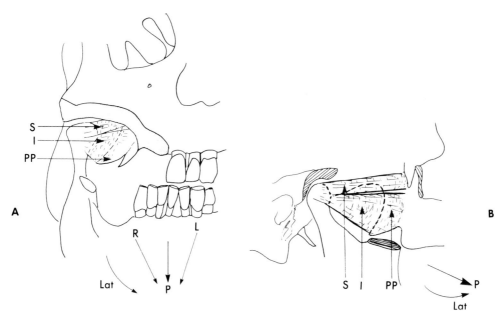

Fig. 7-16. Lateral pterygoid muscle position. **A,** Part of maxilla is removed to show mediolateral relation of lateral pterygoid muscle to mandibular condyle and lateral surface of pterygoid plate. *PP,* Pterygoid plate; *I,* inferior belly of lateral pterygoid muscle; *S,* superior belly of lateral pterygoid muscle; *P,* protrusive movement of mandible; *R,* right; *L,* left; *lat,* lateral movement of mandible. **B,** Zygomatic process and coronoid process are cut away to show anteroposterior relation of lateral pterygoid muscle to pterygoid plate and condylar head. *PP,* Pterygoid plate; *I,* inferior belly of lateral pterygoid muscle; *S,* superior belly of lateral pterygoid muscle; *P,* protrusive movement of mandible. When only one lateral pterygoid muscle contracts, jaw moves along arc *lat* for lateral movement of mandible.

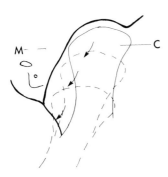

Fig. 7-17. Condylar head *(C)* moves along medial wall of fossa *(M)* when one lateral pterygoid muscle contracts.

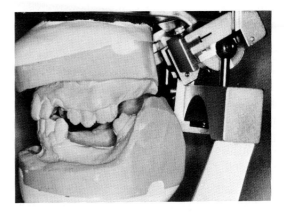

Fig. 7-18. Posterior protrusive contact. With properly recorded condylar inclination, maxillary left first molar contacts mandibular left third molar (in Fig. 7-7). Here, condylar inclination was increased 10°, resulting in no posterior protrusive balance. Because of shallow incisal guidance, increase of only 10° to condylar guidance would result in no posterior contact for articulated casts.

pensating curves generated in an occlusal scheme found on a prosthesis. The anteroposterior and mediolateral compensating curves generated in an artificial dentition to achieve bilateral balanced occlusion are similar in form to the naturally occurring curves of Spee and Wilson but are functionally different. The anteroposterior compensating curve could be considered as a continuous "bulge" in an otherwise flat occlusal plane. If both the anterior and posterior determinants of occlusion are steep, then the compensating curve generated on the RPD can be more pronounced. If the anterior and posterior determinants of occlusion are shallow, then this compensating curve must be shallow. The same theories hold true for the mediolateral compensating curve of the buccal and lingual denture tooth cusps. If the posterior and anterior determinants of occlusion for lateral eccentric movements are steep, then the mediolateral compensating curve can be steep; likewise, when the occlusal determinants are shallow, the compensating curves must be shallow.

The dentist must remember that pure anterior and posterior guidance are the physiologic limits, or border movements, of mandibular function. Any factors (such as extrusion from the occlusal plane, increase in the curves of Spee or Wilson, or increase in buccal or lingual cusp length) that will create steeper guidance than those dictated by the border movements should be considered pathologic interferences. The dentist must work within these limits to develop an individual occlusal scheme for each patient's particular needs that will preserve the remaining dentition.

FRAMEWORK AND DENTURE BASE CONSIDERATIONS. Another factor to be studied on mounted diagnostic casts is how the patient's present tooth and residual ridge relationships will affect framework design and denture base extension. Often, the incisal edges of the mandibular anterior teeth contact the cingula of the maxillary anterior teeth in centric occlusion and glide along their lingual inclined planes in lateral and protrusive eccentric movements. Cusps of the posterior natural teeth occlude on marginal ridges and in fossae and overlap their antagonists on both buccal and lingual surfaces. Mounted diagnostic casts reveal not only static tooth contacts but also continuous tooth posi-

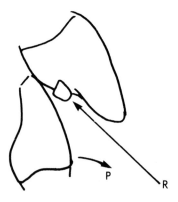

Fig. 7-19. Protrusive contact with cingulum rest. Protrusive movement of mandibular canine *(P)* interferes with cingulum rest *(R)* on maxillary canine.

tions during eccentric movements. The dentist must examine, in particular, all tooth contacts that occur on any proposed abutment teeth for an RPD in centric and eccentric positions. Such an examination will avoid placing portions of the cast framework in areas where they might interfere with the existing or planned occlusion. In the anterior region, the dentist must determine where the mandibular canines or premolars contact the maxillary canines in centric relation, centric occlusion, or both. Placing a rest and minor connector on the lingual surface of the maxillary canine incisal to the contact area of the mandibular tooth could cause an interference in centric occlusion as well as a protrusive or lateral eccentric movement of the mandible (Fig. 7-19). These interfering contacts outside the anterior and posterior determinants have the potential of disrupting neuromuscular activity necessary to proper mandibular function.

Examination of eccentric movements of the teeth may reveal that the mandibular canines (or premolars) may glide along the entire lingual surface of the maxillary canines or that the mandibular teeth may contact the inclines with only part or all of their incisal or cuspal surface. Thus, the dentist considering placement of a rest during the survey and design analysis should consider not only the superior-inferior placement of the rest seat but also its mesiodistal position. Likewise, a minor connector from that rest also has the potential to cause interferences with smooth mandibular movement.

Therefore, the dentist must consider both the thickness and position of any RPD component placed on or near occlusal surfaces of the natural teeth. Canines are one of the most frequent anterior RPD abutments, but, if an incisor must be used for a rest placement, it also must be examined for opposing tooth contact in centric relation and eccentric movements.

Posteriorly, the position of cusp tips in relation to occlusal rest placement must be examined thoroughly. Marginal ridges and triangular fossae of natural teeth are often areas of occlusal contact in centric occlusion. These are the same areas in which rest seats and rests are prepared and located. The rest and its minor connector must be of sufficient thickness to prevent fracture (Phillips, 1973). Consequently, the dentist may find it necessary to modify both the marginal ridge area and the opposing cusp tip clinically by selective grinding procedures to both ensure adequate strength of the cast framework and prevent occlusal interference.

When cusp tips overlap onto opposing buccal and lingual surfaces in occlusion, there exists the possibility of premature occlusal contact with the shoulder of a clasp arm. This potential becomes greater when the survey line is located near the occlusal or incisal edges of the abutment teeth. If this problem exists, either the survey lines need to be lowered, the overlapping cusps need to be reduced, or both procedures need to be performed to provide proper occlusal clearance in function.

INTERRIDGE SPACE. Often, the maxillomandibular space available for arranging denture teeth is markedly reduced. When natural teeth have been missing for many years, the opposing residual ridge expands or extrudes into these voids (Fig. 7-20). This phenomenon is often seen clinically, especially in the area of the residual ridge of the maxillary tuberosity, which expands to occupy the mandibular edentulous space. This is especially true as a consequence of the anterior hyperfunction syndrome (Kelly, 1972; Saunders and associates, 1979). At times both maxillary and mandibular edentulous segments have expanded to almost obliterate any potential space between the dental arches. Clinically, segmental extrusion and its consequences are more likely to occur with early tooth loss. Extractions performed later in

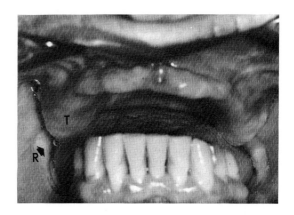

Fig. 7-20. Pendulant tuberosities almost contact mandibular retromolar pads. *T*, Tuberosity; *R*, retromolar pad.

life may not produce such drastic consequences quite as rapidly, yet the long-term effects are much the same.

A rational approach to this clinical problem is to surgically reduce or remove the offending segments. This method of achieving adequate maxillomandibular space and the proper plane of occlusion is becoming more frequently used and popular, but it still remains a procedure that is not commonly performed.

A satisfactory method for adjusting moderately extruded teeth beyond the physiologic plane of occlusion is to reduce the tooth by selective grinding until its excessive length no longer interferes with functional mandibular movements (see Chapter 5). An alternative method, depending on the degree of extrusion, is to place a cast restoration, either an onlay or a full crown. However, when a strategic tooth is excessively extruded, therapeutic endodontic therapy with placement of a cast restoration may be necessary to achieve the tooth's proper position within the proposed occlusal plane. Most often, however, no restoration is necessary to adjust the tooth to the proper plane of occlusion.

Surgical removal of extruded pendulous tuberosities and removal of tissue from the area of the retromolar pad should be performed if the denture bases interfere with each other during physiologic movements. The primary contraindications to any oral surgical procedure are the patient's medical status and the potential for the proposed procedure to cause iatrogenic dental pathosis. Any surgical procedure

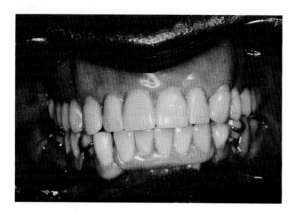

Fig. 7-21. Bilaterally balanced maxillary denture opposing mandibular RPD.

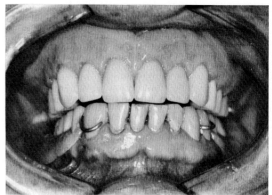

Fig. 7-22. Monoplane teeth are used to develop occlusal scheme that is balanced in centric relation only; there is no eccentric balance.

that would result in an oroantral fistula from an exposure of the maxillary sinus should be thought of as self-defeating and should not be performed. Yet, the alternatives to surgcial intervention are few. If after careful examination of the intraoral conditions, radiographs, and mounted diagnostic casts, there is no possibility of fabricating a prosthesis without causing premature contacts in eccentric movements and oral surgery is contraindicated, then only a few alternatives remain. One possibility is to cover the tuberosities or retromolar pads with a thin cast metal denture base rather than an acrylic resin denture base. The inherent strength of a cast chromium-cobalt alloy allows it to be between 0.5 and 1 mm thick, whereas the acrylic resin must be 2 to 3 mm thick for comparable strength. However, when a metal denture base is used, rebasing these areas when residual ridge reduction occurs is extremely difficult, if not sometimes impossible. A final alternative is to reduce the number of denture teeth on the prosthesis. This is a satisfactory compromise as long as sufficient occlusal contacts are maintained for posterior support of the opposing dentition or prosthesis.

Development of an occlusal scheme for a complete denture opposing a removable partial denture

Creating the proper occlusal scheme for patients treated with a maxillary complete denture opposing a mandibular RPD is extremely important to the success of the prostheses. To establish an appropriate occlusal scheme, the

dentist must consider several patient variables: the number and position of the teeth remaining in the mandibular arch, Angle's classification, condylar guidance, incisal guidance, the curve of Spee, the curve of Wilson, and cuspal inclination.

In complete denture prosthodontics, several occlusal schemes have been proposed and developed that use some or all of these patient variables. Essentially each is either analogous to dentulous occlusions or is a mechanical equivalent. They can be grouped into two major occlusal concepts: (1) balanced or (2) nonbalanced occlusal schemes. A bilaterally balanced occlusion (Gysi, 1929; Jordan, 1978) is developed by using all the variables of occlusion to produce simultaneous tooth contacts in centric and eccentric (protrusive and lateral) movements (Fig. 7-21). A nonbalanced occlusion (monoplane or neutrocentric) is developed by creating bilateral balance in centric relation only, and no interfering contacts are encountered during eccentric movements (no eccentric balance) (Jones, 1972) (Fig. 7-22). Both broad occlusal concepts must be considered when a combined complete maxillary denture is opposed by a mandibular RPD.

NONBALANCED OCCLUSAL SCHEME (MONOPLANE CONCEPT). Using a nonbalanced occlusal scheme (Jones, 1972) in an RPD is most appropriate when the remaining mandibular teeth are or can be modified to produce a relatively "flat" occlusal plane. This occlusal scheme is most often used in patients who have an Angle Class I or III jaw relationship and few remaining mandibular teeth or in patients who exhibit extreme wear of the occlusal surfaces of their remaining teeth. Patients with Angle Class III jaw relations, and many Class I patients, have shallow curves of Spee and Wilson, which permits them to be easily modified to a flat occlusal plane. Patients who have markedly worn occlusal surfaces often obliterate these natural curves completely and sometimes may even establish a reverse curve. In either case, adjusting the remaining naural teeth by selective grinding to achieve a flat occlusal plane is relatively easy for the dentist to accomplish.

BILATERALLY BALANCED OCCLUSAL SCHEME. A bilaterally balanced occlusion may be developed if there are many remaining mandibular posterior teeth or steep curves of Spee and Wilson or if the esthetic or phonetic placement of the maxillary anterior denture teeth will necessitate any degree of vertical overlap. Often, if the patient has both premolars and some molars remaining or has an Angle Class II jaw relationship, it may be necessary to develop a curved plane of occlusion to promote complete denture stability. Anatomic denture teeth arranged to achieve cross arch and cross tooth bilateral balance should be developed in the maxillary complete denture and the mandibular RPD to promote denture stability in eccentric movements.

DIAGNOSTIC STUDY CAST MOUNTING PROCEDURE FOR PATIENTS REQUIRING A MAXILLARY COMPLETE DENTURE OPPOSING A MANDIBULAR REMOVABLE PARTIAL DENTURE. The dentist can know when and how to modify the remaining occlusal surfaces to develop a particular occlusal scheme only when sufficient information is available regarding intermaxillary relationships and the existing occlusal plane. This information can be obtained only if diagnostic casts are mounted on a dental articulator in centric relation at an appropriate vertical dimension of occlusion and the maxillary occlusal rim is contoured intraorally to establish the proper maxillary anterior tooth position for esthetics and phonetics.

Once the maxillary diagnostic cast has been mounted on a dental articulator, using a hinge axis location and face-bow transfer procedure, the posterior portion of both the maxillary and mandibular occlusal rims is adjusted to provide an acceptable vertical dimension of occlusion

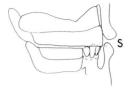

Fig. 7-23. Sibilant, S sounds are used for assessing proper occlusal vertical dimension. When vertical dimension is correct, registration rims will be just short of occlusal contact when S sound is spoken.

with an adequate interocclusal distance. This can be accomplished by adjusting the maxillary occlusion rim to correspond to the previously determined height of the mandibular occlusion rim. The height of the mandibular occlusion rim is initially constructed anteroposteriorly to an arbitrary occlusal plane extending from the marginal ridge of the most posterior remaining tooth to a point approximately halfway up the retromolar pad. The posterior vertical dimension of the maxillary occlusion rim is then adjusted to this mandibular occlusion rim phonetically, using the S sound, so that the occlusal rims barely touch when the patient pronounces words like *scissors* or *seventeen-seventy-six* or counts from 65 to 75 (Fig. 7-23).

The vertical dimension of occlusion established by this phonetic method must be reverified by determining if there is sufficient space between the posterior portions of the occlusal rims at the vertical dimension of rest. Measuring the distance between two widely spaced points on the face at the vertical dimension of rest and subtracting from that the measurement of the occlusal vertical dimension is another acceptable prosthodontic procedure to determine an adequate interocclusal distance. To accomplish this procedure the dentist places a mark on both the tip of the nose and on the chin. The patient is asked to pronounce words with a humming sound, such as *home* or the letter *M*, with the occlusal rims in place. The distance between the points on the chin and nose is measured and recorded during the production of this sound. Production of these sounds places the muscles in a state of minimal tonicity, or the vertical dimension of rest. Swallowing, followed by maximal mouth opening and the patient's lightly touching the lips together, is another method to establish the

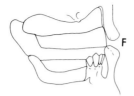

Fig. 7-24. Fricative (labiodental), *F* sounds are used for assessing proper protrusion of anterior portion of wax registration rim. Anterior portion of wax registration rim is correct when edge contacts wet-dry border of lower lip.

vertical dimension of rest. The vertical dimension of rest should be verified by several methods to find a consistent and repeatable position. The patient is asked to close to make maximum contact of the occlusal rims. It is important that the rims make uniform contact throughout their length. The distance between the points on the chin and nose is recorded again while the occlusal rims are in uniform contact. The numerical difference between these two measurements—vertical dimension of rest and vertical dimension of occlusion—is the interocclusal distance. This distance is variable but is between 2 and 5 mm in the average patient.

The vertical length and labiolingual axial inclination of the anterior portion of the maxillary occlusal rim is determined by a combination of phonetics and the proposed esthetic placement of the anterior denture teeth, *not necessarily by the present length of the mandibular anterior teeth*. The esthetic inclination (labiolingual axial inclination) of the maxillary rim is deemed acceptable if the upper lip is properly supported without distorting or obliterating the philtrum, or nasolabial fold. The proper length of the maxillary occlusal rim can be determined by asking the patient to pronounce several fricative sounds, or those words with *F* or *V* sounds in them, such as *fifty-five* or *victory*. The incisal edge of the maxillary occlusal rim is within clinically acceptable limits if it touches just inside the vermillion border of the lower lip when the patient produces these sounds clearly (Fig. 7-24).

During the diagnostic procedure to determine posterior occlusal vertical dimension and maxillary anterior tooth position, the height of the posterior portion of the occlusal rim may not coincide with the length of the anterior

segment; thus a two-step occlusal plane may be present. Remember that the posterior portion of the occlusal rim was adjusted to provide an accepatable occlusal vertical dimension and interocclusal distance; the anterior segment was adjusted for esthetics and phonetics. The difference in height of the rims will be reconciled, usually with a clinical compromise, when the mounted diagnostic study casts are examined on the dental articulator.

After the occlusal rims have been properly contoured, a centric relation recording is made, and the mandibular cast is mounted to the maxillary diagnostic cast.

EVALUATION OF OCCLUSAL PLANE. The diagnostic casts may now be examined to determine: (1) how the remaining mandibular teeth should be modified so that the maxillary complete denture is not dislodged during eccentric movements and (2) what surgical procedures are necessary to provide adequate intermaxillary space for the prosthesis. Modification of the mandibular teeth is made in one of three ways: (1) the mandibular teeth may be adjusted to a flat occlusal plane to develop a nonbalanced occlusal scheme (neutrocentric or monoplane occlusion); (2) they may be adjusted to a shallow curve with a $4^{1}/_{2}$- or 5-inch radius (using a 20° anatomic template) to develop a bilaterally balanced occlusal scheme; or (3) they may be adjusted, at minimum, to a harmonious curve regardless of the size of the radius so that a bilaterally balanced occlusion can be developed.

A nonbalanced occlusal scheme (monoplane occlusion) is often appropriate for the patient, but there are two factors that may preclude the use of a monoplane occlusion. The first consideration is the esthetic and phonetic positioning of the maxillary anterior teeth. If a patient has an Angle Class II, Division 2, anterior tooth relationship or had a deep vertical overlap in the previously existing natural dentition, it is often difficult or undesirable to achieve proper esthetics and phonetics using a monoplane occlusion. In this occlusal scheme, no vertical overlap of the maxillary anterior teeth is permitted. The maxillary denture teeth in these instances usually must be positioned with considerable vertical overlap so that their incisal edges are at the level of or below the middle third of the remaining mandibular anterior teeth. Some re-

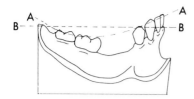

Fig. 7-25. Adjustment of plane of occlusion. If deep curve of Spee exists in partially edentulous mandible, it cannot be adjusted to flat plane *(B-B)*. It must be adjusted to harmonious curve such as *A-A*.

duction of the natural dentition may be indicated to achieve a monoplane (neutrocentric) occlusal scheme (one without any vertical overlap); however, gross reduction of the mandibular teeth to this level would be impossible without pulpal exposure.

The second factor that may preclude the development of a flat or shallow occlusal plane is the presence of a marked curve of Spee in the mandibular natural dentition. Patients who have an Angle Class II jaw relationship frequently have a pronounced curvature of the occlusal plane. Neither modification to a flat plane nor even to a 5-inch radius is usually possible. The only possible solution is to reduce the irregularities in the occlusal plane so that neither cusp tips nor teeth project out of the projected occlusal plane (Fig. 7-25) and use a bilaterally balanced occlusal scheme.

In both of the aforementioned clinical situations, complete denture stability, without compromising esthetics and phonetics, is achieved by developing a bilaterally balanced occlusion.

MODIFYING DIAGNOSTIC CASTS. After the dentist determines that either a nonbalanced (monoplane) or a bilaterally balanced occlusion is to be established, the dental stone teeth on the diagnostic cast are modified for diagnostic purposes.

MONOPLANE (NEUTROCENTRIC) OCCLUSAL SCHEME. The position of the incisal edge of the maxillary occlusal rim can be used as an approximate guide for the modification of the mandibular anterior teeth. Therefore, the mandibular anteriors are ground until no vertical overlap exists. Projecting the proposed occlusal plane posteriorly after anterior tooth reduction to a position halfway up the retromolar pad is

a guide to the maximum height for posterior denture tooth placement.

The simplest method for the dentist to employ when actually modifying the diagnostic cast to a monoplane occlusal scheme is to place a monoplane template on the occlusal surfaces of the teeth to judge whether the teeth have been properly recontoured.

The resultant plane of occlusion should usually divide the interocclusal space equally (or should, at times, favor the mandibular arch) and be approximately parallel with the maxillary and mandibular residual ridges. The plane of occlusion of the remaining mandibular teeth should be adjusted on the diagnostic cast with these principles in mind. Often, however, after optimal diagnostic adjustments are made, certain teeth (or portions of them) on the diagnostic cast will be below the proposed flat plane of occlusion. This deficiency can be made up by planning either (1) to overlay these teeth with metal extending from the RPD framework or (2) to place cast restorations on the teeth (onlays or cast crowns).

BILATERALLY BALANCED OCCLUSION. Diagnostic modifications of the diagnostic cast are also performed if a bilaterally balanced occlusal scheme is desired. A 20° occlusal template is used to help make this adjustment to a $4\frac{1}{2}$- or 5-inch radius. This 20° template is positioned on the diagnostic cast so that it is centered above the mandibular arch. Thin carbon articulating paper can be placed between the template and diagnostic cast and areas of first tooth contact marked on the cast. This will help visualize the areas in which modifications are necessary. The modification of the dental stone teeth is complete when most or all of the incisal edges and posterior cusp tips contact the proposed occlusal plane.

In some instances, no occlusal template can be used effectively to make these diagnostic adjustments. Any patient with a steep curve of Spee or of Wilson will require an individual adjustment to develop an "individualized" occlusion. The steepness of the curve is most often irrelevant to the success or failure of a prosthesis. What is of more importance is the smoothness of the curve. Therefore, any teeth or tooth cusps that protrude above the occlusal plane should be reduced to a level that will create a smooth, continuous anteroposterior and mediolateral curve free of any irregularities.

When the modifications of the occlusal plane have been planned, they can be executed by the dentist intraorally in a stepwise fashion so as to avoid overreduction of a particular tooth. Minimum clinical tooth alterations are the rule rather than the exception. The goal is to obtain a harmonious curve of both the natural and artificial mandibular dentition against which the artifical teeth of the maxillary complete denture can be arranged.

While modifying the diagnostic cast, it is wise for the dentist to select the actual denture teeth that will be used on the RPD. The denture teeth can be arranged, waxed in place, and modified as necessary to conform to the planned plane of occlusion and the occlusal morphologic features of the remaining teeth.

All finished modifications of the dental stone cast should be outlined with a colored pencil so that the amount and location of the reductions can be seen and be more easily reproduced intraorally on the patient's remaining teeth. The modified diagnostic casts are used as a guide to alter the existing occlusal plane before any rest seat preparations, tooth recontouring, or other preparations are performed for the RPD framework. Alteration of the teeth is *never* done after the metal framework is completed. Too often, RPD frameworks are constructed without the dentist's performing a diagnostic mounting and altering the diagnostic casts when indicated. This invariably produces interfering occlusal contacts caused by the components of the RPD framework or by improperly positioned denture teeth.

Summary of the mounted diagnostic cast examination

An analysis of the patient's existing occlusion from mounted diagnostic casts should include a determination of the following:
A. Centric relation and centric occlusion (Fig. 7-26)
  1. Are they separate or coincident positions?
  2. If they are not coincident, what is the amount and direction of slide from centric relation to centric occlusion?
B. Plane of occlusion
  1. Are there extruded teeth?
  2. Does the occlusal plane need modification?
C. Anterior determinant of occlusion
  1. Is incisal guidance present?
  2. Is it discluding the posterior teeth?
D. Lateral eccentric guidance
  1. Is it canine guidance? (See Figs. 7-2 and 7-27.)
  2. Is it group function? (See Figs. 7-3 and 7-28.)
  3. Are there balancing contacts?
E. Present occlusal contacts
  1. Will they interfere with placement of the components of the cast RPD framework?
  2. Will they interfere with the denture base?
  3. Will they interfere with denture tooth placement?
F. Interridge space
  1. Is there sufficient room for retentive latticework of the cast metal framework, acrylic resin denture base, and denture teeth:
    a. Anteriorly?
    b. Posteriorly?
  2. Should oral surgical procedures be performed to provide adequate space for the RPD by:
    a. Maxillary tuberosity reduction?
    b. Mandibular retromolar pad reduction?
    c. Extraction of nonstrategic teeth?
    d. Alveolectomies?
    e. Excision of soft-tissue attachments?
  3. Are there alternatives to oral surgery, such as:
    a. Covering retromolar pad, tuberosity, or both with a thin cast metal base?
    b. Leaving denture base short of its potential extensions?
    c. Compromising esthetics?
G. Complete denture–RPD prosthesis
  1. Is a nonbalanced or a bilaterally balanced occlusal scheme more appropriate?
  2. Must the plane of occlusion be modified to:
    a. A flat plane?
    b. A 20° plane?
    c. A harmonious curve?

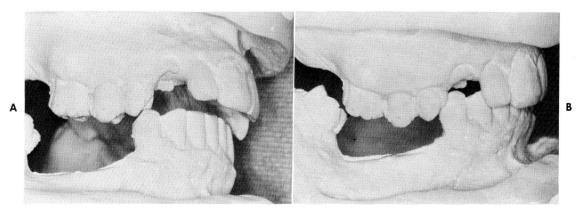

Fig. 7-26. A, Centric relation contact. **B,** Centric occlusion contact. After initial centric relation contact of distal incline of mandibular canine with mesial surface of maxillary premolar, canine tooth "slides" forward into habitual centric occlusion.

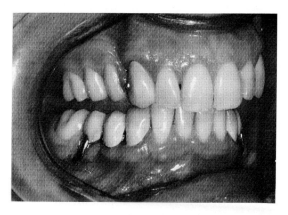

Fig. 7-27. Canine guidance for RPD. Canines disclude maxillary and mandibular teeth in lateral excursive movements.

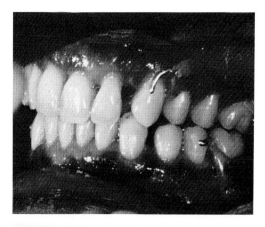

Fig. 7-28. Group function contact with RPD. Maxillary first and second premolars on RPD are in group function contact with natural mandibular first and second premolars.

PLANNING THE OCCLUSION

Once the dentist has gathered the information about the "journey"—the diagnosis—a decision must be made on the "itinerary"—the treatment plan—that is most appropriate for each patient.

Great controversy exists in prosthodontics over which position—centric relation or centric occlusion—is the best maxillomandibular relation at which to fabricate the occlusion for an RPD. When a complete maxillary denture in opposition to an RPD is to be fabricated, centric relation is the position most often used. When a simple cast restoration, such as a full crown, is placed in an occlusal environment that is physiologically sound, centric occlusion is the position of choice (Celenza and Litvak, 1976). The key in deciding which position to restore the occlusion to in an RPD depends on which is the most reproducible position for the individual patient.

An RPD contains elements of both complete and fixed partial denture prosthodontics. In many patients, there are insufficient stable occlusal contacts to maintain a consistent centric occlusion position. However, in other patients the number and distribution of occlusal contacts are sufficient to provide a reproducible position. The dentist must decide on the position at which to restore an occlusion on the basis of what can be practically accomplished while at the same time requiring as little patient adaptation as possible.

Anatomic centric relation position is generally accepted as the position around which the mandible rotates about an imaginary hinge axis. In this position, the mandibular elevator muscles theoretically have their greatest mechanical advantage to close the mandible. Therefore, the muscles should perform the least amount of work when bilateral simultaneous contraction of masseter and internal pterygoid muscles closes the mandible to occlusal contact along this terminal hinge axis position. However, patients rarely function by closing the mandible strictly around the hinge axis. The neuromuscular system functions within a three-dimensional, irregularly shaped space or envelope. The borders of this envelope of motion are referred to as the border positions of mandibular movement. These border positions are the extreme limits to which the mandible will move during normal function. Because of this, the mandible cannot function further posteriorly than centric relation. Therefore, this maxillomandibular position can generally be reproduced, especially after some patient rehearsal (Helkimo and associates, 1971).

Most masticatory muscle function occurs within these borders; however, this function must be related as closely as possible to this theoretical area of maximum efficiency. There is evidence that if there is a marked difference between centric relation and the occlusal position at which prostheses are constructed, occlusally related pathosis can occur (Brill and associates, 1962). Thus, not only is it most practical for the dentist to mount the diagnostic casts in centric relation because of its reproducibility, but also because it is the position in which patients may exhibit the most efficient muscle function.

The dentist must consider two other factors when making the decision to use either centric relation or centric occlusion. The first factor is the number of missing posterior teeth; the second is the existence of any pathosis attributable to premature tooth contacts.

When sufficient numbers of posterior teeth remain that will provide positive occlusal positioning of the mandible at an acceptable vertical dimension in centric occlusion, and when no pathosis exists in this position (that is, no excessive tooth wear, no large mediolateral slides from centric relation, no funneling of the periodontal ligament, or no tooth mobility), centric occlusion may be used as the starting point from which to develop the occlusion. Conversely, centric relation is used whenever there are insufficient posterior tooth contacts remaining to provide a stable mandibular occlusal position. If the diagnostic casts cannot be articulated easily and accurately by the dentist, then the centric relation position must be used.

Restoration of the occlusion in centric occlusion

Centric occlusion may be used as the position of choice when there is a stable maximal intercuspal position free of pathosis.

In partially edentulous arches such as the Kennedy Class III and IV and some Class II situations it is appropriate to consider restoring the occlusion in centric occlusion, because most often sufficicent natural teeth remain to provide stable, consistent, and constant occlusal relationships.

A note of caution should be introduced at this time. Whenever any posterior teeth remain in opposing dental arches, there is always the possibility that one or several cusp tips will initially contact an opposing tooth's inclined planes when the patient closes the mandible along the hinge axis in centric relation. For the patient to achieve a maximum intercuspal position (centric occlusion), these cusp tips must slide down the opposing tooth's inclined planes until stable cusp-to-fossa or marginal ridge contacts are achieved. This deflection can be straight or lateral anteriorly, depending on the inclined planes initially contacted.

Irregular muscle contraction patterns can arise when inclined plane contacts from centric relation to centric occlusion move the mandible from side to side. While the neuromuscular system searches for a stable occlusal position of teeth, the muscles may become fatigued, irritable, and hyperreactive. Constant muscle irritation can create chronic discomfort for the patient (TMJ dysfunction syndrome). In the same way, any interfering contacts or inclined plane contacts encountered from centric relation to centric occlusion may cause muscle disharmony and eventual muscle spasm and pain. Any deflection from centric relation to centric occlusion has the potential for producing muscle instability and TMJ pain dysfunction syndrome (Ramfjord, 1961). Therefore, whenever possible, the dentist should eliminate or minimize any deflective occlusal contacts before patient treatment with a prosthesis is initiated. This is at times a complex task, at other times simple, requiring only minimal tooth alterations.

For example, when all premolars and molars (except for the third molars) are missing and occlusal interferences exist on the mesial inclined planes of the maxillary teeth against the distal incline planes of the mandibular teeth when the patient's mandible is manipulated from centric occlusion to centric relation, it is possible that similar occlusal interferences will occur with all the replacement denture teeth. Consequently, instead of only the third molars' having occlusal prematurities (deflective occlusal contacts), all posterior teeth will exhibit occlusal prematurities. In and of themselves, occlusal prematurities may or may not lead to pathosis. However, it is unwise to assume that because the patient has adapted to third molar prematurities that he or she will adapt to the occlusal prematurities introduced by an RPD.

Deflective occlusal contacts on an RPD do not initiate a neuromuscular reflex arc because of stimulation of affected receptors from an individual periodontal ligament directly but only through movement of the RPD against the abutment teeth. The RPD itself has no periodontal ligament. However, the combination of stress transmitted to the periodontal ligaments of abutment teeth by the prosthesis and the positive mechanical positioning of the mandible by the denture teeth can create muscle imbalance. The adaptability of the individual patient determines whether muscle pathosis will develop. The dentist should not depend on muscle adaptation for determining the success of the RPD.

Freedom in centric relation

A more rational approach to patient treatment is to develop an occlusion in such a way that there will be no interferences from centric relation to centric occlusion and no interfering contacts in lateral eccentric movements throughout the functional occlusal range. Adjustment of this nature will frequently produce what has been described as a *long centric relation* or *freedom in centric relation* (Dawson, 1974). Rather than producing an occlusion that is "locked in" by firm interdigitating point contacts, the dentist produces an occlusal scheme that will allow bilateral simultaneous contacts to occur within a small area. This area of contact will vary in amount between individuals, but it rarely exceeds 1 mm. In all practicality, the vertical dimension of occlusion is the same within this very small area.

Freedom in centric relation allows the dentist to create a small area in which bilateral stable occlusal contacts can be made simultaneously. A precisely developed occlusion with anatomic denture teeth is not recommended, and in most cases it is difficult to fabricate. Likewise, centric relation, because it is registered by guiding the mandible to a hinge axis border position, is not usually a functioning position. In most cases, centric occlusion, or some functional occlusal position, can be permitted to exist 0.5 to 1 mm anterior to centric relation by using this long centric relation concept (Beyron, 1973).

The ideal position for centric occlusion is when the muscular activity of all the muscles of mastication can be kept to a minimum, that is, when the muscles perform as little work as possible to place the mandible in a stable occlusal position. A stable area of contact should be created in the occlusion that will allow some degree of freedom for the muscles to reposition the mandible from centric relation to centric occlusion. When this is done, the objective of producing a noninterfering occlusion will have been met.

Restoration of the occlusion in centric relation

Complete dentures, as well as most Kennedy Class I and II RPDs, require the restoration of all or the majority of posterior occlusal contacts. When the posterior dental arch segments are edentulous, centric relation is the position of choice for developing the occlusion. This applies to most distal-extension RPDs or when a distal-extension RPD opposes a maxillary complete denture. The most stable reproducible mandibular position is centric relation in these instances when so few natural teeth remain.

An additional factor to be considered is the lateral occlusal contacts to be developed. When group function or a bilaterally balanced occlusion is desired, the diagnostic casts must be mounted in centric relation. This is because all eccentric (lateral) movements by definition originate from centric relation. Thus, when the dentist records protrusive or lateral eccentric movements, these can only be accurately positioned and adjusted on the dental articulator and used if the diagnostic casts are first mounted in centric relation. Therefore, in these cases, centric relation should be considered the position in which to mount the diagnostic casts and develop the occlusion. Because of the type and number of occlusal contacts to be restored, centric relation is the only reliable position in which to initially develop the occlusion. However, with many patients it will frequently be appropriate to develop a certain amount of freedom in centric relation (Zarb and associates, 1978).

Lateral eccentric contacts

The decision by the dentist whether to use a group function type of occlusion on an RPD is based on the stability of the remaining natural teeth. If the remaining teeth are not stable and exhibit residual mobility patterns, then a group function type of occlusion should be developed to distribute the masticatory force throughout all the supporting structures of the prosthesis (Isaacason, 1976). These lateral occlusal contacts can occur on either the denture teeth or the remaining natural dentition (Fig. 7-28). Thus, when a group function type of occlusion is used, masticatory force will be distributed to the residual ridges, hard palate, or alveolar bone surrounding all abutment teeth during eccentric movements rather than solely to the alveolar bone around any one tooth. If the remaining teeth and supporting structures show no signs of pathosis and the patient has functioned with these occlusal contacts for a long time, the lateral guidance that the patient exhibits should be retained (Fig. 7-27).

Summary of the maxillomandibular positions used to establish an occlusion for a removable partial denture

Centric occlusion is the position of choice: (1) when stable, maximal occlusal contacts exist with no evidence of pathosis and (2) after any anterior or mediolateral deflections from centric relation have been adjusted.

Centric relation is the position of choice: (1) when there are insufficient occlusal contacts to relate the mandible to maxilla (that is, to relate the diagnostic casts) in a stable, consistent relationship; (2) when eccentric contacts are to be made; and (3) when an RPD opposes a maxillary or mandibular complete denture.

Bilateral simultaneous contact

Regardless of which initial maxillomandibular position, centric relation or centric occlusion, is chosen to develop an occlusion, the natural and prosthetic teeth on both sides of both dental arches must contact simultaneously and with even distribution of force. Bilateral simultaneous uniform contact of the teeth, whatever the decision on eccentric contacts or anteroposterior position of the mandible in the treatment plan, is a fundamental prosthodontic requirement in the development of an occlusion for an RPD.

Vertical dimension of occlusion

The vertical dimension of occlusion is defined as the superior-inferior relationship of the maxilla to the mandible when the natural teeth and prosthetic teeth are in maximum contact. The vertical dimension of occlusion determines to a great extent the patient's morphologic face height. Early tooth loss can affect the morphologic face height adversely during the formative stages, when growth and development are influenced by tooth position.

Throughout a person's life, however, chronic tooth wear affects the vertical dimension of occlusion. However, these aging changes occur slowly, allowing the muscles of mastication and facial expression to adapt to them. In the majority of cases, no adverse sequellae develop from these alterations.

However, as morphologic face height decreases with tooth wear or loss, other intraoral or extraoral changes occur that necessitate the restoration of the occlusal vertical dimension. Some of the initial clinical signs that appear on the face are excessive folding and wrinkling of the skin at the corners of the mouth, producing signs of premature aging. Superimposed on this premature aging change may be the development of angular cheilosis and a *C. albicans* infection (Russotto, 1980). Additionally, the signs and symptoms of the TMJ pain dysfunction syndrome may appear. Besides being esthetically displeasing—this may be the first sign that brings a patient to seek treatment—an excessive decrease in the occlusal vertical dimension may be associated with other pathologic changes in the skin, bones, and muscles.

It is possible to reestablish a functional occlusal vertical dimension for patients who require at least one complete denture. However, it is extremely difficult to attempt to restore an acceptable occlusal vertical dimension with RPDs alone without simultaneous contact of the natural teeth. Any change in occlusal vertical dimension requires that occlusal contact be made over most, if not all, occlusal surfaces of both dental arches. It is not sound prosthodontic practice to construct an RPD that creates a new occlusal vertical dimension on the replacement denture teeth alone while not providing simultaneous uniform contacts on the remaining natural teeth. The excessive occlusal load placed on the abutment teeth and residual ridges by the RPD frequently causes pathologic changes in these areas (residual ridge resorption and increased tooth mobility). In addition, it may create a TMJ dysfunction syndrome. As a general rule, the patient's existing occlusal vertical dimension should always be maintained when an RPD is made. If the dentist elects to alter the occlusal vertical dimension with a prosthesis, he or she must also modify the natural teeth with either cast restorations or by overlaying the occlusal surfaces of the natural teeth with the RPD framework. One of the few times the occlusal vertical dimension can be restored using an RPD alone is when it opposes a complete denture.

TREATMENT PROCEDURES
Restoring the occlusion

The planning for the "journey" to restore the occlusion by using an RPD is completed once the treatment plan is firmly established and recorded. Actual patient treatment—the journey itself—requires that sound prosthodontic principles and practices be used during the treatment that will achieve the goals decided on in the treatment plan. The prosthodontic techniques discussed in the following pages will meet those needs.

Dental articulators

Developing an RPD occlusion or analyzing diagnostic casts requires that these casts be mounted on a dental articulator. The type of dental articulator used depends on its ability to fulfill certain basic requirements. The requirements for a dental articulator are simply those that will allow examination of the anterior determinant (incisal guidance) and posterior determinant (condylar guidance) of occlusion and of how these determinants interact with the plane of occlusion.

The factors of the anterior determinant (incisal guidance) can be studied on any dental articulator that allows the anterior teeth to glide against each other in anterior and lateral directions. It is in the posterior determinant area (condylar guidance) that some dental articulators fall short of closely reproducing the movement of the mandibular condyle in the glenoid fossa. Generally speaking, a semiadjustable arcon-type dental articulator* will be a satisfactory instrument for the dentist to use for either the development of an occlusal scheme on an RPD or the analysis of the patient's existing occlusion. An arcon type of dental articulator is the instrument of choice because it will accept lateral and protrusive eccentric records more easily than a nonarcon type. An arcon (*articulator-condyle*) dental articulator has a freely movable superior and lateral wall that can be adjusted to conform to the protrusive or lateral eccentric record made from the patient (Fig. 7-29). In an arcon instrument, the inclination of the superior wall can be a fairly accurate duplication of the existing structure of the patient's glenoid fossa because of the ease of placement of the superior wall. An accurate setting of the condylar inclination to describe the average slope to the superior wall of the glenoid fossa is significant in planning alterations of the occlusal plane when a shallow incisal guidance is present. On a dental articulator, a reasonably accurate mechanical representation of the condylar guidance and the degree and timing of protrusive and lateral eccentric mandibular movements will greatly enhance the ability of the dentist to produce incisal or canine guid-

---

*Hanau 158-1, Teledyne Hanau, Buffalo, N.Y.; Whip-Mix 8500 series, Whip-Mix Corp., Louisville, Ky.

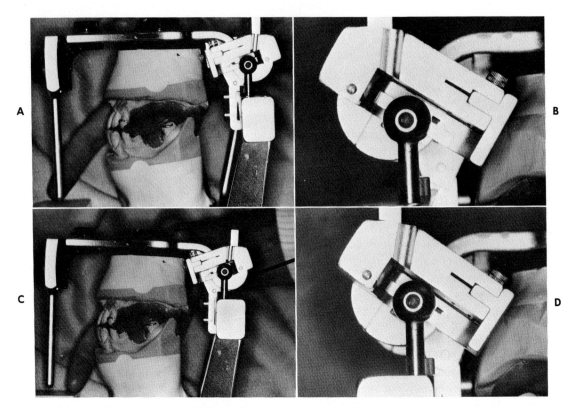

Fig. 7-29. Arcon articulator with protrusive record in place. **A,** Condylar ball does not contact superior wall. **B,** Enlargement of condylar ball. **C,** Freely movable superior wall is moved downward until it just comes into contact with condylar ball, resulting in proper posterior guidance. **D,** Enlargement of condylar ball.

ance, group function, or a bilaterally balanced occlusal scheme in the final prosthesis.

Arbitrary hinge axis location and face-bow transfer technique (Fig. 7-30)

For any technique to be successful, a complete and organized armamentarium is necessary. The armamentarium needed to locate the hinge axis and make a face-bow transfer, includes:

1. Dental face-bow and hinge axis locator
2. Semiadjustable dental articulator
3. Baseplate wax
4. Stick compound
5. Bunsen burner
6. Indelible pencil or red pencil
7. Maxillary diagnostic cast
8. Number 7 wax spatula
9. Scalpel with number 25 blade
10. Mixing bowl and spatula
11. Laboratory plaster
12. Dental articulator mounting plate

The procedure used to locate the hinge axis and make a face-bow transfer is presented in a step-by-step fashion in the following paragraphs.

In the first step, the maxillary cusp tips of the patient's natural teeth are related to the face-bow fork.

Warm baseplate wax or stick compound is placed uniformly on the face-bow prongs. The face-bow fork is centered (in line with the dental midline) over the occlusal surfaces of the maxillary teeth and seated on them to record the occlusal surfaces. The face-bow fork is then stabilized until the material hardens.

The face-bow fork is removed from the patient's mouth, and any excess recording material is removed with a scalpel until just the cusp tips of the teeth remain.

The diagnostic cast is placed in the cusp tip record to check the accuracy of both the record and diagnostic cast. The diagnostic cast should be stable and not rock in the record.

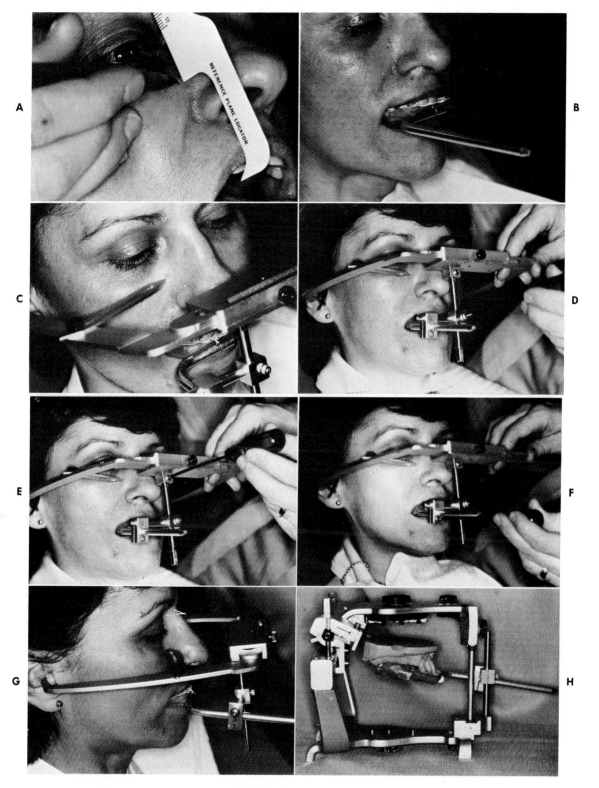

Fig. 7-30. Face-bow technique. **A,** Locating anterior reference point. **B,** Face-bow fork in mouth. **C,** Face-bow and reference pointer in place. **D,** Face-bow secured in place. **E,** Face-bow assembled and all parts secured. **F,** Completing last adjustment. **G,** Lateral view of assembled face-bow; posterior reference point is external auditory meatus. **H,** Face-bow fork and diagnostic cast in place on dental articulator.

The next step is the location of the appropriate hinge axis of mandibular rotation. The hinge axis can be located fairly accurately by using anatomic patient landmarks and reference points. An area 11 to 13 mm anterior to the tragus of the ear on the canthus-tragus line has most frequently been advocated as the location of the center of the mandibular condyles.

By use of this measurement, the mandibular condyle position is marked with a dot from an indelible pencil.

The face-bow fork and record are replaced in the mouth and held securely over the teeth, and the face-bow apparatus is positioned over the face-bow fork. The pointers projecting from the ends of the face-bow are positioned over the dots bilaterally so that both pointers are equidistant from the skin. The face-bow rod is secured to the face-bow by a set screw.

The assembled face bow apparatus relates the maxillary teeth to the rotational centers of the mandibular condyles in both an anteroposterior and a mediolateral position. A third point of reference is used to relate the maxillary teeth to the mandibular condyle hinge axis position inferosuperiorly. The anatomic reference point most commonly used is the infraorbital foramen.

The location of the infraorbital foramen under the eye is palpated, and the pointer on the face-bow is adjusted to this point on the skin and locked into place.

Recently, the ease of completing the face-bow transfer procedure has been facilitated by the use of an "ear" type of face-bow.* This instrument uses specially prepared plastic earpieces attached to both ends of the face-bow; these earpieces are placed in the external auditory meatus of each ear as a means of locating the hinge axis (posterior reference) point. This face-bow system eliminates the need to measure an arbitrary facial point. This type of face-bow assembly is inherently more stable because the earplugs fit snugly in the external auditory meatus, making it easier to hold the face-bow in place while the third point of reference is established and the face-bow fork and rod are secured in place.

*Whip-Mix Corp., Louisville, Ky.

Transferring the face-bow record to the dental articulator is done in several ways, depending on type of face-bow assembly used. The manufacturer's directions should be followed carefully to assure that the procedure is performed accurately.

Technique for mounting study casts
Rationale

All diagnostic casts should be mounted on a dental articulator in centric relation. Maxillomandibular relations, specifically centric relation, must be recorded using a material or materials that will allow an easy transference of the record intraorally to a dental articulator. Several dental materials have been used successfully over the years, and all are equally acceptable when manipulated properly. These dental materials include, in no preferential order, impression plaster, various types of waxes, zinc oxide–eugenol pastes, and more recently, the silicone and polyether elastomers. Regardless of the material used, however, the centric relation position to be recorded should be first determined and rehearsed with the patient so it can be repeated easily.

Rehearsing centric relation

Rehearsal of the centric relation position with the patient is extremely important. Any foreign object placed intraorally, such as a recording medium, changes the patient's perception of the relationship between the maxilla and mandible because of alterations in the sensory feedback system. When the patient has been repeatedly shown where and how to "close," the chances of the dentist's recording this position accurately are considerably increased when the recording medium is in place. Because centric relation is a border position of the mandible and, therefore, one not often used by the patient, familiarity with it will increase the likelihood that the dentist will record it accurately.

Several methods have been used to locate the centric relation position. Various methods are acceptable, but it takes practice and clinical experience for the dentist to feel comfortable with any particular technique chosen.

When any technique is used to record centric relation, it is generally accepted that the initial step in locating centric relation is to deprogram (eliminate sensory input from the periodontal ligament to interrupt muscle memory) the patient's musculature from its habitual centric occlusion position. To prevent any afferent impulses from the sensory receptors in the periodontal ligament, there must be absence of posterior tooth contact. A convenient method to prevent posterior tooth contact is to interpose a material between the anterior teeth; self-curing acrylic resin formed to create a jig (anteriorly inclined plane) is a convenient material (Lucia, 1962). Acrylic resin can be placed on the previously lubricated maxillary central incisors, and the mandible can be guided into centric relation. Closure should be made in the soft acrylic resin to just before posterior tooth contact. After the acrylic resin fully polymerizes, the jig can be trimmed with acrylic burs mounted on a low-speed handpiece. The acrylic resin should be angled posteriorly so that the mandibular incisors will be guided posteriorly as they contact and glide along this inclined plane to centric relation. The acrylic resin jig can be slowly adjusted intraorally using carbon articulating paper and slow-speed acrylic burs mounted in a low-speed handpiece until just short of the first posterior tooth contact. Laboratory plaster, soft aluminized wax,* or other recording media can be placed between the occlusal surfaces of teeth to record the centric relation position. This technique is useful for the novice and is also an extremely valuable technique for use with patients in whom the dentist finds it impossible to successfully manipulate the mandible into centric relation even after the most rigorous training.

Another easy and simple method to deprogram the muscles so that the mandible can be manipulated into a hinge axis closure is to place a cotton roll between the central incisors and have the patient close the mandible firmly in this position for between 5 and 15 minutes. Because of the absence of posterior tooth contact during this time, the muscles will have "forgotten" the reflex control needed to position the mandible in centric occlusion. This deprogramming (interrupting muscle memory) will usually allow the dentist to more easily guide the

*Aluwax, Aluwax Dental Products Co., Grand Rapids, Mich.

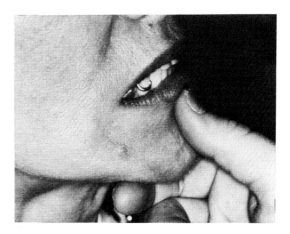

Fig. 7-31. One-handed manipulation is used to guide mandible to centric relation.

mandible to centric relation position along the arc of hinge axis closure.

The patient can be trained to open and close (rotate) the mandible around the hinge axis with some guidance by the dentist. Guidance by the dentist is accomplished by the placing of firm but gentle pressure on the mandible to guide it in a posterior and superior direction. The dentist can achieve a solid grasp of the mandible by placing the thumb on the patient's chin in the region of the incisive fossa below the mandibular incisors and grasping the inferior border of the chin with the forefinger of the same hand. This will allow the dentist to establish secure control of the mandible. Firm control will aid the dentist in manipulating the mandible posteriorly. If the dentist is confident of the placement of the mandible, the patient will be relaxed. This relaxation will be reflected in the relative ease with which the mandible can be guided around the arc of hinge axis closure (Fig. 7-31).

Sometimes patients will be unsure of what the dentist wishes them to do and will protrude rather than retrude the mandible. Different suggestions to the patient can be used to overcome this problem. Asking the patient to relax the mandible while allowing the dentist to "wiggle" the mandible up and down can produce satisfactory results. "Close gently on the back teeth," "Push the upper jaw forward," "Place the tip of the tongue on the back of the roof of the mouth" are all suggestions that the dentist might use to help the patient retrude

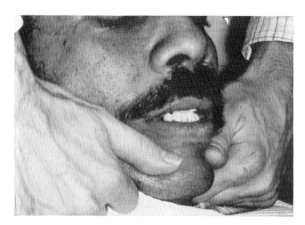

Fig. 7-32. Bilateral manipulation is used for guidance into centric relation.

the mandible to a hinge axis closure. Even though gentle guidance of the mandible most often must be used, excessive force will often cause the patient to resist by producing an undesired protrusive movement. Any untoward reaction of this sort caused by excessive manipulation by the dentist will obviously be counterproductive and lead to an inaccurate recording.

Some patients respond best to posterior and superior guidance when the dentist uses both hands. When this technique is used, the dentist stands behind the patient and places the tips of the fingers along the inferior border of the mandible and the thumbs in the incisive fossa. The dentist then uses a slight superior and posterior pull of the mandible for guidance. The pressure is applied to the mandible gently but firmly, using phrases and words similar to those used in the above technique to guide the patient to the most posterior closure possible (Fig. 7-32).

For many patients, the dentist will easily and quickly detect the easy swinging, hingelike movement of the desired arc of closure of the mandible; for others, time and patience will be required before a repeatable centric relation position can be determined. Regardless of the method used to retrude the patient's mandible into centric relation, the hinge axis closure should be rehearsed until both dentist and patient are sure of the desired position. Once the dentist is assured of closure around the hinge axis, the recording technique is fairly straightforward.

Obtaining centric relation using a wax wafer and a recording medium

When the majority of the teeth are present, a rigid tray is used to confine and direct one of the recording materials in and out of the mouth. The type of tray most often used is made from a wafer of hard wax that is relieved and relined with a free-flowing rigid metallic oxide impression material. The armamentarium needed includes:
1. Hard wax sheets
2. Alcohol torch
3. Compound water bath
4. Scissors
5. Scalpel blade and handle (number 15 or number 11 blade)
6. Registration material (zinc oxide and eugenol paste)
7. Rubber bowl with cold water
8. Mixing pad and spatula

The procedure used is presented in a step-by-step fashion in the following paragraphs.

Half of the hard wax sheet is placed in the preheated compound water bath until it becomes quite soft and pliable. The dentist takes this softened wax wafer to the mouth and presses it gently against the maxillary teeth. After hardening, the wax is removed, chilled in a bowl of cold water, and trimmed on its lateral aspect with a scissors to within several millimeters of the impression formed by the tips of the buccal cusps and incisal edges of the maxillary teeth. When trimming the wax wafer, the dentist should leave a small handle protruding from the wax wafer in the area of the central incisors for ease of placement and removal.

The wax wafer is again softened in the compound water bath, placed intraorally, and held against the maxillary teeth while the mandible is guided into the rehearsed centric relation closure. The patient is cautioned to close the mandible into the wax only to just short of tooth contact. Any occlusal contact has the potential to cause a deflection of the mandible from centric relation. The wax wafer is chilled with air or water intraorally and is gently removed without distortion. Ideally, only cusp tip indentations should exist in the wax wafer. But, because of the curve of Spee, extruded teeth or cusps, impressions of the entire occlusal surface may be made into the wax surface. Impressions of any part of the occlusal surface except for cusp tips must be trimmed away by the dentist, using a sharp scalpel. If left, the occlusal surfaces of the dental stone cast will not accurately fit into the wax impressions of the teeth because of the inherent inaccuracy of the wax as compared to dental stone. Failure of the dental stone cast to fit into the wax wafer invariably occurs because of wax distortion and, equally important, because the wax, being resilient, may flex out of an undercut or irregularity when first removed from the mouth but may not be able to flex back onto the dental stone teeth when returned as a registration tray with another material to complete the centric relation record. The dentist should reverify its position after the wax tray has been trimmed by returning it to the mouth and repeating the centric relation closure into the cut back cusp tip indentations.

The centric relation record can now be finalized so that the mandibular dental stone cast can be related to the maxillary cast by correcting any wax distortions by means of a corrective reline procedure with another impression material. Zinc oxide and eugenol impression material is an excellent corrective reline material. The material is mixed with a stiff-bladed spatula on a mixing pad according to the manufacturer's directions. Then a thin layer (wash) of this material is placed on maxillary and mandibular surfaces of the wax tray. The tray is then positioned onto the maxillary arch, and the patient's mandible is guided closed until just initial tooth contact with the wax tray is made. When the zinc oxide and eugenol impression material is set, the tray is removed from the mouth and the excess wash material is trimmed with a sharp scalpel so that only cusp tip registrations remain. Most impression materials are extremely accurate and, as such, will record the tooth's detailed occlusal surface anatomic features. The corresponding dental stone cast surface rarely reproduces the detailed features that are reproduced by the zinc oxide–eugenol impression materials. To have the diagnostic cast positioned accurately in the centric relation record, all material except for the cusp tips must be removed.

Recording centric relation with record bases and occlusion rims

When fewer teeth are remaining, especially in the posterior dental arches (Kennedy Class I), a wax wafer by itself cannot be used to rec-

ord centric relation. To provide sufficient support for the centric relation record, it is necessary to construct record bases with wax occlusion rims. These record bases and occlusion rims will supply the necessary support to the record to stabilize it during the recording of centric relation and in mounting the diagnostic casts on the dental articulator.

Record bases can be fabricated from either shellac or gutta percha baseplate material or autopolymerizing acrylic resin directly on the diagnostic cast. Autopolymerizing acrylic resin is the preferred material because of its ease of manipulation, its rigidity, and its ability to retain its stability.

The armamentarium necessary for construction of temporary acrylic resin record bases includes:

1. Acrylic resin separating medium
2. Paint brush
3. Number 2 pencil
4. Autopolymerizing acrylic resin
5. Baseplate wax
6. Sticky wax
7. Number 7 and number 31 wax spatulas
8. Bunsen burner
9. Arbor chuck, band and lathe (and/or acrylic resin finishing burs), and slow-speed handpiece
10. Pressure curing unit
11. Petroleum jelly
12. Rubber mixing bowl
13. Laboratory knife

The procedure for making record bases and occlusion rims to record maxillomandibular relations is easy and straightforward; it is presented in step-by-step fashion in the following paragraphs and illustrated in Fig. 7-33.

In the first step, an outline of the extension of the record base desired is drawn onto the diagnostic cast with a number 2 pencil. Because stability is one of the prime prerequisites for record bases, they should not be overextended. Therefore, the mandibular record base outline should extend posteriorly no more than halfway up the retromolar pad and 2 mm short of both the internal and external oblique lines. To connect the left and right posterior distal extensions, the lingual connection should extend from the height of the free gingival margin to within 2 mm of the functional depth of the floor of the mouth.

If large undercuts exist on the residual ridge

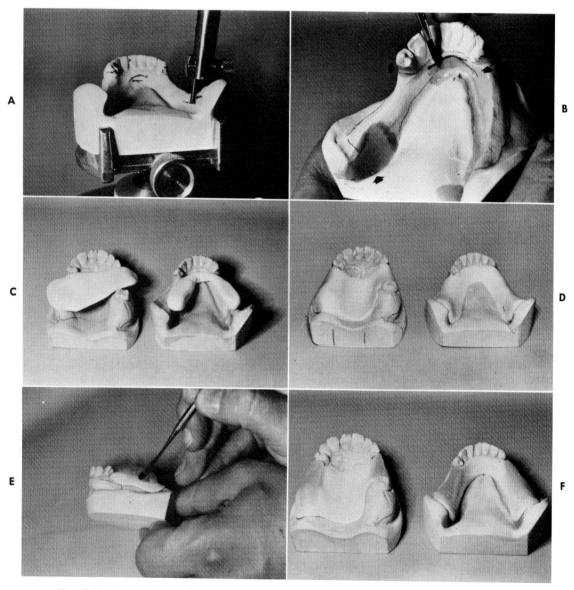

Fig. 7-33. Construction of registration bases for diagnostic mounting. **A,** Tissue undercuts are surveyed on diagnostic cast. **B,** Acrylic resin separating medium is applied. Note that undercuts have been previously blocked out with wax *(arrows)*. **C,** Acrylic resin is made in approximate shape of record bases before doughy acrylic resin is manipulated to desired extensions. **D,** Trimmed acrylic resin record bases are seated on diagnostic casts. **E,** Occlusal wax rims are sealed in place. **F,** Completed temporary record bases and occlusal rims.

or between the teeth, they should be blocked out with wax so that fracture of the diagnostic cast or record base will be avoided when the cured acrylic resin is removed. Any undercuts located on the proximal areas of teeth next to the residual ridges should be especially noted, and block out wax should be applied. The outlined and blocked-out diagnostic cast is then liberally coated with an acrylic resin separating medium* to prevent the acrylic resin from adhering to the dental stone cast.

The outline of the maxillary record base is similar in its intent to the outline of the mandibular cast if not in actual detail. The extension of the maxillary record base is kept 2 mm short of the deepest portion of the buccal vestibule and away from the juncture of movable and nonmovable tissue of the soft palate and palatal rugae. Stability is maximized when areas of muscular movement that would tend to dislodge the record base, such as the buccal vestibule and soft palate, are avoided.

The acrylic resin should be mixed according to the manufacturer's recommended proportions, placed in a glass jar and covered, and allowed to partially polymerize. When the acrylic resin reaches the doughy stage, it can be easily manipulated. Hands and fingers should be lubricated lightly with petroleum jelly to prevent the uncured acrylic resin from sticking to them during the procedure. When used to make the mandibular record base, the acrylic resin can be formed into the shape of a roll with a long constriction in the middle. The two ends of the acrylic resin roll are placed on the distal-extension areas; the middle constriction forms the lingual bar connector. The acrylic resin is pushed with the fingers to the outlined border areas and smoothed with lubricated fingers. Excess acrylic resin should be trimmed with a laboratory knife before the material is fully polymerized. It is much easier and quicker to trim the acrylic resin at this stage than later, when the polymerized material must be trimmed and finished with stones and burs. The acrylic resin record base should only be as thick as needed to prevent its fracture. Usually, 1 to 1.5 mm is a sufficient thickness over the residual ridges, whereas the lin-

*Coe-Sep, Coe Laboratories, Chicago, Ill.

gual bar area must be between 2 and 4 mm thick for strength. A periodontal probe can be used to judge the thickness of the acrylic resin before the material has completely polymerized.

The diagnostic cast should be placed in a rubber bowl with warm water or a pressure curing unit (30 psi for 20 minutes) until the acrylic resin has polymerized. This serves two purposes. The first is to accelerate the polymerization of the acrylic resin and increase its density; the second is to wet the diagnostic cast so that removal of the acrylic resin record base will be made easier. After complete polymerization, the acrylic resin record base can be removed by gently prying it up at the edges in several places with a laboratory knife.

The maxillary record base is constructed in a manner similar to the mandibular base. The partially polymerized acrylic resin is shaped into a thin square or oblong, placed on the prepared diagnostic cast, pushed to the base outline, thinned out, and trimmed.

After removal of the record bases from their respective diagnostic casts, they should be trimmed and finished with acrylic burs mounted in a low-speed handpiece. The record bases can then be polished by buffing the edges with medium and fine pumice on a wet rag wheel, thereby producing even, rounded surfaces. The tissue-fitting surface of the record bases should be checked with the fingers for the presence of acrylic resin nodules. Nodules should be removed with small round burs (number 4) mounted on a low-speed handpiece.

A thin layer of sticky wax is now applied over the center of the residual ridge areas on the record bases to retain the wax occlusal rims more securely. Depending on the extent of the occlusion rim to be constructed, one half or one quarter of a sheet of baseplate wax must be heated thoroughly over a bunsen burner and folded upon itself to form a 7 to 10 mm thick oblong. The baseplate wax should be heated thoroughly so that it will stick together and not have internal voids as it is folded upon itself. The soft baseplate wax oblong is then compressed over the sticky wax on the record base and shaped to form the occlusal rim. In height, the mandibular occlusion rim should extend from the middle of the retromolar pad to the

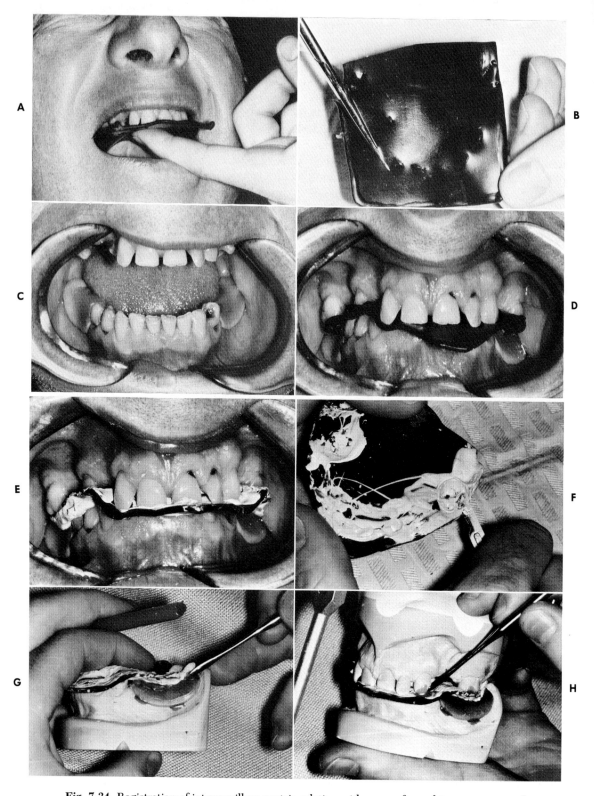

Fig. 7-34. Registration of intermaxillary centric relation with wax wafer and temporary record base. **A,** Softened half sheet of hard wax is placed on maxillary arch. **B,** Wax wafer is trimmed back to buccal cusp tips with scissors. **C,** Mandibular record base in place. **D,** Reheated maxillary wax wafer contacting mandibular record base in centric relation. **E,** "Wash" of zinc oxide–eugenol paste is used to refine intermaxillary centric relation record. **F,** Zinc oxide–eugenol paste is trimmed with sharp scalpel to allow only cusp-tip registration. **G,** Wax wafer and record base are sticky waxed together. Record base had previously been secured to diagnostic cast. **H,** Wax wafer is secured to maxillary cast, which had previously been mounted by use of a face-bow transfer procedure.

marginal ridge of the most anterior remaining tooth. It should be centered over the crest of the residual ridge and be as wide as the natural teeth it replaces, that is, 7 to 10 mm. The baseplate wax on the maxillary record base need only be about 4 mm high posteriorly, and like the mandibular occlusion rim should extend anteriorly to the marginal ridge of the last tooth in the maxillary dental arch. The width of the rim should be the same as that of the mandibular rim, but the maxillary rim should be centered slightly buccal to the residual ridge crest.

Recording centric relation with a single record base and wax wafer (Fig. 7-34)

A single acrylic resin record base and occlusion rim may be used in combination with a wax wafer to record centric relation for a partially edentulous patient. The record base and occlusion rim serves to replace the missing posterior teeth and to provide sufficient contact area for the wax wafer. To accurately mount any diagnostic casts, there must be a sufficient, uniform number of contacts distributed over the entire length of both dental arches to stabilize the diagnostic casts. A record base and occlusion rim in one dental arch temporarily supplies the surface area needed to provide these occlusal contacts.

The procedure used to record centric relation with a single record base and occlusion rim is presented in step-by-step fashion in the following paragraphs.

The single most important step before the recording of centric relation is the verification of the accuracy of the record bases and occlusion rims. Before centric relation is recorded, the record bases must be inspected, both on the diagnostic casts and intraorally. To be clinically acceptable the record bases must: (1) be dimensionally stable on the diagnostic cast, (2) be free of any internal nodules, (3) have borders that are properly extended and contoured to be compatible with the surrounding musculature, and (4) have well-rounded and polished borders. Each record base used to record centric relation must be trial fitted and inspected intraorally for stability, extension, and, in the case of a complete maxillary record base, retention. If the record bases have nodules present, are overextended and displace tissues, or lack sufficient stability and retention, the recording

of centric relation is problematic. Any clinical errors incorporated while recording centric relation will render any of the subsequent RPD procedures useless, since the record will have to be remade using accurate record bases.

The wax occlusion rim on the record base should be heated with an alcohol torch to soften its surface before it is placed in the mouth. The patient is then asked to close the mandible completely to maximum tooth contact (centric occlusion). The teeth in the dental arch opposing the record base and occlusion rim will be forced into the baseplate wax at the vertical dimension of occlusion.

The record base and occlusion rim is then removed, as is the registration of all tooth contacts in the wax rim. This, in effect, places the occlusion rim just barely out of occlusion. To be sure that no occlusal contact with the occlusion rim occurs, the record base should be tried in again. If any occlusal or soft tissue contacts are found, they should be removed.

Two or three shallow notches are then placed into the occlusal rim with a laboratory knife. These notches should diverge occlusally because they will be keyed into the wax wafer.

A wax wafer centric relation record is now made according to the procedure described previously. The zinc oxide–eugenol paste will flow into the wax notches instead of the occlusal surfaces of teeth.

Recording centric relation with opposing record bases and occlusion rims (Fig. 7-35)

Record bases and occlusion rims may also be used together in opposing dental arches to record centric relation. In clinical practice, the mandibular occlusion rim is constructed to a tentative occlusal plane that simulates the naturally occurring plane of occlusion; the maxillary occlusion rim is usually adjusted to the mandibular rim.

The procedure for recording centric relation with opposing record bases and occlusion rims is given in step-by-step fashion in the following paragraphs.

Frequently, some posterior teeth in the maxilla will contact the mandibular occlusion rim constructed to the tentative occlusal plane. The dentist must then adjust the mandibular occlusion rim so that it is just out of contact with the opposing teeth in centric relation. The height

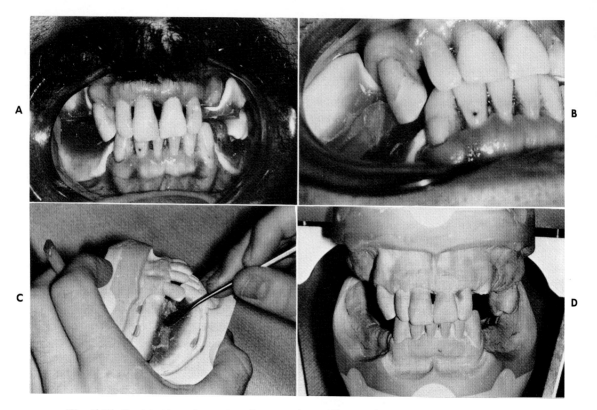

Fig. 7-35. Registration of centric relation with maxillary and mandibular record bases. **A,** Record bases in place. Record bases do not contact at this time. **B,** Intermaxillary registration medium in place. Patient's mandible has been guided to position just before tooth-to-tooth contact. **C,** Record bases are luted together (with sticky wax) after they are luted to cast. **D,** Mounted diagnostic casts.

and contact area of the maxillary occlusion rim are adjusted against the mandibular occlusion rim and any remaining mandibular teeth.

The surface of the maxillary occlusal rim is heated and softened with an alcohol torch. The maxillary record base is inserted, and the patient is asked to close the mandible until the natural teeth touch.

The maxillary occlusal rim is removed, chilled, and trimmed with a laboratory knife so that only slight tooth contacts occur. The mandibular occlusal rim is shallowly notched and returned to the mouth.

At this point the dentist must rehearse the centric relation position with the patient so that a successful registration of this position can be recorded. When both dentist and patient are confident of the position desired, the maxillary record base is returned to the mouth and the patient's mandible is guided into centric relation.

After the rehearsal of centric relation is com-

plete, its actual recording can be made with one of several dental materials. The easiest material to use and one of the most accurate is a zinc oxide–eugenol impression paste. This impression paste should be placed on the occlusal rim that replaces the greatest number of missing teeth. By placing the impression paste on that occlusal rim, the greatest number of contacts with the opposing dental arch will be achieved and the most stable record will be made.

Both occlusion rims must be indexed before centric relation is recorded. The occlusion rim that is to receive the impression paste must have indexes to hold the paste, whereas the opposing occlusion rim should have indexes to key the record bases and occlusion rims together when the diagnostic casts are to be mounted on a dental articulator.

The dentist should first place in the patient's mouth the record base and occlusion rim that replaces the fewest number of teeth. The greatest number of occlusal contacts will be recorded on the occlusion rim that replaces the greatest number of missing teeth. Therefore, this more extensive occlusion rim will receive the recording medium.

A small portion of zinc oxide–eugenol impression paste is mixed and placed on the occlusion rim. The loaded occlusion rim is placed intraorally, and the patient's mandible is guided into centric relation closure.

Once the impression paste has set, the record bases are removed. They can be removed from the mouth separately, but occasionally they will be luted together with the recording medium.

Mounting the diagnostic casts on a dental articulator

After the maxillary cast has been mounted by use of a face-bow transfer procedure, both diagnostic casts should be luted together with sticky wax before the mandibular diagnostic cast is mounted. This is done so that the setting contraction of the laboratory plaster will not alter the relationship of the diagnostic casts to each other. Centric relation records, whether a wax wafer (alone, or in combination with a temporary record base and occlusion rim) or two record bases opposing each other, should be luted to the diagnostic casts and then to each other to form a secure, stable combination that will not be distorted by the setting of the laboratory plaster.

Intermaxillary registration of master casts

The technique for mounting master casts with their respective RPD frameworks is similar to the diagnostic cast mounting procedure. The main difference lies in the relationship—centric relation or centric occlusion—in which the casts are to be mounted.

Adjusting the removable partial denture framework to the existing occlusion

When the master casts are to be mounted in centric occlusion, prematurities on the cast RPD framework must be eliminated in addition to tooth prematurities. The fact that tooth prematurities have been removed does not, of itself, mean that the framework will be without unwanted occlusal contacts that may alter maxillomandibular relations. Warmed articulating

paper or ribbon or occlusal indicator wax may be used to detect these premature contacts on the framework intraorally. The deflective contact can be adjusted, using high-speed instrumentation (diamond or carbide burs) with water either intraorally or extraorally. Burs that are no longer effective for cutting tooth structure may be used. The chromium-cobalt alloy used for the RPD framework is extremely hard and will ruin new burs. The scratch marks left from any adjustments should be smoothed and polished, using rubber finishing wheels graded from coarse to fine. The ultimate objective of these adjustments is to ensure that the natural teeth contact in the same occlusal relationship when the framework is in the mouth as when it is out of the mouth. An RPD framework should not inadvertently alter the occlusal vertical dimension.

Securing the record base and occlusion rim on the removable partial denture framework (Fig. 7-36)

Once the RPD framework has been adjusted, a wax occlusion rim can be secured in the retentive latticework of the framework in the edentulous area. This is done by heating a small amount of baseplate wax over a flame, folding it to form a small rectangle, and then forcing the wax through the retentive latticework onto the master cast. The master cast should have been soaked in slurry water to avoid having the baseplate wax stick to the dental stone. However, the framework should be absolutely dry. As soon as gross shaping of the occlusion rim has been completed with the fingers, the rim can be finished and smoothed with wax instruments. The occlusion rim should extend only as high as the marginal ridges of the teeth adjacent to the edentulous areas and should be no wider than the buccolingual width of these teeth. When the edentulous area is large, the wax occlusion rim should be supported by an acrylic resin record base attached to the cast framework. This will both ensure the stability of the occlusion rim when maxillomandibular records are made and allow the dentist to check the comfort and denture border extensions intraorally.

Making the centric occlusion record

If wax occlusion rims have been placed on the cast framework before the patient arrives,

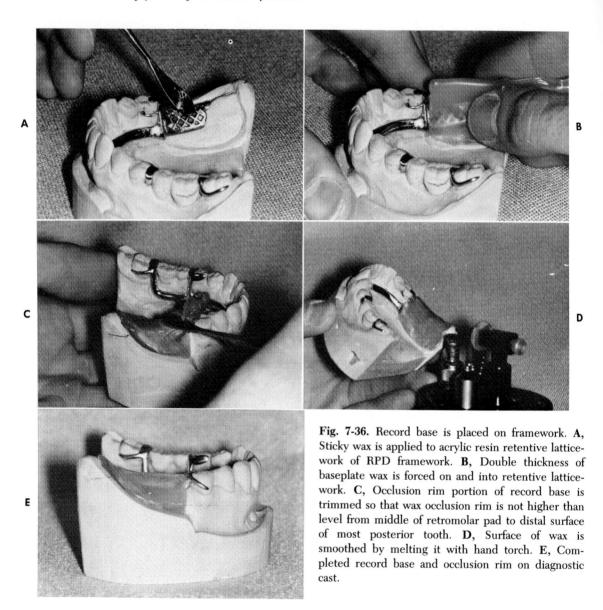

Fig. 7-36. Record base is placed on framework. A, Sticky wax is applied to acrylic resin retentive latticework of RPD framework. B, Double thickness of baseplate wax is forced on and into retentive latticework. C, Occlusion rim portion of record base is trimmed so that wax occlusion rim is not higher than level from middle of retromolar pad to distal surface of most posterior tooth. D, Surface of wax is smoothed by melting it with hand torch. E, Completed record base and occlusion rim on diagnostic cast.

the occlusal surface of the wax should be softened for a few minutes with an alcohol torch. When the wax is soft enough to be easily indented with an instrument, it is inserted intraorally and the patient asked to close the mandible into maximum intercuspation. Occlusal indentations are made into the baseplate wax by the opposing teeth. The framework is removed from the mouth, the wax is chilled, and all occlusal registrations in the wax except for those of the cusp tips are removed with a scalpel. The surface of the wax is again softened, and the framework reinserted intraorally. Similar instructions for closing the mandi-

ble are given to the patient. However, it should be stressed that the dentist must observe the same tooth-to-tooth contact without the framework as with it to ensure that the maximum intercuspal position (centric occlusion) has been achieved.

When two RPDs oppose one another, one of the wax occlusal rims (usually the mandibular) should be indexed by placing V-shaped notches in the wax. This will provide an area for the softer wax on the opposite occlusal rim to flow into. The notches take the place of sulci, so that the softer wax will flow into a keyed area to form a stable record.

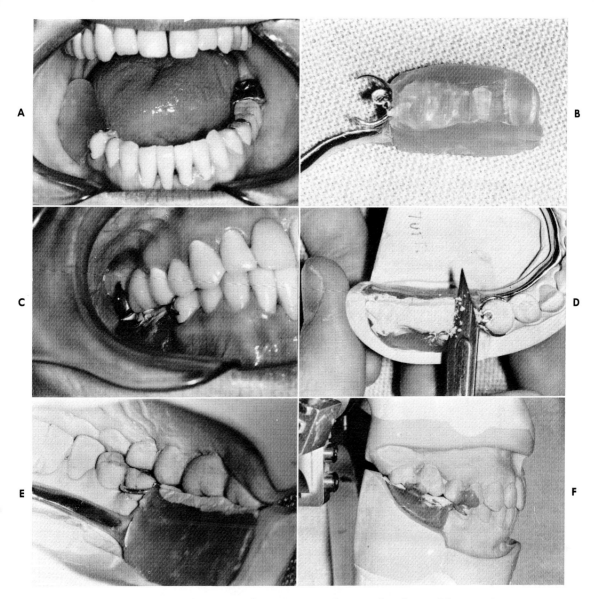

Fig. 7-37. Registration of centric occlusion. **A,** RPD framework and record base in place. **B,** Notched wax occlusion rim. **C,** Zinc oxide–eugenol is used to refine centric occlusion contact. **D,** All contacts except for registration of cusp tips are trimmed away with sharp scalpel. **E,** Casts placed together showing complete seating of maxillary cast into registration. **F,** Mounted casts. All elements are secured with sticky wax.

"Correcting" wax, impression plaster, or zinc oxide–eugenol impression paste should be used to refine the cusp-tip registrations or indexes. Any material that is added, however, should be trimmed away to ensure that only cusp-tip or analogous contact remains (Fig. 7-37).

Making the centric relation record

When master casts are to be mounted in centric relation, one of the several mounting techniques appropriate to the number of remaining teeth can be used. A Kennedy Class III or Class IV RPD mounted in centric relation requires the corrected wax wafer technique. A Kennedy Class II RPD with either a small or no modification space requires the placement of a wax occlusion rim on the cast framework in a manner similar to the wax occlusion rim–wax wafer technique. Record bases and occlusion rims alone frequently can be used for recording a centric relation in Kennedy Class I and many Class II partially edentulous arches, because they will provide a sufficient posterior contact area to stabilize the record even in the absence of anterior tooth contact.

Generally, occlusion rims should be made on wax or acrylic resin record bases that extend to the desired borders of the final RPD. When this is done, the final denture base extension may be checked intraorally for comfort, esthetics, and stability.

All centric relation records, except when a complete maxillary denture opposes a mandibular RPD, must be made at a slightly increased vertical dimension of occlusion so that occlusal contact will not cause a deflection from centric relation to centric occlusion. Frequently, the amount of baseplate wax placed on the framework is excessive. The dentist should trim the wax to the point at which the wax occlusion rim touches the opposing dental arch in such a manner that there is 1 or 2 mm of interocclusal space before any opposing natural teeth occlude (Fig. 7-38).

The occlusal surface of the wax rim can be heated and softened with an alcohol torch, the framework and softened wax inserted intraorally, and the patient's mandible guided to close in centric relation to within 1 or 2 mm before tooth contact. The framework is removed, the wax chilled, and all occlusal surface registrations except for cusp-tip contacts trimmed away with a sharp scalpel. The framework and occlusion rim are reinserted, and the patient's mandible is guided to centric relation closure once again to ensure that the initial wax record was correct. When using this centric relation registration technique, the dentist should "correct" the cusp-tip indentations on the wax occlusion

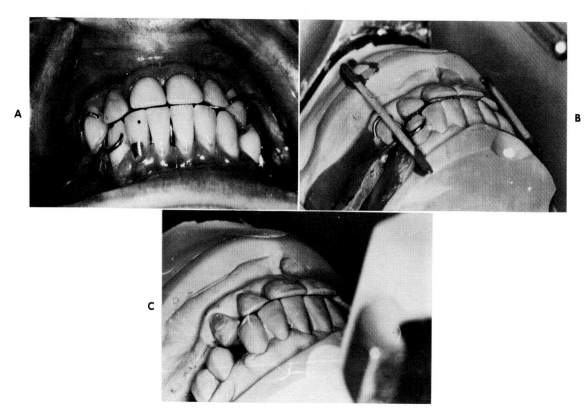

Fig. 7-38. Centric relation recorded at slightly increased vertical dimension of occlusion. **A,** Intraoral registration in place. **B,** Intermaxillary records on diagnostic casts just before mounting. Recording medium is polyether. **C,** Diagnostic casts closed to vertical dimension of occlusion.

rim by using a zinc oxide–eugenol impression paste. A thin layer of impression material (or "wash") is placed on the occlusion rim, the rim is reintroduced intraorally, and the patient's mandible is guided into centric relation. After the material sets, any occlusal surface impression other than those of cusp tips must be trimmed away so that the dental stone casts will seat properly into the record.

When two distal-extension RPDs oppose one another, the unnotched occlusal rim should be trimmed after the initial "soft wax" recording is chilled. To record centric relation, the zinc oxide–eugenol impression paste is then placed on the trimmed unnotched occlusal rim. The dentist must exercise care that the final centric relation record is made just at initial wax contact of the occlusion rims and before occlusal contact of the remaining teeth. A deflective contact on a wax occlusion rim will result in an inaccurate centric relation record, just as a deflective contact would in the natural dentition.

If there are insufficient tooth or wax occlusion rim contacts to ensure a stable centric relation record, then the dentist must use a combination of the wax wafer–record base and occlusion rim technique similar to the technique for mounting diagnostic casts in centric relation.

Making maxillomandibular records for a complete denture opposing a removable partial denture (Fig. 7-39)

When a maxillary complete denture opposes an RPD the maxillomandibular relation recorded by the dentist is always centric relation at an acceptable occlusal vertical dimension. The technique of recording centric relation is similar to the procedure used when two distal-extension RPDs are to be related to each other.

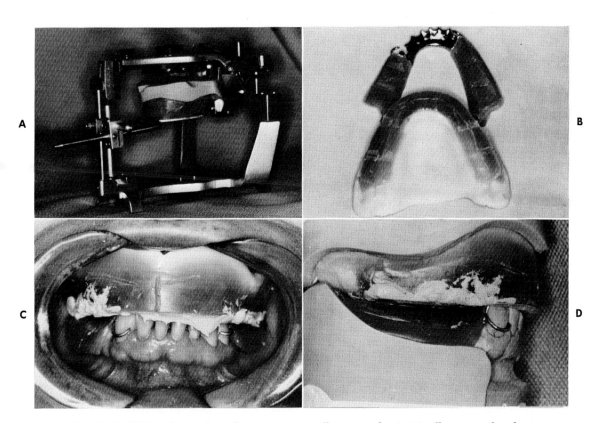

Fig. 7-39. RPD and complete denture intermaxillary records. **A,** Maxillary cast placed on the face-bow registration before mounting on dental articulator. **B,** Record bases are notched (indexed) for receiving recording medium **C,** Zinc oxide–eugenol recording medium in place. **D,** Mounted casts. Registration paste has been trimmed back and rims have been luted together with sticky wax.

The major difference between the two clinical entities is that in the former, the occlusal vertical dimension must be established before the dentist records centric relation. The same procedure is followed as outlined previously when maxillary completely edentulous and mandibular partially edentulous diagnostic casts are mounted.

As in mounting diagnostic casts for diagnosis, the dentist will find it more efficient to adjust the posterior height of the maxillary occlusion rim against the previously determined height of the mandibular occlusion rim. The mandibular occlusion rim is constructed to simulate the height of the proposed posterior occlusal plane and also to be on similar plane as the remaining natural teeth. Thus, because adjustments can be made more easily on the maxillary occlusion rim, adjusting the maxillary rather than mandibular occlusion rim is preferred.

The patient's mandible should be guided by the dentist into the centric relation position during and after the completion of adjustments for the occlusal vertical dimension. When all adjustments are complete, the occlusion rims on both maxilla and mandible should contact simultaneously along their entire length when the patient's mandible is at the established occlusal vertical dimension in centric relation. If there is a premature contact of the occlusion rims in centric relation, it should be removed, preferably from the maxillary rim, and the guided centric relation closure should be repeated. When the occlusion rims have been adjusted for esthetics, phonetics, occlusal vertical dimension, and centric relation, maxillomandibular records can be made. The same prerequisite must be followed for making any centric relation recording; that is, a hinge axis location and face-bow transfer procedure must be performed initially.

Any registration material may be used to record centric relation. An objective in recording centric relation is to complete the relation without disturbing the stability of the record bases. Thus, the material used to record centric relation should be soft enough to prevent displacement of the occlusion rims at first contact but hard enough to withstand distortion when the master casts are mounted on the dental articulator. When centric relation is recorded, the registration medium should be placed on the occlusal surface of the maxillary rim. When the medium is set, there will be multiple contact areas present from both the remaining natural teeth and the RPD wax occlusion rims that will ensure stability during the articulator mounting procedure.

When any occlusion rim is used clinically to record maxillomandibular relations, shallow indexes (notches) are placed in the occlusal surface of the maxillary and mandibular rims. During recording procedures, the mandibular occlusion rim on the RPD framework is always inserted intraorally first. The recording medium is mixed according to manufacturer's specifications and placed on the entire occlusal surface of the maxillary occlusion rim. The maxillary occlusion rim is then inserted, and the patient's mandible is guided into centric relation until even contact of both the mandibular teeth and occlusion rim has occurred with the recording medium just short of wax contact with the occlusion rims. The patient is either asked to maintain this position or is held in this position by the dentist until the recording medium has set. The maxillary occlusion rim and mandibular RPD framework are removed either separately or luted together. To ensure that the master casts are correctly positioned in the recording medium, all material except for cusp-tip contacts or the indexes is cut away with a sharp scalpel. The master cast and occlusion rims are then fitted together and luted in place with sticky wax before the mandibular cast is mounted to the premounted maxillary cast.

Making eccentric maxillomandibular records (protrusive and lateral)

When group function or bilateral balanced occlusion is desired as the occlusal scheme of the prosthesis, recording of protrusive and lateral eccentric movements must be made by the dentist. A number of methods of varying degrees of difficulty using different types of materials have advocated for this purpose. The type of recording material is important in the technique chosen; however, impression plaster, various waxes, or the polyether elastomers are probably the easiest materials to use.

For a protrusive record to accurately reflect the average slope of the superior wall of the glenoid fossa, it must be recorded after the patient's mandible has traveled at least 4 to 6 mm anterior to centric relation (Posselt and Franzen, 1960). This protrusive eccentric movement can usually be approximated when the maxillary and mandibular incisors are in an edge-to-edge relationship. Similarly, a lateral eccentric movement such as that which exists when the incisal or occlusal edges are in contact is desirable when the lateral records are made to ensure that this condylar position is correct.

The techniques for making lateral and protrusive eccentric records are similar to each other and to recording centric relation (Fig. 7-40). The movement must first be rehearsed with the patient so that the desired position can be reproduced. For a protrusive record, the patient should be asked to protrude the mandible until the anterior teeth meet in an edge-to-edge relationship. This position can be achieved readily by having the patient first glide the teeth from centric relation until an incisal edge-to-edge position is reached and then tap the teeth together in this position to create an occlusal awareness of the position. The patient is then asked to close the mandible in maximum intercuspation, open it, and then close it to the incisal edge-to-edge position. The dentist rehearses this sequence of movement with the patient until the desired protrusive position can be found consistently. The right and left lateral eccentric positions are rehearsed in a similar manner to achieve a consistent closure in a lateral edge-to-edge position.

The eccentric record itself is made by placing the recording material on one dental arch and having the patient close the mandible into either the rehearsed protrusive or the right or left lateral eccentric position. The wax wafer method may be used for patients having Kennedy Class III and Class IV partially edentulous arches. For patients with Kennedy Class I or Class II partially edentulous arches, placing impression plaster or injecting a polyether elastomeric impression material on the occlusion rim and adjacent teeth and then directing the patient to close the mandible in the desired position is another acceptable method. This method can produce three eccentric records, a left and right lateral and a protrusive record. The records should be identified to simplify their placement on the master casts when condylar elements on the dental articulator are ad-

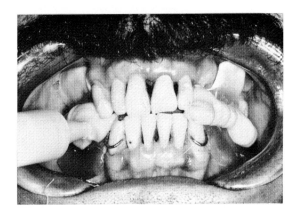

Fig. 7-40. Lateral eccentric records. Polyether material is injected between record bases while patient maintains left lateral position.

justed to these positional records. Adjusting the condylar elements on a dental articulator using these eccentric records should be done by following the specific manufacturer's directions.

Master cast mounting procedure (Fig. 7-41)

In most instances, it is necessary to be able to separate and remove the master cast from its dental articulator mounting. This is necessary for several reasons:

1. When occlusal contacts are created as part of a cast RPD framework, the master cast must be removed from any articulator mounting and sent to a commerial dental laboratory so that it may be duplicated.
2. The occlusion of the finished cast RPD framework must be adjusted to the opposing dental arch on the dental articulator.
3. When the denture base of an RPD is processed with acrylic resin, a small dimensional change invariably occurs that frequently affects planned occlusal contacts. Remounting the master casts on the dental articulator after the prosthesis is processed and correcting the occlusion will eliminate these processing changes.

The armamentarium for completing the mounting procedure includes:

1. Trimmed master cast
2. Laboratory plaster, mixing bowl, and spatula
3. Dental lathe and arbor band or sharp bench knife
4. Petroleum jelly or separating medium

5. Sticky wax or stick compound
6. Number 7 wax spatula
7. Wet-dry medium grit sandpaper
8. Dental articulator
9. Model trimmer

The procedure for mounting the master cast is presented in step-by-step fashion in the following paragraphs.

The technique for making an articulator mounting from which the master cast can be removed and accurately replaced is a simple procedure. The base of the master cast is trimmed flat on a model trimmer. Several widely spaced nonundercut keys or indexes are placed at the junction of the base and sides of the master cast, using either a sharp bench knife or an arbor band mounted on a dental lathe.

The master cast base and keys are then coated with a *very* thin layer of petroleum jelly or similar type of separating medium.

The master cast is attached with sticky wax to the opposing master cast; if the maxillary cast is being mounted first, it is placed in the record face-bow.

A properly proportioned mix of .laboratory plaster (100 g to 30 ml of water) is mixed in a flexible bowl and applied evenly over the base of the master cast and into the keys. Some laboratory plaster should also be placed on the mounting ring of the dental articulator before the dental articulator is closed onto the master cast. The articulator is closed, and any excess laboratory plaster that extends laterally or onto the side of the master cast should be removed before it sets.

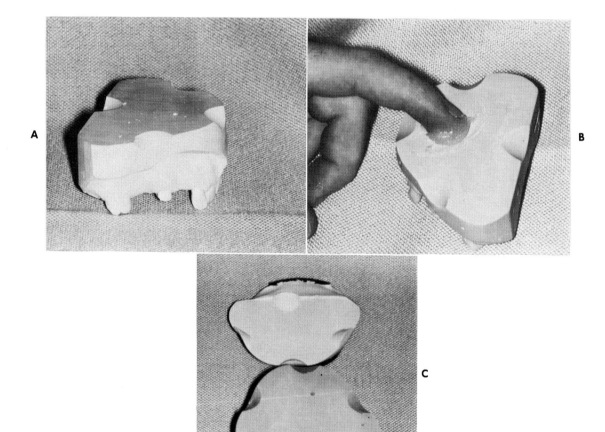

Fig. 7-41. Master cast mounting procedures. **A,** Base of master cast is made flat, smooth, and parallel to occlusal plane. Divergent notches are formed with arbor band. **B,** Thin layer of petroleum jelly is applied to master cast. **C,** Master cast is separated from plaster mounting.

After the laboratory plaster has completely set, any small excess that remains on the side of the master cast must be removed with a laboratory knife so that no laboratory plaster flash remains. If a lip of material remains, it could fracture when the master cast is removed and destroy the accuracy of the articulator mounting. In such a case, the dentist would find it difficult to determine that the master cast was replaced on its articulator mounting in exactly its original position. When the excess flash has been removed, both the master cast and laboratory mounting can be smoothed with water-resistant sandpaper.

Because the master cast lacks mechanical undercuts to hold it securely on its articulator mounting, it must be secured by another means. A small amount of stick compound or sticky wax should be placed at the junction of the dry master cast and the articulator mounting at three or four points. This material will secure the master cast onto the articulator mounting.

Selection of prosthetic replacement teeth

The selection of replacement teeth for an RPD is determined by several factors: (1) the materials against which the denture teeth are to function, (2) the occlusal scheme to be developed, (3) esthetics, and (4) anatomic considerations.

Dental material considerations (Table 7-1)

A factor limiting the useful life of any prosthesis is the wear of both prosthetic teeth and the opposing occlusal surfaces, whether natural or artificial. Dental gold alloys have been found to be the most desirable material to use when the prosthetic teeth are opposed by natural enamel surfaces or other gold surfaces (Mahalick and associates, 1971). Dental porcelain denture teeth become very abrasive after their surface glaze has been lost and can cause considerable wear to any opposing occlusal surface, whether it be a gold alloy, acrylic resin, tooth enamel, or porcelain-fused-to-metal restoration. Acrylic resin denture teeth exhibit considerable occlusal wear in time regardless of the opposing material. However, acrylic resin denture teeth tend to wear opposing materials and dentition least of all. From a practical standpoint, acrylic resin denture teeth are much easier to modify, arrange, and adjust after processing or relining of the RPD. Cast gold occlusal surfaces (or an alloy similar in hardness) are ideal in most situations but are costly and require extra laboratory procedures. Dental porcelain prosthetic teeth opposing dental porcelain prosthetic teeth are acceptable, but in practicality as well as long-term preservation of the opposing occlusal surfaces, acrylic resin denture teeth should be considered the dental material of choice.

Occlusal considerations

When an RPD is to oppose remaining natural teeth or an existing fixed partial denture, the selection of the size and shape of the occlusal surface of the denture tooth and occlusal scheme depends on the size, shape, and posi-

TABLE 7-1
Dental materials selection for replacement denture teeth

	Removable partial denture	
Opposing dental arch	**Primary choice**	**Secondary choice**
Natural dentition (unrestored)	Dental gold alloy	Acrylic resin
Natural dentition or fixed partial dentures	Dental gold alloy	Acrylic resin
Natural dentition or dental porcelain occlusal fixed partial dentures	Acrylic resin	—
Natural dentition with an RPD	Acrylic resin	—
Complete denture with acrylic resin denture teeth	Acrylic resin	—
Complete denture with dental porcelain denture teeth	Dental porcelain	—

tion of the opposing occlusal surfaces. Specifically, the amount of occlusal wear exhibited on the remaining natural teeth will aid in the selection of the cuspal inclination of the replacement teeth. If the existing occlusal surfaces have deep anatomic features and little occlusal wear then anatomic denture teeth with 30° or 33° cuspal inclinations are indicated. Conversely, if the remaining natural teeth are markedly worn, then a replacement tooth with a shallow cuspal inclination or even no cuspal inclines is indicated. The width of the prosthetic occlusal table should roughly coincide with or be narrower than the width of the opposing occlusal surfaces. Other factors, such as the number of replacement denture teeth and the quantity and quality of the residual ridges, have a bearing on the number and width of the replacement teeth, since they affect the load applied by the RPD. There need not be absolute similarity in either width or cuspal inclination of the denture teeth on an RPD. With virtually all RPDs, the occlusal surface morphologic features of the replacement teeth must be individually adjusted to assure a uniform and proper occlusal contact with the existing dentition. In general, replacement denture teeth are manufactured for complete denture occlusions that, essentially, are made with specific requirements as to the compensating curves (0°, 20°, 30°, or 33°) and the arrangement of the teeth anteroposteriorly. It is infrequent that the occlusal surfaces of a manufacturer's denture teeth will coincidently occlude adequately with a natural dentition that has developed specific wear patterns over the years.

When an RPD opposes another prosthesis, whether it be a complete denture or another RPD, the greatest single determining factor for occlusal morphologic features of the replacement teeth depends on the type of occlusal scheme to be developed (that is, bilateral balanced, nonbalanced, or group function) on the prostheses. If a nonbalanced (monoplane) occlusion is planned for a complete denture, then the denture teeth on the RPD would be monoplane (0°). To develop an occlusal scheme on a complete denture that is bilaterally balanced, the dentist must use anatomic denture teeth (20°, 30°, or 33°). If an occlusion is to be developed on opposing RPDs, whether it is group function or centric contacts only, the cuspal

morphologic features, length, and inclination of the remaining dentition should also be considered when the occlusal morphologic features of the replacement teeth are chosen. If a group function occlusion is desired, steep cuspal inclination of the natural dentition will demand steep cuspal inclination of the artifical dentition in order to achieve harmonious and uniform contacts within the functional range. When canine guidance or anterior disclusion is present, any type of anatomic denture tooth may be used, because any eccentric lateral contacts inadvertently produced can be removed by selective grinding in the final prosthesis. See Table 7-2 for a guide to factors that determine the selection of posterior denture teeth.

Esthetic considerations

Esthetic considerations are as important as occlusal considerations in the selection of replacement denture teeth for an RPD. Not only are the maxillary six anterior teeth esthetically important when the patient smiles or talks, but in many patients the first premolars are also visible. In some patients with a broad smile the entire length and breadth of the dental arch from first molar to first molar are noticeable. Therefore, the facial and occlusal shape, occlusogingival length, and shade, as they blend and harmonize with the natural dentition, are three important criteria to be used in the selection of replacement denture teeth for esthetics. The dentist must select a denture tooth that has a similar facial shape to the remaining dentition. Of equal importance, however, is its occlusogingival length. The most natural appearance of an RPD is achieved when a uniform relationship exists between the level of both the gingival sulcus and the cusp tips of the remaining and replacement teeth. The length of the replacement teeth should be similar to the length of the remaining teeth to avoid creation of a stepped relationship between the adjacent natural and artificial dentition. A common esthetic failure usually occurs when an excessively short maxillary premolar is selected adjacent to a natural canine or when that premolar has a flat occlusal table (monoplane tooth).

Anatomic considerations

An additional consideration in setting replacement denture teeth for an RPD is the ef-

TABLE 7-2
Factors that determine the selection of posterior denture teeth

Factors	Anatomic teeth (20° to 33°)	Nonanatomic teeth (0°)
1. Age	Young	Old
2. Health	Good	Poor
3. Residual ridges	Good	Poor
4. Mandibular movements	Coordinated	Uncoordinated, inconsistent movements (Class II, Division 1)
5. Opposing natural dentition	Well preserved, steep cuspal inclines	Poorly preserved, shallow cuspal inclines, severe abrasion
6. Horizontal and vertical overlap	Little vertical overlap little or no horizontal overlap (Class II, Division 2)	Large horizontal overlap little or no vertical overlap (Class II, Division 1)
7. TMJ function	Normal	Abnormal
8. Occlusal scheme	Balanced occlusion	Nonbalanced occlusion
9. Existing artificial dentition	Patient habituated to 20° to 30° teeth	Patient habituated to 0° teeth
10. Better masticatory efficiency	Psychologic and actual	
11. Esthetics	Cusp teeth more pleasing (especially to younger patients)	
12. Residual ridge resorption	Patient more prone to return for treatment because of precise tooth interdigitation	
13. Temporary treatment denture		When changing vertical dimension, centric relation, or occlusal scheme
14. Parafunctional habits		Clenching or grinding, habitual eccentric position
15. Neuromuscular disturbances		Parkinsonism, Bell's palsy, etc.
16. Potential for ridge reduction		Periodontosis, immediate replacement, diabetes, etc.
17. Size discrepancies between the two arches		Necessitates "crossbite"
18. Excisive surgery		Condylectomies, partial mandibulectomy

fect of existing anatomic relationships. The choice of material and length of a denture tooth is also affected by intermaxillary distance, shape of the residual ridges, and structural elements of the RPD framework that will influence the space available for the denture teeth. When space is limited by any of the above factors the material composition of the denture teeth may be limited to acrylic resin. Dental porcelain cannot be modified gingivally to any great extent without removing the mechanical lock (diatoric hole) necessary to bond the denture tooth to the acrylic resin of the RPD. The occlusogingival denture tooth length will be influenced by reduced interarch distance or full and bulging residual ridges. When the patient has these anatomic constraints the dentist may be able to use only an acrylic resin denture tooth as a replacement when developing an occlusal scheme for an RPD.

Arrangement of replacement denture teeth
(Fig. 7-42)

Any technique used to arrange and set the denture teeth requires the appropriate armamentarium, which includes:

1. Selected denture teeth
2. Bunsen burner
3. Alcohol torch
4. Number 2 lead pencil
5. Denture adjustment burs
6. Sticky wax and periphery wax
7. Denture set-up and baseplate wax
8. Articulating paper

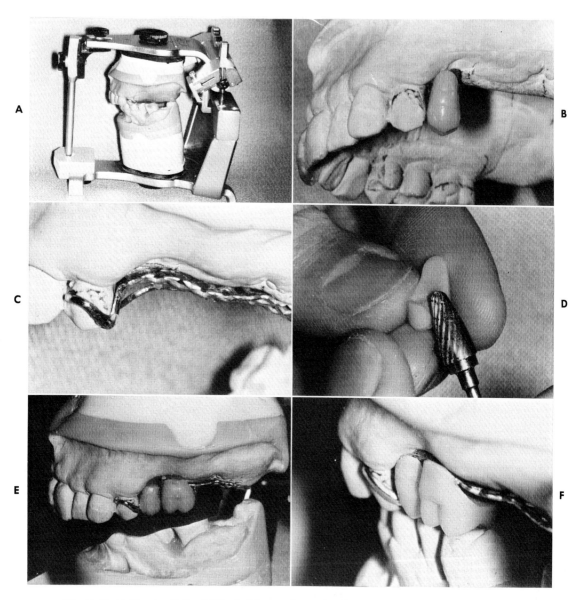

Fig. 7-42. Setting teeth for RPD. **A,** Mounted master cast. **B,** Approximately sized replacement denture tooth is positioned on master cast. **C,** Clasp and minor connector on abutment tooth. Denture tooth must be modified on ridge lap and mesial surface so that it may be in proper contact with abutment tooth mesiodistally and buccolingually. **D,** Modification of mesial surface of replacement tooth with acrylic bur. **E,** Denture premolar and molar arranged in proper esthetic alignment. **F,** The proper labiopalatal placement of molar in relation to opposing dentition.

9. Number 7 and number 31 wax spatulas
10. Low-speed dental handpiece
11. Polishing equipment for acrylic resin and dental porcelain
12. Ward's carver
13. Articulated master casts and RPD framework

The procedure used in arranging and setting denture teeth is presented in step-by-step fashion in the following paragraphs.

Initially, the dentist should arrange the anterior denture teeth with estetics in mind regardless of whether the RPD is to occlude with another prosthesis or an existing occlusion. If, after this is completed, the denture teeth need be moved for functional reasons, they can be shifted labially or lingually.

The posterior wax occlusion rim should be completely removed before the denture teeth are arranged. A very thin strip of soft periphery wax can be placed along the middle of the framework to hold the denture teeth in position while they are initially arranged. The softness of this wax allows the replacement denture teeth to be altered easily. In general, mandibular denture teeth are arranged first when replacement teeth for opposing prostheses are provided.

For esthetic placement, the first denture tooth to arrange is the tooth next to the most anterior remaining natural tooth. Most often the ridge lap area, the mesial surface, or both areas of this tooth must be hollow ground to allow for its proper placement around the minor connector or clasp of the framework. The areas of the tooth to be removed should be marked with a number 2 lead pencil before any reduction is begun. Overreduction of these areas is a common mistake that can be avoided by marking the position that the minor connec-

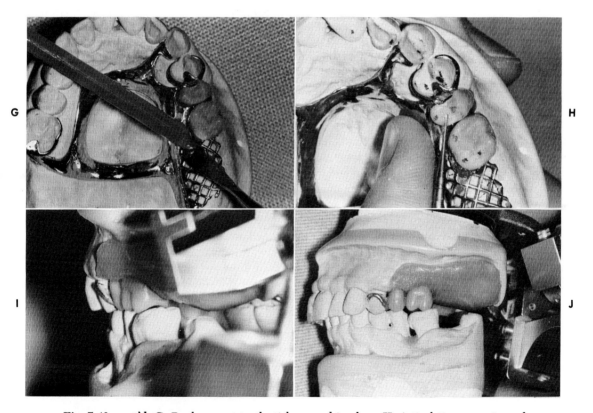

Fig. 7-42, cont'd. G, Replacement teeth sticky waxed in place. **H,** Articulating paper is used to locate initial "high" occlusal contacts, which are then modified to ensure proper occlusal contacts. **I,** Proper occlusal relationships of replacement denture and natural teeth. **J,** Finished set-up and wax-up of RPD.

tors take on the denture tooth and then reducing only this area. The placement of this first denture tooth is critical to esthetics and arch symmetry in both its gingival–cusp-tip alignment and it buccolingual alignment. The use of peripheral vision in viewing the master cast anteriorly will reveal any esthetic disharmony in its buccolingual and occlusogingival placement. By focusing on the dental midline, obvious buccolingual problems will be detected by "the corner of the eye." Similar esthetic errors in a superior-inferior direction are also detected by focusing on one of the natural anterior teeth while looking laterally at the occlusal curve.

When the first denture tooth is properly placed for esthetics, the remaining prosthetic teeth are arranged in periphery wax so that the occlusal curve approximates that of the opposing dental arch and the cusp tips are fairly well aligned within the opposing occlusal fossa. All of the replacement teeth are then secured firmly in place with sticky wax. Sticky wax is used to prevent the denture teeth from being moved when the occlusal surfaces are reshaped by selective grinding to create the desired occlusal articulation.

Thin articulating paper is used to identify the initial denture tooth contacts. Adjustment of these contacts with an appropriate round bur, usually a number 4 or 6 bur mounted in a straight handpiece, is continued until the denture teeth and remaining dentition in the same arch contact simultaneously with the opposing dentition. The occlusal surfaces of the denture teeth should be modified so that they enhance the stability of the denture without unduly destroying the occlusal anatomic features. Preferably, maxillary denture teeth should have the majority of their contacts on the lingual cusp tips so that the forces of occlusion will be concentrated and directed toward the midline. Centric occlusal contacts in the central fossa of the denture can also be created, but this should be done in conjunction with creation of lingual cusp tip contacts. Any contacts buccal to the central fossa will be on inclined planes and should be avoided. Similarly central fossa contacts on the mandibular denture teeth will tend to stabilize the RPD by concentrating forces nearer the midline of the residual ridge. Buccal cusp tip contacts in centric occlusion may be developed but only if there are corresponding fossa contacts and bilateral balanced

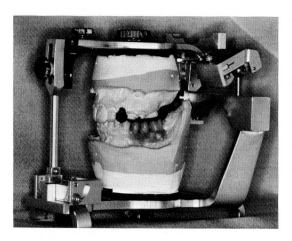

Fig. 7-43. Diagnostic wax-up is made to proper plane of occlusion.

occlusion is desired. Occasionally, because of large occlusal surface morphologic features on the remaining dentition, it may be necessary to develop a flat surface on the buccal or lingual inclines or cusp tips of the denture teeth in order to accept an opposing centric cusp tip. When necessary this is acceptable, but whenever possible the natural teeth should be reshaped to narrow their occlusal table, or the denture teeth should be moved bucally or lingually slightly to achieve a cusp tip to central fossa contact. This small amount of reshaping of a natural tooth rarely causes sensitivity and the slight buccal or lingual movement of the denture tooth is not likely to greatly disturb esthetics. The final goal of centric occlusal contact should be the establishment of point contacts on the denture teeth rather than large, broad areas of occlusal contact.

Group function contacts against an existing dentition are somewhat more difficult to achieve. If they are desired, care must be taken to modify the existing occlusal surfaces so that lateral contacts may also be developed. "Picket fence" occlusal planes must be evened out, and broad flat surfaces on teeth should be adjusted to allow for the proper inclined-plane contacts. Waxing-in the replacement teeth on the diagnostic cast and modifying the opposing dentition on the dental stone cast is an excellent way to determine what changes will be necessary in the opposing dentition before actual treatment is initiated (Fig. 7-43).

To develop a group function occlusion (Fig. 7-44) for opposing RPDs, the dentist must first select the proper replacement denture teeth.

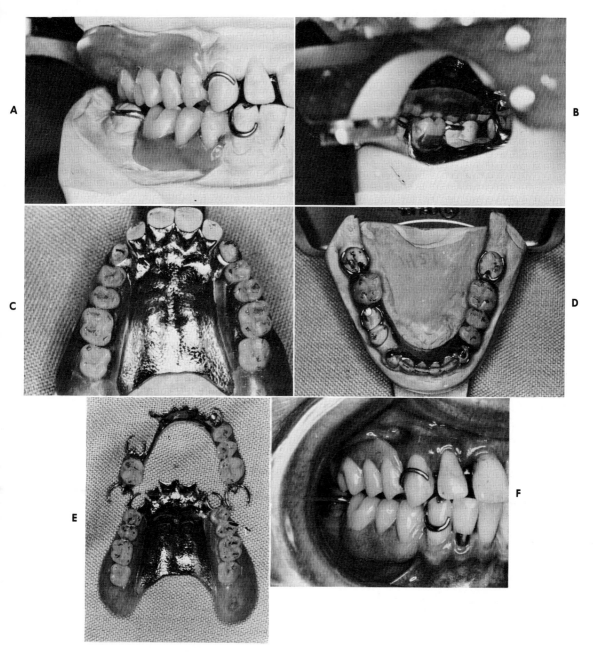

Fig. 7-44. Posterior group function set-up. **A,** Maxillary right first molar and first and second premolars are arranged in group function type of contact with mandibular first molar and premolar. **B,** Maxillary lingual cusps are arranged in central fossae of mandibular teeth. **C,** Group function contacts on maxillary teeth are registered with articulating paper. **D,** Group function contacts on mandibular teeth are registered with articulating paper. **E,** Occlusal contacts on completed RPDs. **F,** Patient in right lateral movement displaying group function contact.

The cusp length and angulation of the denture teeth should have a form similar to that of the remaining dentition. When the denture teeth are arranged, they must be aligned so that the buccal inclines of the buccal cusps of mandibular posterior denture teeth contact the lingual inclines of the maxillary posterior denture teeth in lateral excursions. A hinge axis location and face-bow transfer procedure and centric and eccentric records (protrusive and right and left lateral) are prerequisites for the development of these contacts. A face-bow transfer procedure will provide the correct anteroposterior position of the master casts on the dental articulator so that the arc of rotation on the dental articulator carries the mandibular inclines along the maxillary inclines to coincide with the patient's mandibular movements. The correct condylar inclinations (as determined by the protrusive record) are particularly important if group function contacts are to be developed.

Because most anatomic denture teeth are designed to function with a group function, or a bilaterally balanced occlusal scheme, arranging them for lateral eccentric contacts is not usually difficult. However, these denture teeth are manufactured to function in such a manner that they must be aligned against each other in one specific way. Esthetics and available maxillomandibular space sometimes make this "ideal" tooth arrangement impossible. Then, the dentist must modify the occlusal surfaces of these replacement teeth to achieve the desired goal.

The final denture tooth occlusal contacts should resemble broad lines radiating from the central fossa out onto the lingual inclines of the buccal cusps. The occlusal contacts should not extend the entire way to the buccal cusp tips. Two to 3 mm of occlusal contact should be sufficient to provide the desired group function. A small area of mandibular tooth contact should be seen on the buccal surface just below the buccal cusp tip.

Any balancing side contacts should be eliminated in a group function occlusion to prevent excessive rotational forces on the RPD that will be ultimately transferred to the teeth and supporting tissues. This should be accomplished without eliminating any centric occlusal contacts of the maxillary lingual cusps in the central fossa of the mandibular denture teeth.

A complete maxillary denture opposing a mandibular RPD is one of the most common types of prosthodontic treatment encountered by the dental practitioner because of the chronology of tooth loss. The occlusal scheme developed for this prosthodontic combination falls into two broad categories: (1) a nonbalanced (unilaterally balanced) or (2) a bilaterally balanced occlusion. The bilaterally balanced occlusal scheme is developed by the use of all the variables of complete denture occlusion. This concept is analogous to some occlusions found in natural dentition. The plane of occlusion is curved, both anteroposteriorly and mediolaterally, there is a cusp fossa or cusp-marginal relationship of the opposing dentition, and there are occlusal contacts developed in all eccentric movements. However, there the comparisons and similarities end. The basis of this concept is the belief that simultaneous bilateral cross arch and cross tooth balance help stabilize the maxillary complete denture during functional and parafunctional movements of the mandible.

A nonbalanced (unilateral) occlusal scheme using monoplane denture teeth departs considerably from the traditional concept of bilaterally balanced occlusion. In this concept, the plane of occlusion is flat. No compensating curves are incorporated into the denture tooth arrangement to achieve balanced occlusion. Therefore, in protrusive and lateral eccentric mandibular movements, only one side of the dental arch will contact; thus the term *unilateral balance*. Of course, there is no actual balance except in centric relation. A broad objective is to produce a totally noninterfering occlusion in all eccentric mandibular movements. Proponents of this occlusal scheme believe that it is not necessarily occlusal balance during parafunctional movements but stability during chewing, speaking, and other functional movements that determines the success of the prosthesis.

Monoplane occlusal scheme (neutrocentric occlusion or unilateral balance) (Fig. 7-45)

Arranging denture teeth for either a bilaterally balanced occlusal scheme or a monoplane occlusion (unilateral balance) is relatively straightforward. The first procedure to be performed is the establishment of the occlusal plane by bisecting the interridge distance or, if

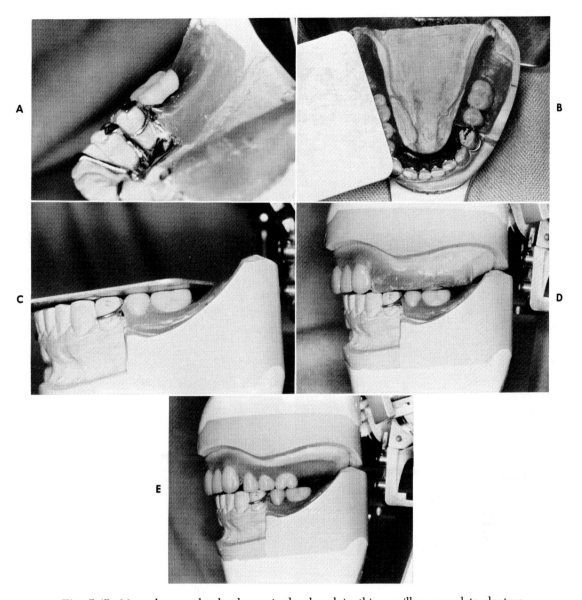

Fig. 7-45. Monoplane occlusal scheme is developed in this maxillary complete denture against RPD. **A,** Nonanatomic molar is placed against minor connector. **B,** Central fossae of mandibular teeth are arranged so that they approximate line drawn along crest of residual ridge. **C,** Cusp tips of monoplane denture teeth aligned against 0° occlusal template.* **D,** Maxillary occlusal rim in place to occlude with established mandibular plane of occlusion. **E,** Completed monoplane occlusal scheme set-up.

---

*Dentsply International, York, Pa.

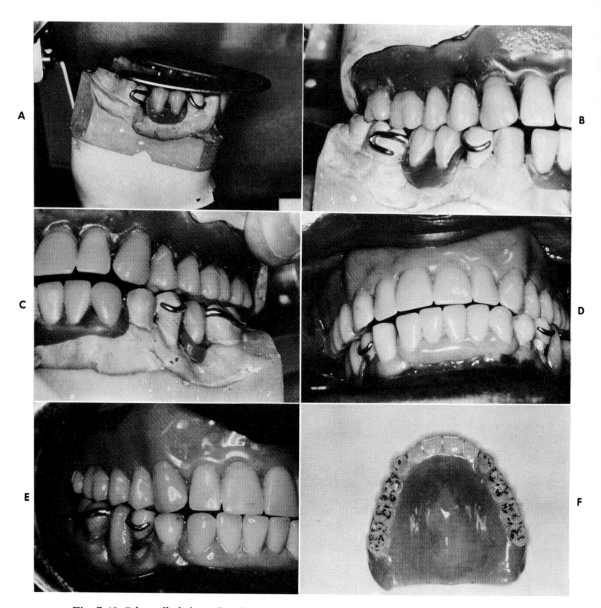

Fig. 7-46. Bilaterally balanced occlusion. **A,** A 20° occlusal template* used to set mandibular denture teeth. **B,** Right working-side contacts. **C,** Corresponding left balancing-side contacts. **D,** Mandibular RPD exhibiting left working-side and right balancing-side contacts. **E,** Protrusive contacts. Note balancing-side contacts posteriorly when patient is in protrusive contact. **F,** Patient made lateral eccentric movements, which were recorded with articulating paper on maxillary complete denture.

*Dentsply International, York, Pa.

that is excessively high in relation to mandibular arch landmarks, lowering it to create an occlusal plane parallel and favorable to the mandibular arch. When a maxillary complete denture opposes a mandibular RPD, this is usually accomplished by setting the mandibular posterior denture teeth on a flat occlusal plane that extends from the middle of the retromolar pad to the distal portion of the remaining natural anterior teeth. This plane will usually be nearly parallel to the mandibular residual ridge. The posterior replacement denture teeth are kept above or slightly lingual to the crest of the residual ridge. The maxillary posterior denture teeth are then set to this mandibular occlusal plane so that the mandibular anterior teeth do not interfere with the maxillary anterior teeth in centric or eccentric movements.

Bilaterally balanced occlusions (Fig. 7-46)

When maxillary denture teeth are set for a bilaterally balanced occlusal scheme, there are two ways of arranging the maxillary denture teeth to the mandibular natural and RPD dental arch.

When the mandibular RPD teeth are first arranged, they are initially modified to conform to the occlusal morphologic features of the remaining natural teeth. For example, if the natural teeth exhibit marked occlusal wear, then the denture teeth should be similarly modified (or a tooth of similar size and cuspal inclination should be selected). The maxillary posterior denture teeth are then arranged in an inclined-plane–to–inclined-plane relationship to achieve point rather than large broad contacts. This will minimize lateral forces placed on the maxillary complete denture and allow cross tooth as well as cross arch balance in eccentric movements after proper occlusal adjustments are made.

A bilaterally balanced occlusal scheme may also be arranged to a cusp-fossa relationship. This type of occlusal relationship is most commonly used when the majority of the posterior teeth in one dental arch are to be replaced with an RPD denture and the decision has been made that a nonbalanced monoplane occlusal scheme is not appropriate.

The mandibular denture teeth should be arranged to an even curve, using a curved template as a guide. Then the maxillary teeth should be arranged in a cusp-to-fossa occlusion

so that the lingual cusps of the maxillary teeth occlude in the central fossa of the mandibular teeth and the buccal cusps of the mandibular teeth occlude in the central fossa of the maxillary teeth. Balancing the occlusion requires interpreting and understanding the Hanau Quint—condylar inclination, compensating curve, incisal guidance, cusp angulation, and plane of orientation—so that the inclines of the cusps of the posterior denture teeth meet simultaneously in all eccentric movements from centric relation (Hanau, 1926). This sometimes requires changing the initially established compensating curve, mediolateral axial inclinations, or both features of the denture teeth several times to achieve balanced occlusion.

Anterior denture tooth position

The position of the maxillary anterior teeth is dictated by esthetics and phonetics, but regardless of the posterior occlusal scheme a deep vertical overlap should be avoided if possible. If it is esthetically necessary to arrange the anterior denture teeth with a deep vertical overlap, it is sound prosthodontic practice to incorporate a 2-to-4 mm horizontal overlap to prevent the "anterior hyperfunction syndrome" (Saunders and associates, 1979) and "tripping" of the complete denture (Fig. 7-47). Most pa-

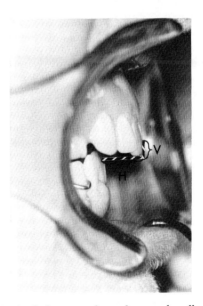

Fig. 7-47. Slight vertical overlap can be allowed if sufficient horizontal overlap of anterior denture teeth can be developed to prevent anterior "tripping" of denture in protrusive movement of mandible. *V,* Vertical overlap; *H,* horizontal overlap.

tients with a large anterior vertical overlap in their natural dentition have had a restriction of large excursive mandibular movements and have become conditioned to a narrow chewing stroke. These patients must be cautioned to avoid mandibular movements that will unseat the maxillary complete denture. They should be advised to incise their food in the premolar rather than incisor areas and to masticate using a vertical motion rather than a lateral grinding, or milling, movement.

Contouring of the removable partial denture base (Fig. 7-48)

The dentist who takes a narrow view of stress distribution might maintain that the denture base serves only to retain the denture teeth on the framework of the RPD. However, the tissue surface of the denture base plays a major role in gaining intraoral support for the prosthesis. The polished surface contour likewise serves to enhance esthetics, provide patient comfort, and aid in resisting the dislodging forces applied to the RPD. Development of both the polished and tissue surfaces, particularly of a distal-extension RPD, requires thought, examination, and care (see Chapter 6).

There are a few simple, general rules for creating the polished surface contour of an RPD. First, the surfaces must be smooth so that they do not aid dental plaque retention. Second, they should simulate, whenever possible, the anatomic features of the tissues that were lost to preserve lip and cheek support for function and esthetics. Third, they must be at least 2 mm in overall thickness for strength with minimum bulk. Fourth, the borders should be 3 to 5 mm thick and well rounded to provide comfort. Thin, knife-edge denture borders should be avoided because they will tend to traumatize both the hard and soft tissues and to fracture more easily.

The armamentarium used in contouring RPD bases includes:

1. Baseplate wax and set-up wax
2. Bunsen burner
3. Alcohol torch
4. Number 7 and number 31 wax spatulas
5. Soft-bristle toothbrush
6. Hard-bristle toothbrush
7. Paper towel
8. Nylon stocking
9. Ward's carver
10. Wax solvent
11. Cotton swabs
12. Flexible plastic sheet (0.001 inch)

The procedure used to recontour RPD bases is presented in step-by-step fashion in the following paragraphs.

To complete the wax-up of the polished surface contour of an RPD, about one quarter of a sheet of baseplate wax is all that is usually needed. Initially, it is heated over the bunsen burner. It is then folded over on itself to form a double thickness about 1.5 cm in width. The still-soft, double-thick rectangle of baseplate wax is placed on the buccal and lingual surface of the master cast in the area of the denture base. The soft wax should extend into the embrasures and onto the facial and lingual surfaces of the denture teeth for about half their length. The bulk of the baseplate wax is now placed, and only a wax-subtraction technique is required to complete the final form of the denture base.

A sharp-ended wax instrument such as a Ward's carver is used to roughly cut the wax from around the gingival margin of the denture teeth. The esthetic length of the denture tooth is established at this point, so care should be taken to remove an amount of wax that is approximately equal to the length of any remaining natural teeth. Using the rounded end of the number 7 spatula, the dentist places a roughly scalloped indentation in the wax about 1 to 2 mm above the crest of the recently established gingiva. This will form the slight depression below the marginal gingiva. Other anatomic concavities, such as the depressions between roots or on either side of the canines can also be roughly delineated with the same instrument if desired.

At this point, the gross removal of excess wax has been accomplished and the rough outlines of the final denture base contours should be discernable. The sharp edges of the sculptured outline are smoothed over and rounded off with a soft-bristle toothbrush. A quick but gentle upward stroke from the replacement teeth toward the buccal sulcus removes any sharp edges from the gingival crest. The same quick, gentle brushing motion (but in different directions) can be used to reduce the sharpness of other areas.

The still-soft wax should be chilled to harden

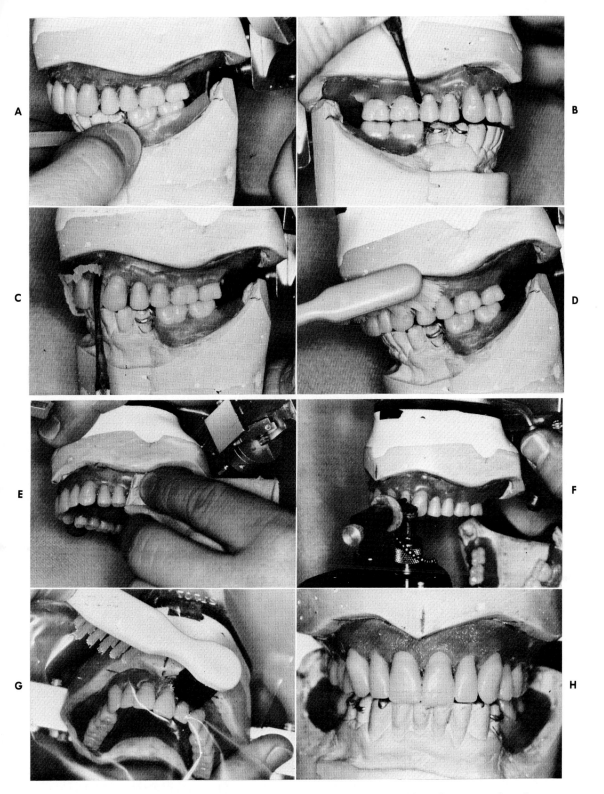

Fig. 7-48. Denture base wax-up. **A,** Narrow, double-thick sheet of baseplate wax is forced between and onto buccal surface of denture teeth. **B,** Gingival and interproximal contours of wax base are established. **C,** Wax is "scalloped" below gingival crest. **D,** All sharp edges of wax are removed with soft toothbrush. **E,** Rounded-off wax is smoothed with paper towel. **F,** Surface of wax is flamed lightly with hand torch to further smooth wax surface. **G,** Stippling, if desired, is placed in wax by tapping it with hard-bristle brush through sheet of plastic. **H,** Completed wax-up. (Length of denture teeth mimics length of remaining natural teeth. Soft-tissue contours are established for labial support.) Usually, gingival papilla should cover collars of teeth and fill interproximal spaces to prevent food impaction and aid in cleaning of RPD.

it. Chilling the wax makes it easier to smooth away any remaining roughness but still retain the basic carved form. A paper towel is used for this smoothing. It can be folded so that pointed ends may be formed to smooth wax around the gingival crest and around any small depressions that are hard to reach. The surface scratches placed by the bristles of the brush are likewise "sandpapered" away, using the flat surface of the towel.

These carving and smoothing procedures will invariably result in the deposition of a thin layer of wax over the denture teeth. This should be carefully removed with wax instruments and finally with a wax solvent on cotton swabs.

If gingival stippling is desired for a more natural-appearing denture base, it should be placed at this time. A sheet of the thin flexible plastic (0.001 inch) used in trial packing dentures is placed over the waxed surface. A hard-bristle toothbrush is used in a tapping motion to indent the wax through the plastic sheet to form small, closely packed indentations in the wax that simulate gingival stippling.

Finally, the wax surface should be highly polished. When the surface of the wax is polished, the processed acrylic resin will be smooth and will only need buffing with a finishing agent. Polishing the wax means removing all scratches, however small. Melting the thin surface skin of the wax with an alcohol torch will achieve this goal. The torch should be kept at a distance from the wax surface and swept rapidly back and forth. It is only a very thin surface layer of wax that need be melted to remove all the scratches. If the wax is melted too deeply it will run, and all anatomic carving will be destroyed.

After the desired finishing of the surface has been carefully done with the alcohol torch, the wax should be chilled and given a final polish using a nylon stocking.

It must be remembered that any heat applied to the wax may cause shifting of the position of the replacement teeth. If these have been held in place with a wax such as sticky wax that is higher in fusing temperature than the baseplate wax, any shifting will be minimized. Also, the labial and lingual surfaces should not be flamed at the same time. In any event, all occlusal contacts should be doubled

checked at this time, and any discrepancies should be corrected.

In preparation for flasking and processing, the baseplate wax must be sealed completely around the metal framework and the border of the denture base must be sealed to the master cast. All wax inadvertently left on the surface of the denture teeth must be cleaned away with wax solvent on a cotton swab.

Occlusal adjustments after processing of the removable partial denture (Fig. 7-49)

When acrylic resin polymerizes, it contracts. Therefore, minor, inadvertent changes in the occlusion of the RPD occur as a result of processing. These changes must be corrected so that the contacts programmed on the dental articulator are maintained. The armamentarium used to do this includes:

1. Sticky wax or stick compound
2. Articulating paper
3. Denture-adjustment burs (number 6 and number 4 round burs)
4. Polishing equipment

The procedure used to adjust the RPD's occlusion after processing is presented in step-by-step fashion in the following paragraphs.

It is important to retrieve the master cast intact after processing so that it can be replaced on its articulator mounting. Therefore, when the RPD is flasked, the master cast should be lubricated so that the laboratory plaster will be easily removed from the base and sides. The base of the master cast should be placed directly onto the bottom of the denture flask before laboratory plaster is flowed into the denture flask. This will help prevent any chips of laboratory plaster from adhering to the base of the master cast.

Residual laboratory plaster is cleaned from the base and sides of the master cast and from around the processed RPD. The base of the master cast is sealed to its articulator mounting with either sticky wax or compound.

The incisal pin on the dental articulator should be returned to its initial position to maintain the original occlusal vertical dimension. The incisal pin is adjusted to its original position so that after occlusal correction it will touch the incisal table when the centric contacts developed during the wax-up will have been reached.

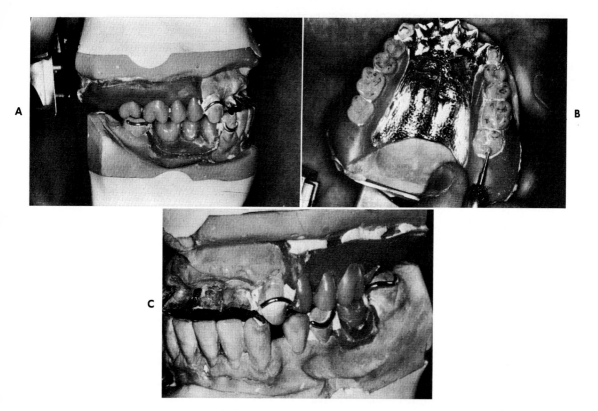

Fig. 7-49. Postprocessing occlusal corrections are made on teeth with casts mounted on articulator. **A,** Processed RPDs mounted on dental articulator. Anterior teeth on maxillary cast have been fractured off. **B,** Premature contacts are identified with articulating paper and adjusted accordingly. **C,** Completed occlusal adjustment.

Articulating paper is introduced between the occlusal surfaces, the articulator is closed in centric relation, and any initial deflective occlusal contacts are registered. Centric occlusal contacts are adjusted first, using smaller and smaller burs until the incisal pin touches the table. Then, using articulating paper of differing colors, the desired lateral and protrusive eccentric contacts (or lack of contacts) are adjusted in similar manner.

When this has been accomplished, the RPD can be removed from the master cast, trimmed, and polished.

CONCLUSION

The "journey" of developing an occlusion for an RPD is completed when two conditions are met. First, the type and position of occlusal contacts planned for the occlusal scheme must actually have been developed and be present. Second, and probably more important, all of the teeth, both natural and prosthetic, must contact bilaterally and simultaneously at the vertical dimension of occlusion.

Diagnosis, treatment planning, and treatment must follow in a logical sequence with particular attention to all detail so that the development of the occlusion will conform to the adaptive limits of the patient.

8 Instructions to the patient

Patient education is one of the most important factors that contribute to the success of removable partial denture (RPD) service. All too often dentists dwell on the technical aspects of RPD treatment and fail to realize that there are other factors that are equally or even more important to an overall successful prognosis. Clinical research has shown that even the most carefully designed, precisely constructed, and biologically oriented RPD may fail unless the patient takes meticulous and continuous care of the oral tissues and the prosthesis (Gomes and associates, 1980). Therefore, the burden of responsibility lies with the dentist to not only educate patients but also motivate them so that they are willing and able to carry out the oral health care procedures prescribed by the dentist. Sincerity and enthusiasm on the dentist's part play an important role in helping to motivate patients to assume the responsibilities that are required of them if successful RPD treatment is to be achieved.

COUNSELING

Patient education should begin during the first visit and continue at each subsequent appointment during treatment. Counseling the patient during the treatment phase provides the dentist ample opportunity to discuss with the patient the many factors that contribute to successful treatment. It is also one of the best methods to establish patient-dentist rapport, which is important to a successful prognosis.

The desires and expectations of the patient should be determined early, during the diagnostic or early treatment phases, because they can lead to a modification in the type or design of the prosthesis and influence the overall prognosis. Most new prosthodontic patients do not know what to expect when they wear an RPD; therefore, the dentist should endeavor to condition the patient for this new experience.

It is much easier to explain the limitations and restrictions of a prosthesis before the patient is treated than it is to try to justify the limitations of the prosthesis after it has been completed.

The reason the patient requires treatment with an RPD should be discussed with the patient before treatment begins. This can best be accomplished by means of mounted diagnostic casts and roentgenograms. Patients should be made to realize that adjusting (habituating) to an RPD is their responsibility. Patience and perseverance are required of the patient during the initial period of habituation in order to learn to adjust to an RPD.

Patients should be apprised of the special problems they will encounter when an RPD is first worn. Some of these are discussed below.

Soreness and discomfort

The patient must anticipate that there may be some soreness and discomfort of the soft tissues or teeth during the first few days. The oral tissues are highly sensitive because of their large numbers of sensory receptors, and it takes time for the tissues to adjust to the pressures placed on them by a new RPD. The patient should be reassured that the dentist will be available to adjust the prosthesis during this annoying and sometimes difficult time.

Coping with a prosthesis

The dentist must always remember that for every RPD there is a certain period of patient adjustment. During this period the patient must acquire the skills necessary to cope with and adjust to this seemingly large, bulky, foreign body in the mouth. This creates a forced learning period for the patient. With an RPD, the patient always has the option of removing it, inspecting it critically, and rejecting it. This ability to remove the prosthesis may retard the rate at which the patient will adjust to it, or, because of a lack of perseverance, the patient may elect not to adjust to it and may ultimately reject it (Zarb and MacKay, 1980). This, in fact, occurs in a high percentage of patients treated with bilateral distal-extension RPDs (Carlsson and associates, 1965). The dentist must remember that wearing a prosthesis is a learned skill in which incentive plays an important part and that wearing an RPD perhaps involves learning at a subconscious rather than conscious level (Berry and Mahood, 1966).

Learning to speak distinctly

The patient may find it difficult to speak distinctly at first, especially if a maxillary RPD covers the anterior portion of the palate. The major connector of the prosthesis interferes with accurate tongue placement for speech articulation because of its position and bulk. However, speech difficulties are usually transitory because the tongue has considerable adaptability. Reading and speaking aloud will assist the patient to overcome this problem.

Learning to eat

Learning to eat is probably the most formidable task the patient must master, especially with a mandibular bilateral distal-extension RPD. The process is usually accomplished through a gradual, conscious learning process. The length of time required to learn to eat with a newly placed RPD will vary with: (1) the number of teeth replaced, (2) the patient's age, (3) neuromuscular control based on adequate sensory input, (4) the type and location of the prosthesis, (5) esthetic considerations, and (6) to a considerable degree, the amount of perseverance and determination of the patient.

Soft foods such as boiled eggs, very tender ground meats, well-cooked vegetables, and cereals should be eaten during the initial habituation period. Toast or crackers should be substituted for soft bread if this food is part of the patient's diet. The patient should be encouraged to take small bites, chew slowly and deliberately, and prolong the time necessary to eat the meal. The patient should be cautioned to incise in the canine premolar region to prevent undue torquing forces on the prosthesis and pressure on the anterior residual ridges. Hard, tough, and sticky foods should be avoided until such time that the patient acquires sufficient neuromuscular control to become proficient with the prosthesis. Such foods tend to dislodge the RPD.

Excessive bulk

The new RPD wearer is usually very conscious of a feeling of fullness and crowding of the tongue because of the increased bulk of the prosthesis. Even the experienced RPD patient will exhibit some of the same feelings, because the new prosthesis may differ from their old prosthesis in size or shape. These changes stimulate sensory receptors, creating a renewed patient awareness of the prosthesis. Patients should be reassured that this will be a temporary situation because the tongue is a very adaptable organ. In a very short time, they should not be conscious of this condition.

Increase in salivary flow

Most new RPD wearers have a transient increase in the amount of salivary flow. Stimulation of the sensory receptors of the mouth (gustatory, tactile, thermal, and pain) characteristically induces increased salivary secretion (Shannon and associates, 1970). A newly inserted RPD acts as a foreign body that stimulates these receptors to secrete excessive saliva. It has also been demonstrated that the highly polished acrylic resin denture base contributes to an increased salivary flow. Fortunately, this condition is usually mild and transitory, and the salivary flow rate returns to normal levels within a few days to weeks.

Increased oral perception

Most dentists will occasionally find a new RPD wearer who cannot tolerate a foreign object in his mouth for whatever reason (physiologic or psychologic). Many times this is a result of an elevated level of oral perception that regards the prosthesis as so foreign and obtrusive that it is offensive to wear. Learning to control and adjust to a prosthesis under these conditions is frequently impossible (Zarb and MacKay, 1980).

MAINTENANCE OF THE ORAL TISSUES
Care of the natural teeth

Several long-term clinical investigations have reported the effects of RPDs on patients.

Some of these patients received complete periodontal therapy before the fabrication of their RPDs and others did not (Bergman and associates, 1971; Carlsson and associates, 1965; Derry and Bertram, 1970; Gomes and associates, 1980; Schwalm and associates, 1977). Carlsson and associates (1965) reported a significant increase over a 4-year period in abutment tooth mobility, gingival inflammation, periodontal pocket depth around the abutment teeth, loss of alveolar bone, and dental carious lesions on the uncrowned abutment teeth. In this study, patients were not instructed in appropriate oral hygiene procedures. Likewise, they were not given frequent recall examinations to detect poor dental plaque control, incipient periodontal and prosthodontic changes, and early stages of dental caries. In contrast to this study, two other longitudinal studies of patients treated with RPDs revealed very different results (Bergman and associates, 1971; Gomes and associates, 1980). In both studies, the patients received complete periodontal therapy before fabrication of the RPDs. They were also instructed and motivated to practice good oral hygiene and were frequently recalled to detect and correct early changes in their periodontal or prosthodontic status. In these studies, no significant changes in the hard and soft tissues were noted during the length of the study. The results of these and other studies indicate that RPDs are an effective treatment modality provided that:

1. The patient is given complete periodontal therapy before treatment with an RPD
2. The patient is placed on a strict oral hygiene regimen emphasizing the need for effective dental plaque control, denture hygiene, and tissue rest (removal of the prosthesis for a specific period daily)
3. The patient can demonstrate effectiveness in maintaining low levels of dental plaque
4. The patient is placed on a frequent, individualized, regular recall program to detect early periodontal and prosthodontic changes
5. The dentist provides the necessary periodontal and prosthodontic therapy as well as dental caries control to maximize the longevity of both the periodontal supporting apparatus and the RPD (Gomes and associates, 1980)

Patient education

All patients, especially those requiring removable prostheses, should be introduced to dental treatment by means of a regimented oral hygiene program. This program should be initiated during the first visit and continued during each successive visit throughout treatment and the recall and maintenance phase. The etiology of dental disease, dental caries, periodontal disease, and residual ridge reduction should be discussed. Patients should know that bacteria and their by-products plus fermentable carbohydrates and a susceptible tooth surface are the prime etiologic factors in the production of dental caries. In addition, bacteria (gram-negative species and motile forms) are an important etiologic factor in the pathogenesis of gingival and periodontal disease. The etiology of residual ridge reduction and its sequelae must be explained to each patient treated with a removable prosthesis (Atwood, 1971; Plotnick and associates, 1975; Tallgren, 1972). Dentists must also educate their patients in the role that dental and denture plaque play in the pathogenesis of dental disease.

Dental plaque

Adequate dental plaque control is perhaps the single most important factor in the success of any RPD. Dental plaque is a salivary precipitant that forms every 24 hours. It is not caused by food but is the matrix attached to a tooth in which the fermentable carbohydrates found in food are retained. Dental plaque forms a nidus for bacteria that, in using carbohydrates for their growth, produce acids and enzymes that precipitate dental disease. These bacteria cause either a demineralization of the tooth surface that leads to dental caries or a progressive inflammatory process in the gingival sulcus that leads to periodontal disease.

Dental plaque is instrumental to calculus formation, because calcium salts deposit on dental plaque, which hardens to form dental calculus. Supragingival and subgingival calculus should be removed periodically during therapy and recall, because it harbors bacteria that contributes to the destruction of the gingival tissues.

Brill and associates (1977) reported in a study of 13 patients who wore RPDs that there was a statistically significant increase in dental plaque formation on all abutment tooth surfaces. They found that the tooth surface between the clasps and the free gingival margin revealed a conspicuous increase in dental plaque formation and retention. Their findings also revealed that greater amounts of dental plaque formed on the proximal surfaces of abutment teeth adjacent to the RPD base than on the buccal surfaces of the teeth. Gomes and associates (1980) reported that even when a strict recall program was made part of a therapeutic treatment sequence with RPD patients, these patients could not maintain a dental plaque–free condition. This was in spite of the fact that the prosthesis could be removed and the teeth were accessible to cleaning. The areas of greatest dental plaque accumulation (distal, proximal, and interproximal areas) should be pointed out to the patient with disclosing solution as areas that require special attention during their oral hygiene procedures. Patients should know that the ultimate success of an RPD is predicated on a plaque-free mouth.

Methods of dental plaque control (Fig. 8-1)

USE OF THE TOOTHBRUSH. The most universal method of effective dental plaque removal is for the patient to use a toothbrush. As part of an office dental hygiene control program, the patient should be requested to brush his or her teeth in the presence of the dentist or dental hygienist. The patient should be given a toothbrush and requested to brush in his or her customary manner for the customary amount of time. Next the patient should be given a disclosing tablet or solution and instructed in its use. The patient should rinse his or her mouth with water to remove any excess stain and should then be given a hand mirror. The dentist or dental hygienist should demonstrate any remaining areas of dental plaque stained by the disclosing solution. A demonstration of the most effective methods of removal of these areas of dental plaque is then performed. Oral hygiene aids, in addition to the use of a toothbrush, are dental floss, gauze, or four-ply knitting yarn. The patient should be encouraged to continue the daily use of disclosing solution until the most effective technique to remove dental plaque has been mastered. The disclosing solution should then be used once a week to determine the effectiveness of the patient's oral hygiene procedures to remove dental plaque.

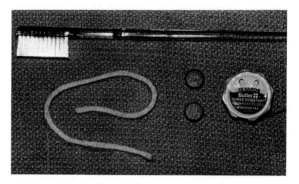

Fig. 8-1. Armamentarium for oral physiotherapy and dental plaque control should include soft synthetic toothbrush, disclosing wafers, unwaxed dental floss, and four-ply synthetic knitting yarn. Additional hygiene aids may be required for some patients to promote optimal oral and periodontal health.

If the patient's toothbrushing technique is adequate for effective dental plaque removal, no change in the technique is indicated other than to demonstrate the most effective way to remove residual dental plaque. If the patient has no organized toothbrushing technique, then a demonstration of an effective toothbrushing technique, such as the Bass technique, is required.

When the Bass technique (sulcular brushing) is used, the toothbrush should be held at approximately a 45° angle to the tooth at a level that allows the bristles to enter the gingival sulcus for a distance of between 2 to 3 mm. The brush should be moved in a vibratory motion using a short stroke in this area and should then be removed from the gingival sulcus (Bass, 1954). All facial and lingual surfaces of the teeth should be brushed in this manner to establish a brushing pattern for the patient. The patient should be encouraged to brush at different angles over the remaining tooth surfaces to remove residual dental plaque.

Although there is conflicting clinical evidence in the periodontal literature regarding the type of toothbrush that is most effective for dental plaque removal, there is sufficient agreement among periodontists that a soft, round-ended nylon bristle (0.007-inch diameter) of uniform length is an effective toothbrush when used with the Bass technique. The soft bristles tend to enter the gingival sulcus effectively and atraumatically. They also flatten out on the tooth surface and therefore contact a greater surface area than does a hard-bristled toothbrush, leading to increased mechanical efficiency. The soft bristles, when properly used, will clean not only the tooth surface but also the gingival sulcus and will provide physiologic stimulation to these tissues without irritation. Ideally, the natural teeth should be thoroughly brushed after each meal and before bedtime.

USE OF DENTAL FLOSS. A daily toothbrushing routine can effectively remove dental plaque from the buccal, lingual, and occlusal surfaces of the teeth; however, it will not remove dental plaque from the proximal surfaces of the teeth. The proper use of unwaxed dental floss is an effective oral hygiene aid in cleaning these areas. The dentist should demonstrate the use of dental floss to the patient. The floss should be gently inserted between the proximal surfaces of the teeth by moving it back and forth through contact areas of the teeth. Once the dental floss passes through the contact area, it should be moved up and down several times against the proximal surfaces of the adjacent teeth, between the contact area and gingival col, until these surfaces are free of dental plaque. The use of dental floss should not cause the interproximal gingival tissues to hemorrhage or become irritated. Ideally, dental floss should be used daily as part of a complete oral hygiene program.

USE OF FOUR-PLY SYNTHETIC KNITTING YARN (Fig. 8-2). Dental plaque tends to accumulate on the proximal surfaces of the teeth adjacent to the RPD base, resulting in an increased incidence of dental caries and gingival irritation. The patient must make a special effort to keep this area free of dental plaque. Dental floss can be used to clean this surface. In addition, four-ply synthetic knitting yarn, because of its soft texture and its slightly greater bulk, is an excellent material for cleaning these inaccessible areas (Levin, 1979). The knitting yarn is used in a fashion similar to dental floss.

Dental caries control

Carlsson and associates (1965), in a 4-year longitudinal study on patients treated with RPDs, reported a 75% incidence of dental caries of the uncrowned abutment teeth. In view of these findings, it would seem that most patients treated with RPDs should be considered as having a high dental caries risk. However,

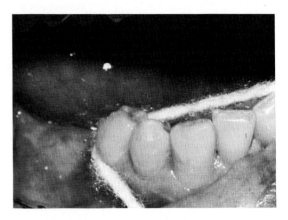

Fig. 8-2. Four-ply synthetic knitting yarn is used to clean distal surface of abutment tooth adjacent to edentulous space.

Carlsson's group did not recall their RPD patients for dental plaque control or periodontal therapy during the period of the study, which probably increased the incidence of dental caries. In a similar longitudinal study, Gomes and associates (1980) instituted recall and dental plaque control measures on a 6-month basis. In this study, the incidence of dental caries was only 11% and the incidence of periodontal disease was low.

These findings point again to the fact that regardless of the type of prosthetic restoration used to treat a patient, ultimately it is the patient's ability to maintain a mouth free of dental plaque that will lead to its success or failure. Zarb contends that when dentists prescribe a fixed partial denture for a patient, they do so on the basis of the patient's ability to maintain an effective level of dental plaque control (Zarb and MacKay, 1980). Yet dentists often prescribe an RPD for a patient who cannot demonstrate an acceptable level of dental plaque control. According to the results obtained from a multitude of long-term and short-term clinical studies of RPDs, patients who wear a prosthesis appear to have a greater risk of developing dentogingival disease than those who do not. However, treating a patient with an RPD does not in itself cause dental caries or periodontal disease.

Both the dentist and patient must assume their individual responsibilities for the success of prosthodontic treatment. The dentist's responsibility is to use sound clinical judgment in deciding whether to restore a mutilated dentition and how this can be accomplished with the least amount of long-term damage to the patient. The patient must understand that in the majority of cases the impact of prosthodontic treatment can be minimized or magnified by the patient's motivation and ability to maintain a mouth free of dental plaque (Zarb and MacKay, 1980).

It is established clinical practice that application of topical fluoride is an effective method for reducing the incidence of dental caries because it makes the teeth more resistant to demineralization. Stratemann and Shannon (1974), working with 96 orthodontic patients, reported that daily self-applications of a water-free 0.4% stannous fluoride gel provides a very high level of protection from dental caries, even in patients with a high dental caries risk. The amount of protection provided appeared to be predicated on the degree of cooperation shown by the patient. The procedures recommended for the use of a water-free 0.4% stannous fluoride gel are as follows:

1. The patient should rinse his or her mouth thoroughly with water after brushing the teeth before bedtime.
2. Fluoride gel should be placed on a thoroughly wetted toothbrush and brushed onto all surfaces of the teeth.
3. The patient should attempt by oral movements (sucking and pursing the lips) to force the fluoride gel into the interproximal spaces between the teeth.
4. The patient should wait with the fluroide gel on the teeth for 1 minute before expectorating. The mouth should not be rinsed for 2 hours after application of the fluoride gel.

Care of the soft tissues covered by the removable partial denture

Numerous articles in the dental literature report that RPDs abuse the mucoperiosteum and associated soft tissues unless adequate measures are instituted for proper care of both the tissues and the RPD (Gomes and associates, 1980; Jones, 1976; Miner, 1973).Consequently, it is the dentist's responsibility to inform the patient about the measures that should be undertaken to help prevent this tissue abuse.

There is not a concensus of opinion among dental educators as to the need for tissue rest under a prosthesis; however, continuous RPD wearing is a chief etiologic factor in the development of denture stomatitis beneath a prosthesis (Renner and associates, 1979; Steffel, 1968; Tautin, 1978). The tissues that are covered by the prosthesis do not receive the normal stimulation supplied by contact with the tongue and cheeks. This causes stagnation of the blood flow to the denture-bearing tissues, reducing their capacity for repair and regeneration. Parasitism with *Candida albicans*, the patient's oral hygiene practices, parafunctional habits (bruxism or clenching), denture trauma, over-the-counter reliners, systemic alterations, and dietary deficiencies are the other major contributing factors in the production of denture stomatitis under the tissue-fitting surface of an RPD (Renner and associates, 1979). RPD stresses or occlusal forces as well as parafunctional habits often place excessive pressure on the denture-supporting soft tissues. This pressure interferes with the tissue circulation and subjects the tissues to abuse by the prosthesis. Each of these factors alone or in combination can have an adverse effect on the health of the tissues covered by the prosthesis. The tissue reaction may range from simple increased vascularity, as evidenced by a change in tissue tone and color, to inflammatory reactions with or without ulceration to *C. albicans* infection to, when the process is chronic, hypertrophy of the tissues (that is, papillary hyperplasia).

To promote optimal and continuous health of the tissues covered by the prosthesis and help prevent the formation of denture stomatitis, patients should be instructed to leave the RPD out of their mouth for a 6 to 8 hour period each day (Tautin, 1978). It is not important which period of the day the prosthesis is left out of the mouth. What is critical to oral tissue preservation is that the soft tissues are not covered by the RPD continuously and that the tissues are permitted to rest a definite amount of time during each 24 hours. Patients treated with an RPD that does not replace missing anterior teeth (Kennedy Class IV) are more likely than other patients to follow these instructions, because esthetics and the risk of social embarrassment are not involved.

Many patients find that the most convenient time to leave the prosthesis out of the mouth is

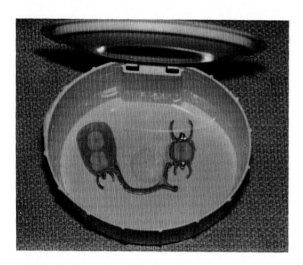

Fig. 8-3. RPDs should always be placed in tap water or immersion-type chemical denture cleanser when they are left out of mouth longer than 30 minutes. Denture bath makes convenient container for soaking dentures.

at night while they are sleeping. This interval furnishes not only an adequate rest period for the tissues, but also an optimal time for use of a chemcial cleaner (alkaline peroxide solution) to clean and freshen the prosthesis (Budtz-Jorgensen, 1979). When removed from the mouth for 30 minutes or longer, RPDs should always be placed in water (Fig. 8-3). If an RPD is permitted to dry out, the acrylic resin portion of the prosthesis may undergo dimensional change caused by dehydration, which could alter the fit of the prosthesis.

Parafunctional habits (bruxism or clenching) are conditions for which the patient may be instructed by the dentist to wear an RPD at night. Parafunctional habits subject the underlying tissues to destructive occlusal forces. The splinting effect of an RPD on the teeth will often help to distribute the occlusal forces over a larger number of teeth and thus reduce the amount of force transmitted to the individual teeth.

Another situation in which the patient might be instructed to wear an RPD while sleeping occurs when a Kennedy Class I RPD opposes a maxillary complete denture and the patient refuses to sleep or cannot sleep comfortably without wearing the maxillary complete denture. Clinical experience has shown that rapid resorption of the maxillary anterior residual ridge and abuse (epulis formation and hyper-

trophy) of the soft tissues beneath the maxillary complete denture are almost inevitable when a maxillary complete denture opposes only natural mandibular anterior teeth without a functional RPD (Kelly, 1972; Saunders and associates, 1979).

Patients who are reluctant to sleep without their RPD, for whatever reason, should be encouraged to remove it at a convenient time during the day. These patients must be advised that they need to exert an extra effort to practice meticulous oral hygiene, including thorough soft-tissue massage and tissue rest by leaving the RPD out of the mouth for 6 to 8 hours every 24 hours, if an optimal state of health of the tissues covered by the prosthesis is to be maintained.

Thorough cleaning and massage of the oral tissues covered by an RPD are an essential part of a total patient oral hygiene regimen. Some of the materials and methods that can accomplish this are discussed below.

Use of a toothbrush

Probably the easiest and most convenient method of cleaning and massaging the soft tissues covered by an RPD is by means of a soft nylon, multitufted toothbrush. Gentle brushing of the tissues with a toothbrush removes dental plaque and food debris that adhere to the mucoperiosteum and stimulates the flow of blood through the tissues. Although the normal epithelial response to RPD wearing is one of keratosis (Turck, 1965), Markov (1967) found that keratinization of the edentulous tissues increased with toothbrush physiotherapy. Increased keratosis of the covered tissues may result in better tissue tolerance to the prosthesis. Patients wearing an RPD should be encouraged to brush and cleanse the supporting soft tissues as well as the teeth daily to remove dental plaque and food debris. It would be preferable if the patient removed accumulated food debris after each meal, but often this is impractical.

When RPD patients use inadequate or ineffective oral hygiene procedures, inflammation of the marginal gingiva is a common finding (Carlsson and associates, 1965). The free gingival margins beneath a lingual plate or areas where components of the RPD framework (such as indirect retainers or retentive arms for bar clasps) are particularly susceptible to gingival inflammation if dental plaque is allowed to accumulate. Another common site of gingival irritation is on the proximal surface of the abutment teeth adjacent to denture bases. These susceptible areas should be pointed out to patients, and the importance of the proper cleaning and massage of these tissues should be emphasized. It should also be emphasized that when a patient is on a regular recall maintenance program and practices effective plaque control, gingivitis can be eliminated (Gomes and associates, 1980).

The dentist should realize that there is a danger that some patients may be overenthusiastic with toothbrush massage. Patients should therefore be encouraged to proceed carefully at first so as to avoid traumatic injury to the soft tissues. Having the patient demonstrate toothbrush massage of the soft tissues under the supervision of the dentist should be encouraged.

Use of a washcloth

Another method of cleaning and massaging the soft tissues is by means of a washcloth. Patients who have difficulty holding or using a toothbrush to properly brush the soft tissues may be able to clean and massage them more effectively by means of a moist washcloth. The washcloth should be moistened and placed over the forefinger of either hand, and the gingival and supporting tissues should be scrubbed thoroughly with the cloth (Fig. 8-4).

Use of chewing gum

Chewing gum can also serve as an adjunctive method to clean and massage the soft tissues when the RPD is removed from the mouth.

The patient should soften several pieces of sugarless chewing gum under warm water to form a soft bolus. The bolus should be large enough so that when it is placed in the mouth it will contact a large soft-tissue area while the patient chews. The bolus should be moved around in the mouth so that it will contact as much of the tissues covered by the RPD as possible. Chewing gum for 5 to 10 minutes a day usually provides adequate stimulation for the soft tissues. If the patient wishes, the chewing gum may be stored in a container with a flavored mouthwash to allow it to be used several times.

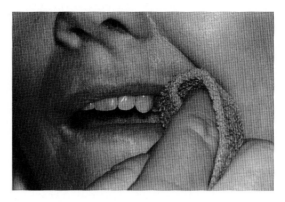

Fig. 8-4. Moistened washcloth is used to cleanse and massage soft tissues covered by RPD.

Motivation of the patient

Perhaps the greatest challenge that confronts the dentist is the need to motivate patients to practice effective daily oral hygiene procedures. Long-standing patient habits are not easily modified or changed, and the dentist must realize that it is very difficult to upgrade the level of oral hygiene practiced by patients. The results of the longitudinal study by Gomes and associates suggest that even when patients are given constant reinforcement of dental and denture plaque control measures on a regular recall basis, they tend to increase their effective level of plaque removal only for the first few weeks after the recall visit and then return to their old habit patterns. Very few patients exhibited a marked improvement in dental plaque removal during the 2-year study (Gomes and associates, 1980). The following are some techniques and procedures that the dentist can use to help motivate patients to improve the daily care of their mouths.

1. The dentist should, above all, be enthusiastic and sincere in his or her approach to patients. The dentist must firmly believe what he or she tells them.
2. Patient education and reeducation is very important to a successful long-term prognosis. The better informed the patients are and the higher their dental IQ, the more likely they will be to practice effective oral hygiene.
3. Patients should be encouraged to brush and floss their teeth in the dentist's office during the treatment phases and at subsequent recall visits. This permits the

dentist to point out areas in which a patient is not effective in dental plaque removal and to demonstrate that he or she is truly interested in both the patient and the patient's oral health.

4. The dentist should work with each patient to develop a daily routine that makes an oral hygiene program convenient.

5. Patients should be recalled periodically to remotivate them (Roberts, 1980). The frequency of recall should not be based on a standard time period (such as 1 year), as is frequently suggested. Instead, the frequency of recall of a patient treated with an RPD should be based on: (1) the patient's demonstrated ability to remove dental and denture plaque; (2) the patient's periodontal status and need for active periodontal maintenance; (3) the rate of residual ridge resorption, which will determine the need to correct the prosthesis; and (4) the type of prosthetic treatment that the patient has received (Gomes and associates, 1980).

CARE OF THE REMOVABLE PARTIAL DENTURE

Meticulous care by the patient in the use and cleaning of an RPD constitutes an important prerequisite to successful long-term RPD service (Wagner, 1971).

Use of the removable partial denture

Patients should understand that a great amount of effort and skill is required to make an RPD function within the patient's biologic environment. If the precision fit of the prosthesis is altered, irreparable damage to the oral tissues could result. Patients should therefore be encouraged to care for the RPD as they would a valued possession. Although an RPD is constructed to withstand masticatory forces and, with proper care and maintenance, should last several years, it can be bent or broken by careless patient handling.

Patients should be cautioned about dropping the prosthesis or carrying it in their purse or jacket pocket. They should be taught the correct method of insertion and removal of an RPD, which should always include the use of gentle finger pressure to seat the prosthesis on the teeth. Inserting the RPD by placing it in the mouth and biting it into place is a hazard-

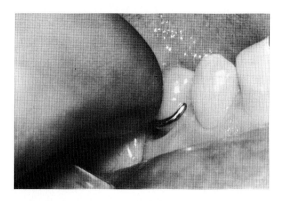

Fig. 8-5. Force used to dislodge RPD should be applied only to shoulder of clasp arm and not to clasp tip to avoid distortion of retentive clasp arm during removal of RPD.

ous procedure that can bend the prosthesis. When the prosthesis is removed, it should be grasped with the patient's fingers around and under the denture base. If the direct retainers are used to remove the RPD, the dislodging force should be applied only to the shoulders of the clasp arms (Fig. 8-5). This is especially important when the retentive arm is made of platinum-gold-palladium 18-gauge wrought wire rather than cast metal. If the RPD is removed by grasping the tip of the retentive arm, the force required to dislodge the prosthesis could cause distortion of the clasp, with a resultant loss of retention.

The retentive arms of a clasp on an RPD tend to loosen during use (Benson and Spolsky, 1979). If the patient can function comfortably with the retentive arms in this loosened condition, as is often the case, he or she should be encouraged to do so, because this will reduce the destructive forces created on the abutment teeth by the direct retainers.

The patient should be instructed to return to the dentist if adjustments of the RPD are required. RPD adjustment by the patient should be discouraged.

Cleaning the removable partial denture

Dental plaque that accumulates on dentures has the same basic structure as dental plaque found on the natural teeth (Miner, 1973; Theilade and Budtz-Jorgensen, 1977). Dental plaque that accumulates on the tissue surface of the RPD is a contributing factor in the pathogenesis of denture stomatitis (Budtz-Jorgensen, 1974, 1978a). Neill (1968) has indicated that dental plaque acts as a matrix for the deposition not only of stains derived from the breakdown of food substances and tobacco but also of calcium salts, resulting in calculus formation on the prosthesis. Plaque probably is also a major cause of the odor often found on an RPD.

Patients must be educated about the importance of a routine denture-cleaning regimen for their prosthesis (Budtz-Jorgensen, 1979), because an RPD should only be considered clean when it is free of dental plaque, food debris, calculus, and exogenous discoloration. A convenient time to do this is during the 24-hour adjustment appointment. During this visit, patients should be instructed to clean the RPD by using one of several acceptable methods: (1) mechanical denture cleansing with a denture brush or ultrasonic agitation or (2) chemical denture cleansing. When a mechanical device such as a brush is used to clean an RPD, it must not abrade the acrylic resin. Wear of the acrylic resin will be minimal if a brush has long bristles and if the diameter of the bristles is small (Wictorin, 1972). A common method of cleaning a prosthesis is to use a denture brush of this nature with soap and water or just plain tap water. This technique is effective in removing discoloration and denture plaque when used meticulously (Theilade, 1958).

The dentist should place the RPD in a disclosing solution after one of the above cleaning methods has been used and should point out to the patient the remaining areas of accumulated dental plaque. Patients should be encouraged to use a disclosing solution daily in this manner until they locate the areas of dental plaque that are the most difficult to remove. This should be part of a routine denture-cleaning regimen. The disclosing agent should be used on the prosthesis once or twice a week, corresponding to the times when a disclosing agent is used on the natural teeth.

Methods of cleaning a removable partial denture

BRUSHING. The majority of people clean their prosthesis by brushing it with soap and water or a commerical dentifrice. It has the advantage of rapid cleaning and is an effective method of removing dental plaque, food debris, and discoloration from the prosthesis (Theilade, 1958). Its major disadvantage is that it is an ineffective method of cleaning the in-

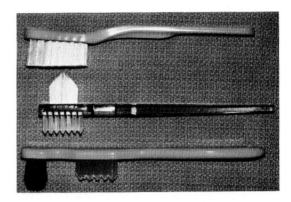

Fig. 8-6. Three different types of denture brushes may be recommended for cleaning RPDs.

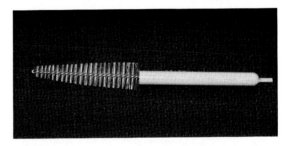

Fig. 8-7. Fixed bridge and clasp brush should be recommended for cleaning inner surfaces of clasps on RPD.

accesable areas present on most RPDs.

The type of brush and cleanser used to clean the prosthesis should be selected very carefully, because this mechanical method of cleaning can cause severe abrasion of the acrylic resin portion of the RPD if the wrong denture brush or cleaning agent is used. Short, stiff-bristle toothbrushes or denture brushes should be avoided, because they can abrade acrylic resin even without the use of an abrasive agent in the hands of a patient who is a vigorous brusher. A medium, synthetic toothbrush with long, round-ended bristles of small diameter or a soft denture brush is generally considered the most suitable for cleaning an RPD and should be recommended for this purpose (Fig. 8-6) (Wictorin, 1972). The wear of the acrylic resin is usually negligible under conditions of prolonged brushing if the proper brush is used and the abrasive is not too coarse (Pipko and El-Sadek, 1972). Because it is difficult to clean the inner surfaces of the clasp assembly with a denture brush, a bridge or clasp brush (Fig. 8-7) should be used for this purpose.

Abrasive cleaners or household cleaners or abrasive soaps should not be used, because they can scratch and abrade the polished surface as well as alter the fit of the tissue surface of the RPD. Most patients, however, like to use a commercial paste or powder to clean their dentures. All commercial pastes and powders contain abrasive agents that will wear the acrylic resin. Commercial products that contain insoluble calcium carbonate as the abrasive should be discouraged because of their high abrasiveness. A product containing soluble sodium bicarbonate is less abrasive and more desirable (Wictorin, 1972). Although most of these products may not materially affect the RPD, they are abrasive to some extent and will increase the wear or dull the surface of the prosthesis with prolonged use, leading to increased dental plaque retention. Facial soap or sodium bicarbonate will not affect the surface of acrylic resin to any significant degree and should be considered the cleaning agents of choice for use on an RPD. The occasional use of a commercial denture cleaner can be recommended for those patients who tend to accumulate stains on their prosthesis.

Patients should brush both the polished and tissue surfaces of the RPD. Brushing in several different directions is usually a more effective way to clean the RPD than is brushing in just one direction.

The RPD should be brushed after each meal and before bedtime. If during the day the patient cannot brush the prosthesis after a meal, he or she should be encouraged to take the RPD out of the mouth and rinse it under running tap water. The patient should also rinse the mouth with water to flush out any food particles that may be present.

An RPD, when brushed with soap and water, becomes very slippery and difficult to hold. The prosthesis should always be brushed over a basin that has been partially filled with water to avoid breakage or damage to the RPD if it should be accidently dropped. The patient should hold one half of the RPD in one hand while the other half is being brushed. The RPD should not be held in the palm of the hand while it is being cleaned, because if it slips the patient will instinctively close the hand, which could result in bending the prosthesis. Hot tap water should never be used on

the RPD, because this could cause a dimensional change of the acrylic resin.

CHEMICAL (IMMERSION) METHODS. Another method of cleaning an RPD is by means of commercial immersion-type chemical denture cleaners. This method of cleaning can serve as an adjunct to the brushng method and is often preferred by handicapped or geriatric patients who are not able to clean their prosthesis adequately by brushing. Immersion-type denture cleaners may be classified into four types: (1) the alkaline peroxides, (2) the buffered alkaline hypochlorites, (3) dulite organic or inorganic acids, and (4) enzymes.

ALKALINE PEROXIDE CLEANERS. Alkaline peroxide cleaners are the most common type of commercial immersion cleaners used today. There are a large variety of these products available on the commercial market. They are convenient to use, have a pleasant taste, and do not harm or have a deleterious effect on the metallic or acrylic resin portions of the RPD (MacCallum and associates, 1968; Neil, 1968).

Alkaline peroxide cleaners usually consist of powders containing alkaline detergents, which reduce surface tension. They also contain chemicals such as sodium perborate or percarbonate, which release oxygen when they come in contact with the RPD in water. The large number of oxygen bubbles released exert a mechanical effervescent cleaning action on the prosthesis.

These cleaners are effective on immature dental plaque or light stains if the RPD is soaked in them daily for 6 to 8 hours or overnight (Mac Callum and associates, 1968). However, they are not considered effective for short immersion periods of 15 to 30 minutes (Anthony and Gibbons, 1958; Nickolson and associates, 1968). The alkaline peroxides are effective stain-removing agents but are only as effective as soap and tap water in removing microbial plaque. They are indicated primarily for patients who have new RPDs and clean their dentures daily. These cleaners do not effectively remove heavy stains or calculus from a prosthesis.

BUFFERED ALKALINE HYPOCHLORITE CLEANERS. Hypochlorites or commerical bleaches are very effective denture-cleaning agents because of their ability to dissolve mucin or other organic compounds associated with the formation of dental plaque on an RPD. They are effective in removing stains and calculus on a prosthesis because they dissolve the organic matrix that binds these substances to the surface of the prosthesis and thus permit the deposits to be easily removed by brushing. The hypochlorites are also bactericidal and fungicidal.

Hypochlorites have one major disadvantage: they will tarnish and corrode cast chromium alloy frameworks and the gold-plated nickel pins of porcelain anterior denture teeth (Backenstose and Wells, 1977). To overcome the corrosive effect of the hypochlorites on the metal components of an RPD, glassy phosphates such as sodium hexametaphosphates must be added to buffer the hypochlorite solution. Anthony and Gibbons (1958) suggested that a glassy phosphate such as Calgon and Calgonite, which are available at any grocery store, seems to provide sufficent protection for the metal parts to allow the use of hypochlorite solutions for cleaning purposes. They recommended that a cleaning solution of 1 teaspoonful of Clorox, or a similar hypochlorite, and 2 teaspoonfuls of Calgon in a half a glass of water is an efficient and safe cleaner for an occasional overnight immersion; however, they stated that this cleanser is not indicated for routine use with any prosthesis constructed with base metals (nickel or other alloys of chromium). Because hypochlorite solutions are effective in removing dental plaque on RPDs, soaking the prosthesis for 6 to 8 hours or overnight once a week in a buffered hypochlorite solution can be recommended for those patients who tend to accumulate large amounts of stain or calculus deposits on their prosthesis. Because the metal components of an RPD will tarnish or corrode very rapidly if exposed to an unbuffered hypochlorite solution, patients must understand that the prosthesis must never be placed in a hypochlorite solution unless a glassy phosphate has been added. They should also stop using the buffered hypochlorite cleaning solution and notify the dentist if any darkening of the metal portions of the RPD occurs. A prosthesis with aluminum or stainless steel components should never be placed in a buffered hypochlorite solution.

ACID CLEANERS. Dilute organic or inorganic acids are another type of chemical cleaning agent that can be used for cleaning an RPD. The occasional soaking of the RPD in vinegar (5% acetic acid) can be recommended for those patients who accumulate persistent stains and calculus deposits on their prosthesis. Acid cleaners such as a 5% hydrochloric or 15% phosphoric acid will cause corrosion of the metallic portions of an RPD; however, Sunoo (1969) found that various concentrations of acetic acid produced little change in the microstructure of chromium alloys. Although dilute acids do not attack the organic matrix that binds stains and calculus deposits to the prosthesis, they do dissolve the inorganic portions of these deposits and enhance their removal by brushing.

ENZYME CLEANERS. A relatively recent approach to dental plaque control on an RPD is the use of enzymes to break down the glycoproteins and mucoproteins and the mucopolysaccharides of dental plaque. MacCallum and associates (1968) reported that denture cleaners based on a chelating agent with a mixture of enzymes were effective in removing stains, mucin, and heavy deposits from an RPD. Connor and associates (1977) reported that a dual enzyme cleaner was more effective in dental plaque removal than a peroxide commercial cleaner after 8 hours of immersion. In a more recent study, Budtz-Jorgensen found that enzyme-based denture cleaners, using a 15-minute immersion period, caused a significant reduction in the amount of denture plaque (Budtz-Jorgensen, 1978b).

Enzyme cleaners are bactericidal, fungicidal, and nontoxic, and no harmful effects on denture materials have been reported with their routine use. Although the enzyme cleaners at this time are still considered an experimental approach to control of dental plaque on a prosthesis, some of them have recently been introduced commercially and may prove to be an important method of denture plaque control.

ULTRASONIC (ELECTRONIC) CLEANING. Ultrasonic, or electronic, denture cleaners for use in the home have been available for several years on the commercial market as an aid to cleaning RPDs. These units do not produce true ultrasonic waves but use electronic energy waves that pass through a specially prepared cleaning solution to produce a vibrating action. They are reported to remove calculus, stains, and odors from a prosthesis.

Meyers and Krol (1974) in an investigation of eight patients who showed moderate to heavy calculus deposits on their RPDs, reported that a sonic-action denture cleaner was effective in removing calculus and stain from these prostheses. In another study, Nickolson and associates (1968) reported a dramatic difference between the effectiveness of the sonic cleaning device with water compared with its use with cleaning agents. They concluded that under the conditions of that study the cleaning of an RPD is related to the chemical activity of the solutions and has little relationship to the vibratory activity of the cleaning devices. Ultrasonic cleaning, by itself, is not an effective method to render an RPD plaque free, because it does not significantly reduce the number of microorganisms that can be cultured from the prosthesis (Grun and Engelhardt, 1976). It therefore does not appear that the electronic denture cleaners offer any great advantage over the combined brushing and immersion method of cleaning an RPD.

COMBINED BRUSHING AND IMMERSION METHOD. The most efficient method of cleaning an RPD is to combine the brushing and immersion-type chemical cleaning methods. Combining these two methods uses the advantages of both to clean the RPD. Ideally, patients should be instructed to brush their prosthesis after each meal and before bedtime and soak the denture in a chemical cleaner while they are asleep. This method should be recommended as the method of choice for the majority of patients treated with RPDs.

PERIODIC MAINTENANCE

Educating the patient to the necessity of regular periodic maintenance should not be left until the insertion appointment; it should be emphasized early in the treatment phases and reemphasized during subsequent appointments. Patients should realize that not only do they now have a commitment to maintain their oral health and comfort, but they also have a financial investment in the RPD that could be lost if they do not return to the dentist for regular periodic evaluation and maintenance visits.

The dentist should establish a definite recall system for the patient (Gomes and associates, 1980; Roberts, 1980). Most patients should be recalled at intervals of between 4 and 9 months, depending on the patient's: (1) dental caries susceptibility, (2) periodontal status, (3) rate of residual ridge reduction, and (4) type of prosthesis.

The following should be elements of periodic recall and maintenance regimen:

1. An oral prophylaxis should be performed as well as an evaluation and reinforcement of oral and denture hygiene procedures.
2. The teeth should be examined for new dental carious lesions.
3. The gingival and periodontal status of the patient should be evaluated. A radiographic examination of the periodontium should be made, if necessary, once a year.
4. The soft tissues covered by the RPD should be examined for evidence of oral pathosis.
5. The stability and retention of the RPD should be evaluated. Rotation of a distal-extension RPD around the abutment teeth indicates the need for relining. Patients should be advised that the denture-supporting structures are constantly undergoing change (residual ridge reduction) that usually is not recognized by the patient because of the oftentimes slow and gradual process of residual ridge resorption. Relining of the RPD will help to reduce the destructive forces transmitted by the prosthesis to the teeth and associated soft tissues and lengthen the life span of the prosthesis.
6. The fit of the RPD should be evaluated, and the required repairs or adjustments should be made.
7. The occlusion of the teeth should be examined and corrected if required.
8. Dental plaque removal and denture cleanliness should be reemphasized.
9. The prosthesis should be polished to produce as smooth a surface as possible on both the metal and the acrylic resin surfaces. This should be a routine procedure during each recall appointment.
10. The patient should be given any other adjunctive treatment and scheduled for another recall appointment.

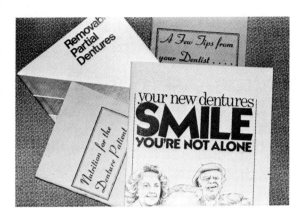

Fig. 8-8. Photograph of a few of the many booklets available at minimal cost that can be used for patient education.

WRITTEN INSTRUCTIONS

Written instructions help to reinforce the role that the patient must play in caring for the oral structures and the new RPD. They also provide the patient with a source of knowledge for future reference. The written instructions should be concise and easily understood and should describe the important points covered during the counseling sessions with the patient. There are several booklets available at minimal cost that can be used for patient education (Fig. 8-8); however, the dentist should make certain the information contained in the booklets does not conflict with the oral instructions previously given to the patient. The dentist who chooses to prepare his or her own set of written instructions can be assured that the instructions will conform with those previously recommended to the patient during counseling.

9 Removable partial denture insertion and postinsertion adjustment procedures

Section 1: Removable partial denture insertion

The purpose of the insertion appointment is twofold: (1) to provide the final psychologic evaluation of the patient to receive the completed prosthesis and (2) to insert and adjust the prosthesis so that it will function in harmony with the hard and soft tissues of the oral cavity.

The dentist must allow sufficient time for this appointment to perform both phases of the insertion procedure satisfactorily in a stepwise, unhurried manner. More complex removable partial denture (RPD) designs require longer insertion appointments. For example, a completely tooth-supported mandibular Kennedy Class III RPD will usually require a short appointment of 30 to 60 minutes. Opposing distal-extension RPDs replacing most of the posterior teeth or involving over six abutment teeth will require a much greater dentist effort and appointment time. The dentist should never rush this appointment, because there are too many details to cover, and the acceptance of a new prosthesis will be enhanced if postinsertion discomfort is minimal (Bauman, 1979).

DENTIST'S EVALUATION OF THE PATIENT'S PSYCHOLOGIC ATTITUDES TOWARD DENTAL PROSTHESES

A psychologic evaluation of the patient should begin at the diagnostic appointment and continue throughout treatment, leading up to the insertion of the prosthesis. The dentist's evaluation of psychologic factors and ability to assist the patient in overcoming problems are one of the key factors of successful prosthodontic rehabilitation of the patient.

Dentists have recognized that there are numerous factors that will influence patients' acceptance of their prostheses. A considerable body of knowledge has been published in recent years regarding the psychologic factors important in accommodating to dental prosthetic restorations (Strauss and associates, 1977; Cinotti and associates, 1972). Some patients have a high dental IQ, perhaps because they have had regular dental examinations and treatment for years. They appreciate the benefits of a healthy oral cavity. They know dental terminology, such as *periodontal disease, dental caries,* and *ceramic crowns,* and they understand the need for continual dental care. Conversely, some patients lose teeth, and their reasons for seeking dental care at this time are not genuinely motivated. It could be that their children have pressured them into having prosthodontic replacements, the company they work for has begun to provide them with dental insurance, or they are lonely and bored. The patient with a low dental IQ will react much differently to an RPD than the patient with a high dental IQ. The patient with a high dental IQ will usually be highly motivated to replace missing teeth. The patient who goes to the dentist only to satisfy family members or because he or she can get something for nothing will often be a poor and unappreciative dental patient.

The dentist must constantly evaluate the attitudes of patients during the treatment phases of RPD service. Each patient's perception of prosthodontic treatment will be different. The pessimistic patient must be encouraged, whereas the overly optimistic patient must be cautioned concerning the difficulties that may arise in the use of the prosthesis. The exacting patient may require detailed explanations

264

about the problems involved in using and adapting to the prosthesis.

Cinotti, Grieder, and Springob (1972), in their book, *Applied Psychology in Dentistry,* stated:

Essentially, acceptance of dentures is an educational and retraining process on the part of the patient. Disorientation, difficulty in concentration, excessive loquaciousness, preoccupation with certain ideas, and emotional lability will also present difficulties. . . . Motivation may be lacking for a variety of reasons, including nonacceptance of the disability of his oral mechanism and a reactive depression in the face of the realistic problems that being edentulous presents. . . . The dentist can present to the patient a philosophy on learning to adapt to new dentures. . . . Life consists of a series of problems. What counts is not the fact that problems are present but how effectively one handles them. If one is motivated to master and enjoy his prosthesis, he will.

We encourage the reader to study this important aspect of prosthodontic treatment in more detail in the textbooks and articles found in the dental literature (Bliss, 1951; Colett, 1955b; Epstein, 1970; Ramsey, 1970; Silverman, 1958).

INSERTION PROCEDURES

A routine, sequential approach should be followed for insertion of completed partial dentures. It should include the following:
1. Final inspection of the prosthesis before insertion
2. Seating of the RPD framework
3. Assessment of acrylic resin denture base adaptation
4. Assessment of peripheral extension of the denture base
5. Establishment of occlusal harmony
6. Instruction of the patient in the use and care of the prosthesis (see Chapter 8)

Final inspection of the removable partial denture

The dentist's meticulous attention to the details of the laboratory phases is an important factor in the successful treatment of a partially edentulous patient. The dental laboratory procedures involved in the waxing-up, packing, processing, and finishing of the prosthesis can introduce inaccuracies that will preclude an ac-

curate fit of the RPD intraorally. Imprecise workmanship by the dental laboratory technician can also contribute to a poor finish and polish of the RPD. A poorly finished RPD might not interfere with the fit of the prosthesis, but it would be unacceptable because of the poor impression it would make on the patient. The RPD must be inspected by the dentist before the insertion appointment. This inspection should include an examination for the deficiencies discussed below.

Nodules of acrylic resin on the tissue surface of the prosthesis

When air is trapped during the setting of a dental stone cast, small voids or porosities are left in the cast that may not be visible on the surface (may be subsurface) of the master cast. When acrylic resin is cured against a master cast under heat and pressure, these subsurface voids collapse and become filled with acrylic resin (Fig. 9-1). When the RPD is deflasked, the acrylic resin may be covered with surface nodules. These small tissue-surface nodules of acrylic resin, if left on the RPD, act as a source of irritation to the mucoperiosteum, causing pain and tissue trauma. The easiest way for the dentist to locate these nodules is to run a finger over the tissue side of the prosthesis. Once identified and marked with a pencil, the nodules can then be removed with a vulcanite scraper or a small, round acrylic bur mounted in a slow-speed handpiece. This procedure is continued until the tissue surface is free of all artifacts. The tissue surface of the prosthesis should not be polished but should be left as it was cured against the master cast.

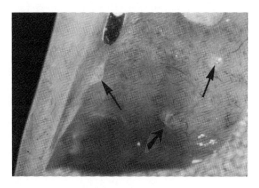

Fig. 9-1. Nodules of acrylic resin that fill in voids in master cast should be removed before insertion of RPD.

Porosity in the acrylic resin caused by poor packing procedures or a rapid curing cycle (Fig. 9-2)

Surface and internal porosity in the acrylic resin caused by poor dental laboratory procedures reduces both the quality and ultimate strength of the completed RPD. When the surfaces of the acrylic resin cannot maintain a high surface luster because of porosity, it will be difficult for the patient to keep these surfaces free of dental plaque. The surface pores will act as a nidus for dental plaque accumulation. The only way to correct porosity defects in the acrylic resin portions of an RPD is to rebase the entire prosthesis.

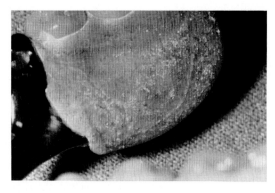

Fig. 9-2. Porosity in acrylic resin indicates poor packing or curing procedures.

Fractured teeth

Each denture tooth on an RPD, whether acrylic resin or dental porcelain, should be closely inspected for fractures that may have occurred during the processing or finishing procedures (Fig. 9-3). Under masticatory stress, a minutely fractured dental porcelain denture tooth will break and shear off, whereas the fracture line of a minutely fractured acrylic resin denture tooth will persist and fill with food stain. In either event, all fractured teeth should be replaced with new denture teeth before the RPD is inserted.

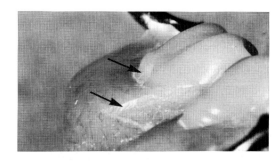

Fig. 9-3. Denture teeth and acrylic resin denture base should be inspected for fractures, which should be repaired.

Crevices at the denture tooth–acrylic resin junction

If the junction of the denture tooth and acrylic resin denture base is improperly contoured and finished after processing, any crevices left in this area will become a potential site of food entrapment or unsightliness because of food stain accumulation (Fig. 9-4). The junction of the denture tooth and acrylic resin of a prosthesis should be carved in a manner similar to that of the skin–nail bed junction found on the fingers.

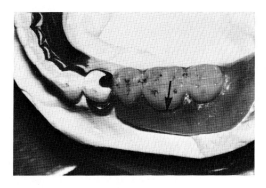

Fig. 9-4. Crevices at denture tooth–acrylic resin junction create food traps.

Untrimmed acrylic resin–cast metal framework finishing lines

When acrylic resin joins the components of an RPD framework, that junction should be a butt (90°) joint with no overlap of the acrylic resin onto the metal framework. Any acrylic resin that has flowed over the metal framework will appear thin and jagged (Fig. 9-5). If this acrylic resin is allowed to remain, it will interfere with the proper placement of the RPD and be both a source of irritation to the sensitive intraoral tissues and a food trap. Also, the patient will find it difficult to keep the RPD clean and stain free. All acrylic resin flash should be removed with finishing burs or finishing chisels and polished so that there is a smooth, continuous transition between the two materials.

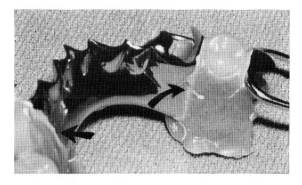

Fig. 9-5. Acrylic resin overlapping metal past finishing line may be indication of poor wax-up or processing procedures.

Destruction of acrylic resin peripheral contours

The acrylic resin borders should be an exact duplication of the border anatomic features recorded by the corrected (altered) cast final impression. Care should be taken not to overly smooth and polish these areas (Fig. 9-6). Excessive use of coarse pumice abrasive on the borders of the RPD will destroy the anatomic contours and the fit of these borders to the patient's intraoral anatomic features. Loss of border fit will encourage food entrapment underneath the RPD.

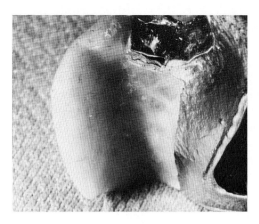

Fig. 9-6. Periphery of acrylic resin denture base has been overtrimmed, overfinished, and overpolished, destroying original contours.

Poor finish and polish of the removable partial denture

The final step in the evaluation of a prosthesis before the insertion appointment is the general inspection of the finish and polish of the polished surfaces. The acceptance of an RPD by the patient is based on the new prosthesis looking clean, well contoured, and meticulously finished (Fig. 9-7). A poorly finished and polished prosthesis will adversely affect the patient's attitude toward the dentist and diminish patient-dentist rapport. The polished surface contours should have a smooth, high luster appearance without surface blemishes.

The dentist's attention to detail during these steps before the patient's appointment for insertion of the RPD will go a long way toward ensuring that the insertion phase will proceed smoothly for both the dentist and patient. When the RPD is completed, it can be stored until the insertion appointment in a plastic bag partly filled with mouthwash and then heat sealed. This will keep the prosthesis moist to prevent dehydration and warpage of the acrylic resin until the prosthesis is inserted.

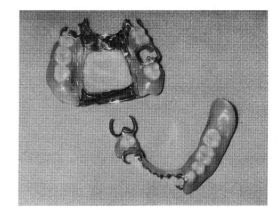

Fig. 9-7. Well-finished and polished prosthesis is pleasing to patient.

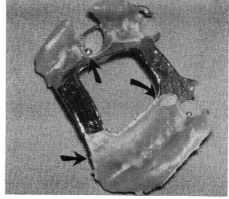

Fig. 9-8. Acrylic resin was cured into undercuts and on major and minor connectors and clasp assemblies.

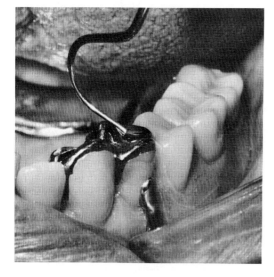

Fig. 9-9. Explorer is used to check seating of occlusal rests.

Seating of the removable partial denture framework

For the majority of patients, the cast metal framework is tried in and adjusted to fit the abutment teeth before the insertion appointment. This is usually accomplished after the casting has been completed and before the corrected (altered) cast impression is made. Now, the completed RPD should be carefully inserted into position on the abutment teeth. If there is considerably more resistance to seating the prosthesis than in seating the framework alone, it is necessary to investigate the reason for this resistance. Various errors may have been introduced during the dental laboratory procedures that will alter the accuracy of the cast metal framework. During processing of the acrylic resin, one or more of the following problems may have developed:

1. Clasp assemblies or other components of the framework may have been bent or distorted.

2. Acrylic resin may have been cured into undercuts adjacent to the abutment teeth, preventing the uniform seating of the prosthesis (Fig. 9-8).

3. Overpacking the prosthesis with acrylic resin may have resulted in a layer of acrylic resin flash covering part of the metal casting. The junction of the metal–acrylic resin finishing lines should be inspected for that possibility.

When the RPD has been inserted on the abutment teeth as far as possible, a sharp dental explorer or dental floss can be used to check for the complete seating of the occlusal rests (Fig. 9-9). Tooth contact of the shoulders and terminal ends of the retentive arms can be checked in the same manner (Fig. 9-10). The dental explorer must be sharp enough to enter any small space between tooth and rest or tooth and clasp.

If the occlusal rests on the prosthesis do not seat completely in their respective rest seat

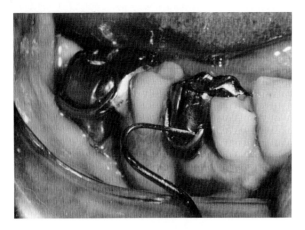

Fig. 9-10. Explorer is used to check terminal ends of clasps.

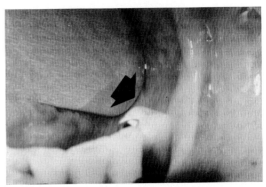

Fig. 9-11. Sharp mylohyoid ridge can be painful when pressure is placed on ridge during function.

preparations, the dentist must determine if minor adjustments of the framework will allow complete seating of the rests. A minor discrepancy in the cast metal framework can be identified and corrected as outlined in Chapter 6. If incomplete seating is not caused by the cast metal framework, then the processed acrylic resin portion of the prosthesis may be at fault. If major faults in the acrylic resin denture bases are identified that prevent the complete seating of the RPD, they must be corrected by relining or rebasing procedures. Refer to Chapter 10 for details of relining and rebasing.

Assessment of acrylic resin denture base adaptation

When the cast metal framework has been fully seated satisfactorily, the dentist should proceed to fitting the acrylic resin portions of the prosthesis. An accurately fitting acrylic resin denture base is a primary consideration in both the comfort and acceptance of an RPD. Excessive pressure from the prosthesis on any of the primary support areas or even minor pressure on relief areas over a period of time can cause irritation of the mucoperiosteum that covers the bony structures of those areas. During mastication, especially in a tooth-tissue–supported RPD, the acrylic resin denture base moves slightly because of differential tissue displaceability. Functional stresses combined with denture base movement will cause irritation of the mucoperiosteum.

There are several reasons that the denture base can cause pressure in areas that cannot

accept pressure. One of the major causes of excessive pressure is that dimensional changes occur in the acrylic resin denture base during the processing procedures. The corrected (altered) cast can be an almost perfect reproduction of the anatomic structures of the oral cavity, but the dental laboratory procedures of waxing-up, flasking, packing, processing, and finishing may introduce inaccuracies that must be eliminated by the dentist before and during insertion of the prosthesis.

In addition to the technical inaccuracies inherent in the processing of the denture base, another reason for a painful response to pressure is the presence of a sharp or irregular bony residual ridge with a thin mucosal covering. A sharp or irregular bony ridge may also occur in some patients whose ridges have a relatively thick mucosal covering. For instance, residual ridge resorption may result in a sharp mylohyoid ridge (Fig. 9-11). The mucoperiosteum covering the mylohyoid ridge is usually thin, with a minimally thick connective tissue layer; therefore, there is little or no cushioning effect from this tissue when a load is applied from a prosthesis. When the denture base moves slightly under masticatory load, the mucoperiosteum is caught between two hard structures, the acrylic resin denture base and the sharp, bony mylohyoid ridge. The resulting mucosal entrapment can cause a severely painful patient response. Therefore, all pressure from the denture base must be eliminated over the mylohyoid ridge or any other sharp, bony areas.

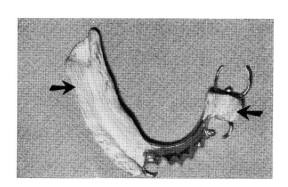

Fig. 9-12. PIP applied to acrylic resin base of mandibular RPD. Note brush marks.

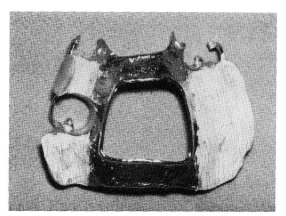

Fig. 9-13. PIP applied to acrylic resin base of maxillary RPD.

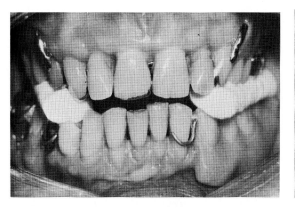

Fig. 9-14. Patient closing mandible onto cotton rolls.

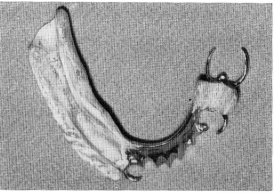

Fig. 9-15. PIP flattened on external oblique ridge, which is a primary stress-bearing area, should not be relieved.

The use of pressure indicator paste (PIP) is one means of determining the accuracy of adaptation of the acrylic resin denture base to the denture-bearing tissues. The PIP is evenly applied to the tissue-fitting surface of the prosthesis with a stiff, short, coarse-hair brush. A coarse brush is essential because it will leave thin brush marks on the acrylic resin surface that will flatten out under pressure. An even, thin layer of PIP is applied so that a good registration of pressure areas will be attained (Figs. 9-12 and 9-13). The RPD is then inserted, cotton rolls are placed between the teeth, and the patient is asked to close the mandible lightly onto the cotton rolls (Fig. 9-14). The dentist may use finger pressure in lieu of cotton rolls. The patient should not be allowed to occlude directly on the teeth, because

the final occlusal adjustments have not been completed. Interceptive occlusal contacts will appear as pressure areas on the tissue side of the RPD. These pressure areas will appear directly underneath an interceptive occlusal contact; thus, a false interpretation of the reason for the pressure area would be recorded.

Correct interpretation and adjustment of pressure areas indicated by the PIP are important. For example, when a mandibular bilateral distal-extension RPD uses the external oblique ridge as a primary stress-bearing area, the PIP will be flattened on the buccal flange area when the patient bites down on the cotton rolls. (Fig. 9-15). In this instance, the buccal periphery covering the external oblique ridge should not be adjusted or reduced, because this would cause a major loss of support for the

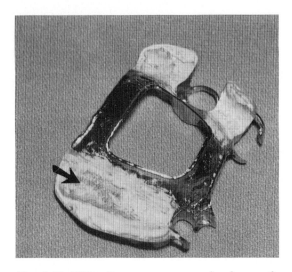

Fig. 9-16. PIP indicates pressure on alveolar maxillary ridge, a primary stress-bearing area that should not be reduced.

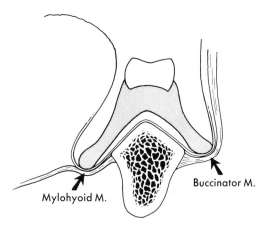

Fig. 9-17. Muscles unseat RPD when borders are overextended.

prosthesis. The dentist must remember the fundamental prosthodontic principles involved in support from the primary and secondary stress-bearing areas and the relief areas of an RPD. Relief areas, such as the median raphe, sharp mylohyoid ridges, and sharp residual ridges, should be reduced judiciously, to prevent overreduction of the denture base. Indications of general pressure on primary stress-bearing areas, such as the crest of the residual ridge of the maxillary arch, are normal, and these areas should not be reduced (Fig. 9-16).

After an area has been judiciously reduced with acrylic burs, the tissue side of the RPD is recoated with PIP and reseated under finger pressure or cotton rolls. Adjustments are made by the dentist until displacement of PIP appears only in the primary stress-bearing areas. There should be little or no paste distortion in secondary stress-bearing areas and none on areas that require relief or are not stress bearing (incisive papilla, tori, mylohyoid ridge, crest of the mandibular residual ridge, median raphe, etc.).

Assessment of peripheral extension of the denture base

The peripheral borders of the RPD base have a direct bearing on the retention and stability of the prosthesis intraorally.

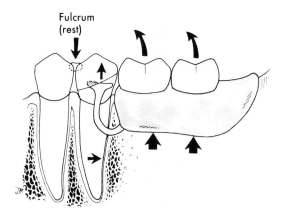

Fig. 9-18. Distal-extension RPD with overextended peripheries (*short, wide arrows*) creates torque on abutment teeth.

Overextension of the denture borders of an RPD will have several deleterious effects:

1. The muscles and frena, when displaced, will tend to dislodge the RPD during function (Figs. 9-17 and 9-18). The clasp assemblies will transfer this stress to the abutment teeth, with a resultant torquing of the tooth. This can cause irreversible damage to both the teeth and associated periodontal tissues. These forces are especially destructive when the borders of a bilateral distal-extension RPD are overextended. The longer the distal-extension

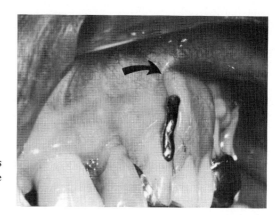

Fig. 9-19. Overextended periphery *(arrow)* displaces muscle and tends to unseat denture and create sore spots.

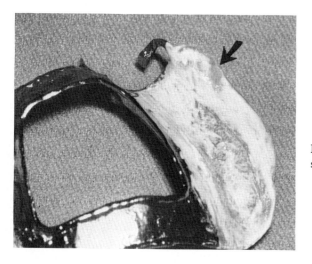

Fig. 9-20. PIP wiped out on periphery by pressure of muscles.

base, the longer the lever arm and the more destructive the stresses on the periodontium of the abutment teeth will be if the denture base is overextended.

2. Overextension can cause ulceration, pain, and swelling of the vestibular tissues. If this condition is not corrected for an extended period of time, redundant tissue will form in the vestibule as a response to chronic irritation.

3. Impingement on the muscles of mastication will interfere with muscle function during mastication and speech production (Figs. 9-19 and 9-20).

Underextended peripheral denture borders will cause the following problems:

1. Support for the prosthesis will be insufficient to resist masticatory stresses. The retromolar pads and buccal shelf area to the external oblique ridges must be covered by the denture base to obtain maximal support for the RPD.

2. Food will collect under the tissue surface of an RPD and be a cause of constant annoyance to the patient.

3. The prosthesis will exhibit a lack of stability. Denture borders that are insufficiently extended onto the residual ridge will not satisfactorily resist lateral or horizontal stresses. Therefore, this lack of stability will place excessive lateral stresses on the abutment teeth.

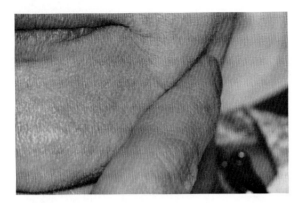

Fig. 9-21. Palpation of buccal flange of mandibular pad determines overextension in relation to outer border of external oblique ridge.

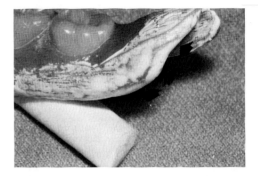

Fig. 9-22. PIP is wiped off distobuccal border when border is overextended into masseter muscle area *(arrows).*

There are several methods that the dentist may use as an aid in determining whether the denture bases are extended correctly:

1. The dentist may observe directly and intraorally the denture borders of the RPD. The patient is instructed to open the mouth just wide enough for the dentist to observe the denture borders. Overextension is usually easily detectable, because the mucosal tissues will be displaced by the denture border's pressing into the soft tissues. Underextension can be observed by very lightly deflecting the border tissues with the fingers and then letting the tissues return slowly to their relaxed position.

2. The dentist may use external palpation with the index finger. This is an especially effective method, which uses applied pressure on the outside of the face over the region of the external oblique ridge. When the buccal flange of a mandibular RPD is overextended in this area, the dentist can feel that border extending out beyond the external oblique ridge (Fig. 9-21).

3. For areas that are difficult to observe, the dentist can apply PIP to the RPD borders. The RPD is then placed in the mouth, several drops of water are placed on the patient's tongue, and the patient is asked to swallow. Any areas of overextension will be visible where the wax or paste has been flattened or displaced by

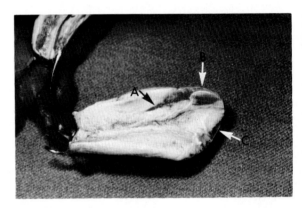

Fig. 9-23. PIP indicates pressure on *(A)* mylohyoid ridge and overextension of *(B)* retromylohyoid, or distolingual, and *(C)* distal buccal borders.

muscle action. The use of PIP is especially effective on the distobuccal border of the mandibular RPD, which is controlled by the masseter muscle (Fig. 9-22). Pressure on the mylohyoid ridge, distolingual border, and distal border during function is seen in Fig. 9-23.

The most common areas of overextension of a maxillary RPD are the tissue side of the distobuccal flange, the denture border contiguous to the malar process, and the area of the hamular notch, where the prosthesis may interfere with the pterygomandibular raphe or pterygoid hamulus.

Determination of pressure areas that occur during the insertion and withdrawal of an RPD as a result of soft-tissue and bony undercuts is important. The use of PIP is an effective means to disclose these undercut areas. Common undercut areas are located inferior to the mylohyoid ridge, in the canine and premolar fossae, and in the retromylohyoid space. Recent extraction of either maxillary or mandibular anterior teeth will leave bony undercuts in the incisive and canine fossae. The RPD base must be adjusted correctly to allow the prosthesis to be inserted and withdrawn over undercuts without damaging the mucoperiosteum. Adjustment of the prosthesis to provide adequate relief so that the RPD can be inserted and withdrawn without tissue damage is accomplished in two ways. The first is by selective grinding of the tissue-fitting surface of the denture base over the undercut area; the second is by compression of the mucoperiosteum and its subsequent relaxation when the RPD is inserted. If either of these methods fails to allow the prosthesis to be inserted and withdrawn in a nontraumatic manner, vertical reduction of the denture flange may be indicated.

Replacement of the anterior residual ridge with an acrylic resin denture base is necessary when considerable residual ridge resorption has occurred. The acrylic resin esthetically replaces missing bone by recontouring the anterior residual ridge area to support the facial muscles. Altered cast impression procedures are not feasible for registering the anterior dental arch segment; therefore, the impression that registers the anterior edentulous area is made with irreversible hydrocolloid. This material (alginate) will not accurately register the dynamic state (width or depth) of the labial frenum and vestibular tissue. To determine whether the denture border is properly contoured, the dentist must retract the lip and move it to the left and right while observing the movement of the frenum into the acrylic resin notch. The acrylic resin notch may need additional width or depth modification to accommodate the labial frenum. The patient's facial profile should be examined by direct observation from both the frontal and profile views to determine if the lips are properly supported in repose and function. Areas in which there is excess vertical height and bulk can be reduced with acrylic burs. Areas of undercontour can

first be restored by the application of baseplate wax to deficient areas to increase contour; then, when both dentist and patient are satisfied, new acrylic resin can be processed to the existing denture base. The acrylic resin polished surface should be contoured correctly to harmonize with the labial contours of the residual ridge and tapered properly to blend with the contour of the mucosal tissues anterior to the abutment teeth.

Establishment of occlusal harmony

Occlusal harmony is a prerequisite for successful long-term treatment of the partially edentulous patient. The destructive effects of interceptive occlusal contacts are many and varied and may include one or all of the following:

1. Temporomandibular joint (TMJ) pain
2. Ulceration of the mucoperiosteum immediately under the interceptive contact
3. Trauma to the periodontium of the abutment teeth
4. Trauma to abutment teeth
5. Masticatory difficulties and inefficiency
6. Denture instability on the side opposite the occlusal interference
7. Nonspecific patient discomfort.

Occlusal equilibration of natural teeth and rests for RPDs has been previously discussed (see Chapter 5). Denture-tooth arrangement for the prosthesis should be accomplished in accordance with sound prosthodontic principles and practices. At the try-in visit, the maxillomandibular relationships and the esthetic and phonetic arrangement of the denture teeth are verified. Therefore, the occlusal adjustment of the RPD following processing of the denture bases should involve only minor processing changes. Many of these processing changes can be corrected with a laboratory remount of the prosthesis before removal of the master cast.

Various clinical methods can be used for determining interceptive occlusal contacts:

1. Direct observation of teeth during closure
2. Use of articulating paper (Figs. 9-24 and 9-25)
3. Use of occlusal indicator wax (Figs. 9-26 through 9-29)
4. Use of a new interocclusal record and remounting of the prosthesis on a dental articulator (Figs. 9-30 through 9-35).

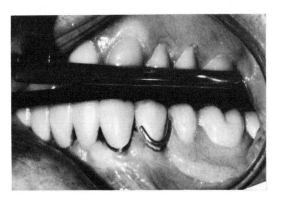

Fig. 9-24. Patient is asked to close mandible onto articulating paper with tip of tongue positioned up and back.

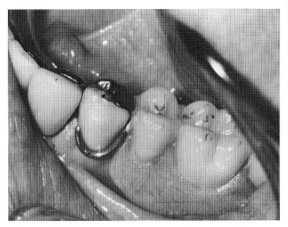

Fig. 9-25. Occlusal contacts distributed on natural and denture teeth.

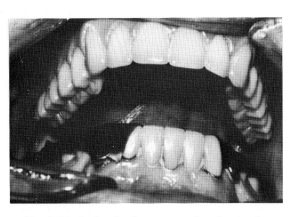

Fig. 9-26. Occlusal indicator wax placed on occlusal surface of RPD.

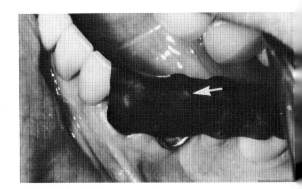

Fig. 9-27. Perforation in wax indicates interceptive occlusal contact.

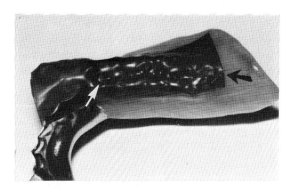

Fig. 9-28. Perforations are located on first premolars and second molar *(arrow)*.

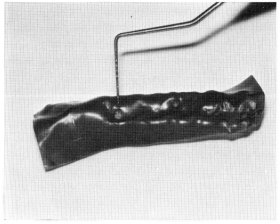

Fig. 9-29. Perforation completely through wax indicates heavy premature contact.

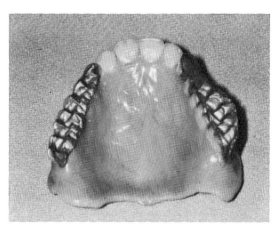

Fig. 9-30. Centric jaw relationship record should be made before remount impression.

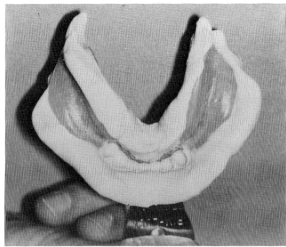

Fig. 9-31. Alginate impression with RPD imbedded in impression for remount procedures.

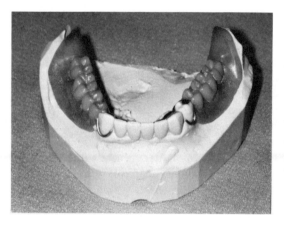

Fig. 9-32. Plaster cast and RPD is recovered from impression.

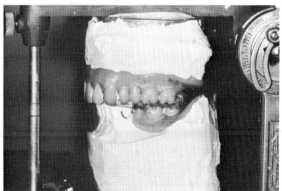

Fig. 9-33. RPD is mounted on articulator using centric jaw relationship record.

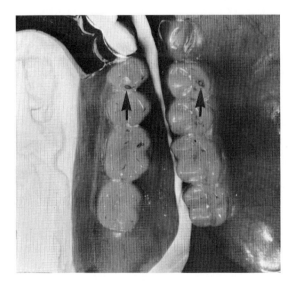

Fig. 9-34. Carbon articulating paper is used to determine interceptive occlusal contacts on premolars *(arrows)*.

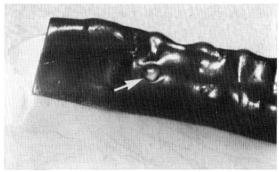

Fig. 9-35. Interceptive occlusal contact is demonstrated using occlusal indicator wax (same contact as in Fig. 9-34).

Occlusal adjustment of a single removable partial denture

Gross occlusal disharmonies can be determined by direct observation of the occlusion when the patient closes the mandible into centric relation. When the occlusion is checked by direct observation, it is necessary that the prosthesis be firmly seated on the denture-bearing areas when the teeth occlude. Therefore, the dentist must maintain the RPD in position (especially if it is a bilateral distal-extension RPD), because it may be displaced slightly when the mouth is opened. To prevent even a slight displacement of the denture, the dentist places his or her index fingers bilaterally on the buccal polished surface contours of the denture base. The patient is instructed to place the tip of the tongue on the posterior portion of the palate and then to close the mandible slowly. The patient will usually achieve centric relation when he or she uses this tongue position when retruding the mandible. The dentist should observe the contact of both the denture teeth and the natural teeth as the patient closes the mandible into maximum intercuspation. Any minor interceptive occlusal contacts can be corrected by selective grinding adjustments, which are made after the contacts are marked with articulating paper. If gross premature occlusal contacts are noted, a new interocclusal (centric relation) record must be recorded. The RPD is remounted on a dental articulator, and the necessary occlusal corrections are made by selective grinding at an acceptable vertical dimension of occlusion.

Occlusal adjustment of opposing maxillary and mandibular distal-extension removable partial dentures

The same procedures used to adjust the occlusion for a single RPD can be used for opposing RPDs. However, when the occlusion is observed intraorally, the less retentive of the two RPDs should be maintained in position with the index fingers. In most instances, new interocclusal (centric relation) records are required so that the RPDs can be remounted on a dental articulator to perfect the occlusion.

This is especially true if the dentist feels that in eccentric movements the occlusion should be rechecked for interfering balancing-side contacts.

Following any occlusal adjustment, the anatomic features of the artificial teeth should be restored to maximum efficiency by redefinition of the grooves and embrasure spaces and repolishing of the teeth.

Procedures for remounting the prosthesis

The master cast most likely was destroyed when the RPD was finished and polished. Therefore, to obtain an accurate remount cast to correct occlusal disharmonies, it will be necessary for the dentist to make an intraoral irreversible hydrocolloid (alginate) impression of the prosthesis correctly positioned on the supporting tissues. The remount cast will include both the natural teeth and the prosthesis, which can be mounted on a dental articulator against a dental stone cast of the opposing dentition by means of a new centric relation record. Correction of major occlusal discrepancies might require the dentist to remove the denture teeth from the prosthesis, reset the same or new denture teeth, schedule another patient try-in visit, and reprocess the RPD. Minor occlusal disharmonies can be corrected by selective grinding, reestablishment of the occlusal anatomic features, and repolishing of the denture teeth.

If there are no observable premature contacts when the patient occludes, articulating paper is used to determine if there are any deflective occlusal contacts. Using occlusal indicator wax is another method of registering major interceptive occlusal contacts. The goal in occlusal adjustment is to eliminate all deflective occlusal contacts and provide evenly distributed, simultaneous balanced occlusal contacts on both the natural teeth and denture teeth at the vertical dimension of occlusion. Occlusal harmony is an important aspect of the RPD service. It is necessary in order to maintain the health of the periodontium and residual ridges and for patient comfort during mastication and deglutition.

Section 2: Postinsertion adjustment procedures

Postinsertion problems can cause a myriad of difficulties for both patient and dentist. Even when meticulous care is taken by the dentist during all procedures involved in making the prosthesis, many unforeseen problems arise when the patient is becoming habituated to a new RPD. These problems, however, are minimized when a sequential insertion procedure, as described in section 1, has been followed by the dentist. The problems associated with becoming habituated to a new RPD can be classified under four major headings: (1) comfort, (2) function, (3) esthetics, and (4) phonetics.

No one of these four areas is more important than another, but each patient may be willing to accept an inadequacy of the prosthesis in one area to achieve near perfection in another. However, even if the patient is willing to compromise one aspect of the prosthesis to achieve a better result in another, there are fundamental principles governing the fabrication of the prosthesis that cannot be compromised. An example of this would be an attempt to improve the esthetic result by increasing the vertical dimension of occlusion. In this instance, fundamentals of muscle physiology would be violated, thereby precluding successful prosthodontic rehabilitation of the patient.

Postinsertion problems can arise as a result of one or a combination of these four factors. The dentist must approach the patient's complaints and solve them in a logical, systematic manner. For example, the etiology of a TMJ dysfunction for a patient using an RPD may be caused by one or more of eight different factors:

1. Inadequate interocclusal distance
2. Centric occlusion not in harmony with centric relation
3. Interceptive occlusal contacts
4. Referred pain from an abutment tooth
5. Arthritis
6. Denture trauma
7. Overextension of the distobuccal border of a maxillary RPD
8. Patient parafunctional habits

COMFORT

Areas of tissue trauma may develop the first day or several days after the insertion of an RPD. Table 9-1 lists the various potential patient complaints of pain associated with a new prosthesis.

A generalized soreness over the crest of the residual ridges can be caused by patient habits, such as clenching or bruxing. The patient with a parafunctional habit such as bruxism usually has an underlying emotional problem or excessive stress that has led to the habit. To detect parafunctional habits, the dentist should engage patients in casual conversation and observe their mannerisms. Usually when patients clench their teeth together firmly, the dentist can observe a marked, prolonged contraction of the masseter and temporalis muscles. Severe emotional problems, a causative factor in bruxism, are beyond the scope of the dentist to diagnose and treat. Such patients should be made aware of the problem and encouraged to see their family physician. A letter should be sent to the physician explaining the patient's physical problem and the possible emotional relationship.

A differential diagnosis of a burning sensation is determined by the location of the problem. The most common area for a localized burning sensation to occur is the anterior hard palate, which receives its sensory innervation through the anterior palatine nerve. The anterior palatine papilla (incisive papilla), which is just lingual to the maxillary central incisors, covers the exit of the anterior palatine nerve from the incisive foramen. Pressure on the incisive papilla can occur when an RPD is first inserted, or it can occur subsequently under occlusal loading. Usually the incisive papilla will appear reddened because of the pressure from the prosthesis. Reduction of the pressure on the incisive papilla by selective grinding of the denture base will usually correct any anterior burning sensation. A burning sensation located on the posterior hard palate is corrected by reduction of pressure over the posterior palatine foramen.

Tongue and cheek biting is more prevalent when monoplane (0°) posterior denture teeth are used than when other types of denture teeth are used. Monoplane posterior denture teeth can easily be arranged with no horizontal overlap. This lack of horizontal overlap allows the soft tissues of the tongue and cheeks to become trapped between the denture teeth during mastication or swallowing, leading to pain-

TABLE 9-1

Patient's postinsertion complaints about discomfort and their causes

Complaint	Cause
Tissue trauma	
In vestibules	Overextended denture borders
On the posterior limit of maxillary RPD	Posterior palatal seal too deep
	Sharp posterior denture border
	Overextension on highly mobile soft palate
Single areas of tissue trauma over residual ridges	Interceptive occlusal contacts
	Inaccurately fitting denture base
	Acrylic resin nodules
	Movement of denture on bony eminences
	Thin mucosal covering
Generalized soreness over residual ridges	Vertical dimension of occlusion too great; inadequate interocclusal distance
	Inaccurately fitting denture base
	Parafunctional habits (such as bruxism)
	Nutritional deficiencies
	C. albicans infection
Pain at distobuccal denture border	Impingement on masseter muscle during function
Pain under lingual bar or at lingual peripheries	Overextension of lingual denture border
	Lingual bar too low, impinging on lingual frenum or floor of mouth
	Deflective occlusal contacts
Pain and swelling of gingival tissues	Lingual denture borders too close to teeth
	Pressure on lingual gingival tissues
	Lack of adequate oral hygiene
Painful abutment teeth	Interceptive occlusal contacts on abutment teeth
	Interceptive occlusal contact on one or more denture teeth
	Rest or clasp exceeding physiologic limits of abutment tooth tolerance
	Interceptive occlusal contact on rests
	Unstable denture bases
	Insufficient interocclusal distance

Adapted from Morstad, A.T., and Petersen, A.D.: J. Prosthet, Dent. **19:**126, 1968.

ful ulcerations. The problem can be corrected by reducing the lingual or buccal surfaces of the maxillary or mandibular denture teeth, allowing the unaltered opposing denture tooth to hold the soft tissues away from the occlusal surfaces of the teeth.

Lip biting is generally caused by improper placement of mandibular teeth in relation to the maxillary teeth. Usually, recontouring the labial surfaces of the mandibular canine teeth will eliminate the problem. Observation of patient can determine whether lip biting is caused by habit. Counseling can often correct the problem.

It is often necessary to differentiate between an allergic reaction caused by denture materi-

als and an irritation that is caused by an ill-fitting denture, avitaminosis, or inadequate oral hygiene. An allergic reaction may be primarily suspected when all tissues, tongue, cheeks, and denture-bearing areas that come in contact with the acrylic resin denture base or metal framework are fiery red. However, true allergic reactions are extremely rare. In contrast, an ill-fitting denture, avitaminosis, monilial infection, or poor dental hygiene will cause redness only in the denture-bearing areas. This is a fairly common problem.

There are at least eight causes for TMJ pain. If pain occurs in the TMJ initially or shortly after the RPDs are first inserted, the cause may be either a reduced vertical dimension of oc-

TABLE 9-1

Patient's postinsertion complaints about discomfort and their causes—cont'd

Complaint	Cause
Burning sensation	
In anterior hard palate and anterior residual ridge areas	Pressure on anterior palatine foramen
In maxillary premolar to molar area	Pressure on posterior palatine foramen
In mandibular anterior residual ridge	Pressure on mental foramen
Tongue, lip, or cheek biting	Overclosure (that is, excessive interocclusal distance)
	Posterior denture teeth set with no horizontal overlap
	Posterior denture teeth set too far buccally or lingually
	Posterior teeth set too far distally
	Improper position of anterior teeth
	Patient habits
Fiery redness of all tissues contacted by RPD	Denture base allergy (rare)
	Excessive residual acrylic resin monomer
	C. albicans infection
Redness of denture-bearing areas	Ill-fitting RPD
	Avitaminosis
	C. albicans infection
	Inadequate oral and denture hygiene
TMJ pain	Insufficient vertical dimension of occlusion
	Centric occlusion not in harmony with centric relation
	Interceptive occlusal contacts
	Referred pain from sensitive abutment tooth
	Arthritis
	Trauma
	Patient habits (such as, bruxism, clenching)
	Overextension of distobuccal border of maxillary prosthesis

clusion (absence of adequate interocclusal distance) or centric occlusion that is not in harmony with centric relation. When properly diagnosed, either of these errors is correctable by the dentist. However, pain caused by arthritis or trauma is more difficult to diagnose and treat. Arthritic pain or pain caused by trauma usually has a previous history and will not require treatment with a new prosthesis.

FUNCTION

Table 9-2 lists the numerous functional complaints arising after the patient has used an RPD for varying periods of time. This table presents several recurring reasons for the complaint. They include:

1. Insufficient retention of the prosthesis and denture border overextension
2. Incorrect occlusal vertical dimension
3. Interceptive occlusal contacts

Insufficient retention and denture border extension

Bilateral distal extension RPDs are inherently less stable than most other types of RPDs because there are no posterior abutment teeth that can be used for retention and support. The remaining natural teeth must be used judiciously for retention or the physiologic limits of the periodontium will be exceeded. The abutment tooth's capacity to be maintained over a prolonged period of time is seriously compro-

TABLE 9-2

Patients' postinsertion complaints about function and their causes

Complaint	Cause
Instability of prosthesis	
When not occluding	Insufficient engagement of retentive areas by arms of direct retainers
	Insufficient number of retentive abutment teeth
	Overextension of RPD borders
	Hypermobile tissues displaced when impressions were made now rebound
When incising food	Insufficient engagement of retentive areas
	Poor support under anterior denture teeth
	Incorrect incising habits of patient
When masticating food	Interceptive occlusal contacts
	On individual teeth
	On one side of dental arch
	In premolar area
	Poorly designed clasp assemblies
	Redundant tissue on residual ridge
	Centric occlusion not in harmony with centric relation
Interference	
Swallowing	Posterior denture teeth set too far lingually
	Distolingual border (retromylohyoid area) of mandibular RPD overextended
	Distolingual border (polished surface) of mandibular RPD too thick, interfering with pterygomaxillary ligament and palatoglossal muscle
	Distal border of maxillary RPD too thick
	Distal border of maxillary RPD overextended
	Excessive or insufficient vertical dimension of occlusion
Gagging	
On insertion of RPD	Overextension of maxillary RPD
	Posterior border of maxillary RPD too thick
	Distolingual border of mandibular RPD too thick
	Psychologic rejection of prosthesis
	Inadequate retention of RPD
Delayed (2 weeks to indefinite time after insertion)	Inadequate posterior palatal seal, allowing saliva under maxillary RPD
	Lack of retention, allowing saliva under prosthesis
Teeth contacting during speech	Excessive vertical dimension of occlusion (insufficient interocclusal distance)
Deafness	Insufficient vertical dimension of occlusion (excessive interocclusal distance)
Functional problems with no specific symptoms	Incorrect vertical dimension of occlusion
	Interceptive occlusal contacts
	Incorrect centric relation
	Psychologic rejection of prosthesis

Adapted from Morstad, A.T., and Petersen, A.D.: J. Prosthet. Dent. **19:**126, 1968.

mised by excessive overloading from this type of prosthesis. If the RPD dislodges during function, the temptation for the dentist is to deepen the retentive undercut for the retentive arm of the clasp assembly and bend the retentive arm into the deepened undercut. Not only will this place a greater stress on the abutment tooth and ultimately on the periodontium, but also half-round cast clasps cannot be adjusted edgewise to increase or decrease the retentive potential of a cast clasp (Henderson and Steffel, 1981). A more prudent approach is to examine the denture base extensions by using disclosing wax during function to determine if they are overextended and thus causing the RPD to dislodge. Properly extended denture borders and intimate denture base-tissue contact minimize the retentive requirements of an abutment tooth. Over the long-term after the habituation period, it is ultimately neuromuscular control rather than the influence of the direct retainers that is the key to successful RPD retention.

Incorrect occlusal vertical dimension

An incorrect vertical dimension of occlusion is more often associated with problems of complete dentures rather than with those of RPDs because of the inherent subjectivity involved in determining this dimension. However, the functional problems associated with an inappropriate occlusal vertical dimension in an RPD are the same as those of a complete denture and will create similar patient difficulties.

An incorrect vertical dimension of occlusion can be caused by:

1. Surveyed abutment tooth crowns' being too long or short occlusogingivally
2. Multiple natural tooth loss and muscle shortening, which cause intrusion of teeth with reduced vertical dimension of occlusion and morphologic face height
3. Extensive occlusal abrasion and wear, which cause a decreased vertical dimension of occlusion
4. An RPD's opposing a complete denture constructed at an incorrect vertical dimension of occlusion

Meticulous care is required by the dentist both to determine and reverify the records of facial dimension to establish an acceptable vertical dimension of occlusion and to construct the prosthesis to this predetermined occlusal vertical dimension.

Interceptive (deflective) occlusal contacts

The occlusion of an RPD is adjusted before and during the insertion phase of patient treatment. However, occlusion is a dynamic, not a static, entity. Under masticatory pressure, the natural teeth shift and denture bases adapt to the resilient denture-bearing tissues. The result of these changes, coupled with continual residual ridge reduction, is that interceptive occlusal contacts continue to recur for the majority of patients as long as the prosthesis is used.

Interceptive occlusal contacts are the most frequent causes of instability of an RPD during its functional use. One interceptive occlusal contact on one side of the dental arch can cause the RPD to be displaced from the tissues on the opposite side of the dental arch and

give the patient a "rocking" sensation. Occlusal adjustment is an ongoing maintenance procedure that must be performed at all recall visits. It is a necessary procedure to maintain the continued oral health of all patients treated with RPDs.

Swallowing and gagging

Problems associated with swallowing can be caused by a number of factors. One is the overextension of the mandibular denture base in the retromylohyoid space or the polished surface contour of the prosthesis in that region's being too thick. A maxillary RPD may cause swallowing difficulties if it is overextended posteriorly or if its posterior border is excessively thickened. An increased or grossly decreased vertical dimension of occlusion can also contribute to patient swallowing difficulties. Placement of posterior denture teeth in lingual version is another possible cause of swallowing problems.

The problems associated with swallowing can also cause physiologic gagging on insertion of the prosthesis. However, if a gagging problem is absent immediately after insertion of the RPD and the physiologic gagging occurs several weeks to months following insertion, salivary entrapment under the prosthesis may be the cause. An imperfect posterior denture border seal or malocclusion may cause the RPD to allow saliva to enter between the mucoperiosteum and the prosthesis, triggering the patient's gag reflex.

Food collection on the borders

Proper contouring and tapering of the peripheral borders is important to prevent collection of food on the borders. However, there are some peripheral borders that must be left thick to fill in space and support the facial musculature. Such is the case when the maxillary distobuccal vestibule is wide.

Food can adhere to the denture if it is poorly contoured or not polished or if the patient has a diminished salivary flow. A decreased salivary flow may be caused by aging, medication, or irradiation. Patients with ulcers who are taking propantheline bromide (Probanthine) usually have less saliva and have to compensate by drinking more fluids when eating. High polish of acrylic resin will cause chewing gum to stick to the surface. Usually,

TABLE 9-3

Patients' postinsertion complaints about esthetics and their causes

Complaint	Cause
Upper lip distorted or unsupported	Anterior denture teeth placed too far lingually
	Maxillary anterior denture base too thin (unsupported) or too thick (distorted)
Excessive anterior denture tooth display	Occlusal plane established too low
	Cuspids and lateral incisors arranged with excessive prominence
	Lack of adequate "smile line"
	Anterior denture teeth too large for dental arch segment
	Vertical dimension of occlusion excessive (interocclusal distance insufficient)
Fullness under nose	Maxillary anterior denture base too thick or overextended
Poor esthetics: anterior artificial teeth not in harmony with natural teeth	Incorrect size and position
	Incorrect characterization
	Poor color selection
	Poor blending of acrylic denture base with natural gingivoalveolar anatomic features
	Patient expectations too great

Adapted from Morstad, A.T., and Petersen, A.D.: J. Prosthet. Dent. **19:**126, 1968.

removal of the high polish with flour of pumice and a rag wheel will correct the problem.

Functional problems with no specific symptoms

If the patient states that the RPDs do not feel right but has no specific symptoms, the dentist may suspect that an incorrect occlusal vertical dimension, incorrect centric relation or other malocclusion, maladaptation to the prosthesis, or some combination of these problems is the cause. Time spent by the dentist in reevaluating the occlusal vertical dimension, recording new interocclusal records, and remounting the prosthesis to correct the difficulties will be well spent and will save the patient a great deal of distress.

ESTHETICS

Replacement of anterior teeth with an RPD presents esthetic problems that are particular to a patient treated with an RPD but are less of a factor in fixed partial denture or complete denture prosthodontics. Esthetic problems are especially pronounced for the patient with a short, active upper lip who displays a large amount of tooth and residual ridge when smiling. Common patient complaints about esthetics are given in Table 9-3.

Contouring the acrylic resin to taper and blend harmoniously with the natural tissues in both color and morphologic characteristics requires a considerable effort by the dentist. Matching anterior denture teeth with natural teeth requires proper attention to shade control, characterization of the contours of the denture teeth to harmonize with the natural teeth, and correct denture tooth positioning. Correct lighting in the dental operatory is an important factor in shade selection, because the incidence of refraction of light by the natural teeth will not be the same as that for artificial teeth.

A poor esthetic result in an RPD can be caused by the same factors as are present in a complete denture:

1. The occlusal plane is established at a level that is either too low or too high
2. The cuspids and lateral incisors have too much prominence and are not sufficiently rotated in the dental arch
3. Incorrect labiolingual and axial inclination and denture tooth position are used
4. The dentist fails to create an adequate "smile line"

The patient's expectations of the esthetic result may be far beyond the ability of the dentist. Often older people will request that verti-

TABLE 9-4

Patients' postinsertion complaints about phonetics and their causes

Complaint	Cause
Whistle on *S* sounds	Too narrow an air space on the anterior part of palate
Lisping on *S* sounds	Too broad an air space on anterior part of palate
Indistinct *TH* and *T* sounds	Inadequate interocclusal distance
T sounds like *TH*	Maxillary anterior denture teeth set too far lingually
Indistinct *F* and *V* sounds	Improper position of maxillary anterior teeth (either vertically or horizontally) in relation to lower lip

Adapted from Morstad, A.T., and Petersen, A.D.: J. Prosthet. Dent. **19:**126, 1968.

cal wrinkles of aging radiating out from the lips be eliminated. This would often require that the teeth be placed too far labially. Plastic surgery is usually the only way to eliminate these lines. Patient counseling and close attention to the patient's desires can often lead to successful treatment of unhappy, discouraged patients. There is a challenge in restoring patients to an esthetically acceptable result. Although some patients are emotionally disturbed and will never accept loss of their teeth, others, with proper treatment and care, can be successfully restored.

The dentist must develop an appreciation for good artistic reflection to achieve maximum esthetic results in RPD prosthodontics.

PHONETICS

The majority of RPDs will not produce any appreciable adverse effects on patient speech patterns or sounds. However, the loss of maxillary anterior teeth or extensive loss of maxillary posterior teeth will change the anatomy of the maxillary dental arch. Replacement of the missing teeth, major connector placement, dental arch form, and denture base contour can either detract from or enhance the ability of the patient's tongue to function effectively in the production of speech sounds.

It is difficult for the dentist to determine the source of speech problems at the try-in stage because:

1. The prosthesis is new for the patient.
2. The tongue and lips do not assume the same position when in contact with wax as they do against a finished and polished acrylic resin denture base.

Phonetic problems associated with RPD treatment and their probable causes are listed in Table 9-4.

Whistling on *S* sounds can indicate that the anterior part of the tongue is being crowded by the maxillary premolars, which constricts the tongue groove necessary to carry expelled air down the center of the palate. This forces the air to whistle through a smaller than normal space. By addition of a ridge of acrylic resin to the palatal portion of the prosthesis in this region, the flow of air will be cut down and the whistling stopped. Lisping on *S* sounds may indicate too small an air space or improper tooth position functionally related to the mandibular anterior teeth. Therefore, the palatal portion of the prosthesis must be thinned or the denture teeth repositioned.

When *TH* and *T* sounds are indistinct, there is usually inadequate interocclusal distance. This can be corrected by thinning the maxillary prosthesis or both maxillary and mandibular denture bases lingually and also by reducing the lingual surface of the premolars. If the *T* sounds are similar to the *TH* sounds, the anterior denture teeth have been positioned too far lingually.

In normal *F* and *V* sound production, the maxillary anterior teeth contact the "wet-dry" line of the lower lip at its highest point. If these sounds are indistinct, the maxillary incisors must be repositioned either vertically or horizontally to their proper positions.

10 Rebasing, relining, and repairs

This chapter deals with reestablishing function for an existing removable partial denture (RPD) that may no longer fit or function in the way in which it was originally intended. This loss of function may be caused by: (1) residual ridge resorption, (2) loss or modification of abutment teeth, (3) mucosal damage or change, (4) fracture of one or more of the various components of the RPD, or (5) deterioration of the denture teeth or denture base of the prosthesis. A number of techniques are explained and illustrated in an effort to present the best or most expedient means of reestablishing function.

RESIDUAL RIDGE REDUCTION AND THE REMOVABLE PARTIAL DENTURE

An RPD that no longer fits or functions properly may be discovered by the dentist at a routine recall examination, but more often than not it is the patient who will seek help from the dentist because of some sort of discomfort. The fracture of some portion of the RPD framework, denture teeth, or acrylic resin denture base is usually obvious, and this subject is dealt with later in this chapter. More insidious, however, is residual ridge reduction (RRR), which occurs with considerable variation in time and rate and directly affects the function of the RPD (Plotnick and associates, 1975).

There are several variables related to the rate of RRR: (1) time (2) availability of viable bone cells, (3) local biochemical factors, (4) systemic biochemical factors, and (5) prosthodontic load factors (Atwood, 1979). The prime feature of this disease process is the chronic and continuing reduction in the size of the residual ridges, which in many individuals continues until death (Tallgren, 1972). RRR occurs most rapidly in the first 6 months to 2 years following extraction of the teeth and thereafter proceeds at a slower pace until death (Atwood, 1979; Carlsson and Persson, 1967; Tallgren and associates, 1980). Dentists must rely on the bony base of the residual ridge to provide the support for an RPD. However, because this bony base is constantly changing as a result of RRR over an indefinite period of time, even the most well-constructed prosthesis will become unserviceable and require constant attention to maintain comfort, function, and esthetics. RRR is a multifactorial process with a large number of variables. In each RPD patient, these variables exist in a unique combination that will determine that patient's rate of RRR. If the variables change, the rate of RRR may change (Atwood, 1979). The sequelae of RRR for any given patient who has been treated with an RPD may include (1) loss of intimate mucosal fit of the tissues to the prosthesis; (2) loss of articulation and occlusal harmony; (3) mucosal damage (such as ulceration, inflammation, or hypertrophy); (4) altered relation of the clasps on the abutment teeth, leading to increased abutment tooth stress; (5) fracture of components of the RPD; and (6) signs and symptoms of the "anterior hyperfunction syndrome" (Saunders and associates, 1979).

The loss of function of an RPD as a result of changes in the bony support of the prosthesis will vary depending on the type of partially edentulous arch. The prosthodontic load factors vary in each patient and in each partially edentulous arch. These factors include (1) amount, frequency, duration, and direction of the applied load; (2) force per unit area; (3) amount of occlusal contact area; (4) amount of denture-bearing area; (5) type of mucoperiosteum; (6) cancellous bone–dampening effect; and (7) traumatic prosthodontic factors (Atwood, 1979). However, there is a certain pattern to RRR, depending on the classification of the partially edentulous arches.

Tooth-borne removable partial denture (Kennedy Class III)

In general, any given patient who has well-healed residual ridges (extractions more than 24 months ago) and is treated with a Kennedy Class III RPD will require the least amount of alterations to the RPD to restore function and receive the longest patient service. Because the prosthodontic load factors are applied to the abutment teeth rather than to mucoperiosteum overlying the labile residual ridges, the tooth-borne prosthesis will have the least amount of RRR. Therefore, the tissue-fitting surface of this type of RPD, whether in maxilla or mandible, will require the least amount of correction to maintain its servicability. Most corrections of the tooth-borne prosthesis need to be made for reasons of esthetics or denture hygiene.

Maxillary distal-extension removable partial denture (Kennedy Class I)

The Kennedy Class I maxillary RPD is borne by both tooth and tissue, with many of the prosthodontic load factors applied to the mucoperiosteum and underlying residual ridge. In spite of this, a patient with well-healed residual ridges who is treated with a maxillary distal-extension RPD will need only occasional RPD correction. This has been found to be especially true when the hard palate rather than the residual ridges is used to support the RPD. Palatal support can be accomplished by use of a wide palatal strap or a complete-palate major connector.

Mandibular distal-extension removable partial denture (Kennedy Class I)

The Kennedy Class I mandibular RPD is the prosthesis that most often requires correction to restore function because of the ravages of RRR. This type of RPD derives some of its support from the residual ridges; therefore, the prosthodontic load factors applied to the residual ridges through and by the prosthesis are the greatest of any type of RPD. All other factors being equal, the denture-supporting area of a maxillary RPD is roughly 1.5 to 2 times that of a mandibular RPD. Plotnick and associates (1975) have reported that the greatest change in the mandibular residual ridge in patients treated with mandibular bilateral distal-extension RPDs occurs when this prosthesis is opposed by a maxillary complete denture; the next amount of change occurs with opposition by a maxillary RPD; the least amount occurs with opposition by natural teeth. When RRR occurs in the mandibular arch of patients treated with a bilateral mandibular distal-extension RPD opposed by a maxillary complete denture, a combination of signs and symptoms occurs that the dentist must be aware of. Kelly (1972) has described the "combination syndrome" as follows: (1) RRR in the anterior maxilla, (2) downgrowth of the maxillary tuberosities, (3) formation of papillary hyperplasia over the hard palate, (4) extrusion of the mandibular anterior teeth, and (5) mandibular residual ridge resorption. In addition, Saunders and associates (1979) have described other associated changes that are often noted in these patients: (1) loss of occlusal vertical dimension, (2) occlusal plane discrepancy, (3) protrusive repositioning of the mandible, (4) poor adaptation of the prostheses, (5) epulis fissuratum formation on the maxillary anterior residual ridge, and (6) retrograde periodontal changes. When a patient is treated with this type of RPD, the patient and dentist must be aware of the magnitude of changes that can occur and of the fact that these changes may occur rapidly when RRR proceeds quickly.

Obviously, in any given clinical situation if the patient is treated with an RPD soon after extraction of the teeth, changes in the morphologic features of the residual ridges are of a greater magnitude than in a patient with well-healed residual ridges. The rate and amount of RRR are greatest for periods of up to 2 years after extraction of teeth and then progressively lessen with time (Carlson and Persson, 1967; Tallgren, 1972).

PROCEDURES FOR REESTABLISHING FUNCTION FOR A REMOVABLE PARTIAL DENTURE

The dentist may perform one or several of the following procedures to reestablish function for an RPD: (1) relining of the tissue surface of the prosthesis, (2) rebasing of the prosthesis, (3) reconstruction of the prosthesis using the existing cast framework, (4) simple and complex repairs, and (5) restoration of an abutment tooth under a clasp.

Relining and rebasing

In the vast majority of refitting procedures, relining an RPD is the most expedient treatment. Relining of a prosthesis is the process of adding new base material (usually acrylic resin) to the tissue surface of an RPD to restore the fit of the prosthesis to the mucoperiosteum.

Rebasing of an RPD is normally limited to clinical situations in which: (1) the denture base acrylic resin is esthetically or functionally unacceptable, (2) substantial denture flange extension is necessary, or (3) denture teeth must also be replaced on the RPD during the refitting procedure. For Kennedy Class I mandibular distal-extension RPDs in which there is severe residual ridge resorption, rebasing is frequently necessary for one or all of these reasons. Rebasing procedures involve replacing the entire denture base with new base material to restore not only the tissue surface but also polished surface contours and to provide mechanical retention for new denture teeth if they are needed.

Factors to be considered

PATIENT EXAMINATION RESULTS. The patient's mouth must be in a state of health. Areas to be evaluated by the dentist are: (1) anatomic features of the residual ridges in both the mandible and maxilla (clinical and radiographic examination required), (2) mucoperiosteum (masticatory mucosa), (3) mucosal tissue (border tissues), and (4) periodontium.

If the results of the patient examination reveal injury to the soft tissues associated with the RPD, the dentist's usual tissue-recovery procedures should be followed to return these tissues to optimal health before relining or rebasing of the prosthesis is done. Tissue-recovery procedures may involve: (1) tissue rest, (2) use of tissue-conditioning materials, (3) construction of temporary prostheses, (4) nutritional counseling, and (5) surgical procedures.

For the patient who cannot or will not leave the RPD out of the mouth before the relining impression procedure is done, tissue-conditioning materials may be used as an adjunct to return the mucosal tissues to a noninflamed state of health. The same indications and contraindications that apply to the use of the tissue-conditioning materials for complete dentures apply to their use with RPDs.

ABUTMENT TEETH AND THE FIT OF THE REMOVABLE PARTIAL DENTURE FRAMEWORK. The RPD framework must adequately fit the abutment teeth, with all of its components in good condition (that is, all clasp arms intact, occlusal rests of adequate thickness, and major connector fitting properly) before any relining or rebasing procedure is done. To determine the accuracy of fit and the correct position of the RPD framework, it must be reseated in its original terminal position (Figs. 10-1 and 10-2). When the framework of the prosthesis is correctly oriented on the abutment teeth, the dentist should depress the distal-extension denture bases. When RRR has been severe, the RPD will rotate about an imaginary fulcrum line between the two occlusal rests or proximal plates of the terminal clasps. When this rotation occurs, the dentist will observe any indirect retainers anterior to this fulcrum

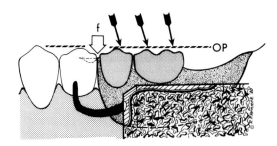

Fig. 10-1. Normal direction of forces of occlusion in distal-extension RPD. Note intimacy of fit of RPD on residual ridge. *f*, Fulcrum; *OP*, occlusal plane.

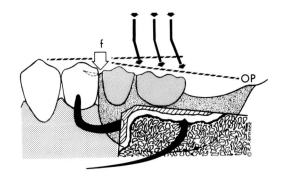

Fig. 10-2. Loss of alveolar supporting structure and rotation around fulcrum at rest seat. Occlusal plane is depressed and inclined posteriorly. Occlusal rest is rotated out of seat, and there is loss of intimacy between RPD and residual ridge. *f*, Fulcrum; *OP*, occlusal plane.

line that are not in their terminal position and the anterior portion of occlusal rests that are slightly rotated out of their rest seats. When rotation of the prosthesis occurs, the dentist will also notice that the inferior portion of the lingual bar major connector will impinge on the lingual mucosal tissues. If the tissues have been chronically irritated, there will be hypertrophied tissue formed at this portion of the major connector (Fig. 10-3). These rotational forces will also cause destructive torquing forces on the abutment teeth. The dentist may observe radiographic changes associated with this or discover increased mobility of the abutment tooth.

FIT AND CONDITION OF THE DENTURE BASE. When a distal-extension RPD requires refitting, a space will exist between the distal-extension denture base and the mucoperiosteum when the occlusal rests and clasps are seated in their terminal positions (Fig. 10-4). The amount of RRR that has occurred can be gauged by use of a diagnostic wash of alginate on the tissue-fitting surface of the RPD. The thickness of the alginate in the various areas of the distal-extension base, as determined by a periodontal probe marked in millimeters, will determine the amount of RRR. When using an alginate wash for diagnosis, the dentist must be careful to orient the framework to the abutment teeth in its terminal position and not load the distal-extension base while the material is undergoing gelation. The dentist should check the borders of the RPD for proper extension into all anatomic locations so that a maximum area of support for the prosthesis is obtained during the relining procedure. The physical condition of the denture base must be evaluated. If it is found acceptable, the denture base can be used as the matrix for new acrylic

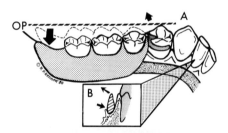

Fig. 10-3. When residual ridge resorbs under distal-extension RPD, there is rotation at fulcrum *(arrow)*, which causes lower portion of lingual bar to press into lingual tissue *(B)* and also creates destructive forces on abutment tooth *(A)*. Occlusal plane *(OP)* is also depressed.

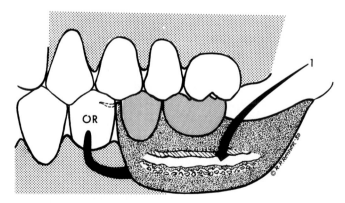

Fig. 10-4. When RPD refitting is needed, space exists under RPD when occlusal rests and indirect retainers are seated properly. *1,* Potential space between denture base and residual ridge; *OR,* occlusal rest.

resin. If, however, the denture base is porous, has fractured, or is unesthetic, the entire acrylic resin denture base must be changed by use of a rebasing rather than a relining procedure. This procedure will also require the dentist to reset or replace denture teeth on the RPD.

OCCLUSION. The occlusion of the RPD must be carefully examined when the mouth is closed and again when the occlusal rests are completely seated. As the dentist observes the occlusion when the RPD is in correct orientation to the abutment teeth rather than in maximum intercuspation, several differences will be noted. There will usually be deflective occlusal contacts from one position to another, a reorientation of the plane of occlusion inferiorly, and, in many instances, anterior traumatic tooth contact (Saunders and associates, 1979). In most prostheses that require relining or rebasing, occlusal equilibration must be completed after the relining procedure in order to have the natural teeth and the denture teeth on the RPD absorb an equal share of the masticatory load (Hindels, 1957). That is, both the natural and prosthetic teeth must occlude simultaneously and evenly at the occlusal vertical dimension.

When there has been extrusion of opposing dentition, irregular wear, shifting of teeth, or reorientation of the occlusal plane (in the case of a maxillary complete denture), it is usually necessary to selectively grind the opposing dentition and possibly change some or all of the denture teeth on the RPD being relined or rebased. In most cases of severe residual ridge resorption beneath a mandibular bilateral distal-extension RPD, the articulation and occlusion are so altered that either new denture teeth must be used or the existing ones, if still usable, must be repositioned on the denture base. If this were not done, the posterior denture teeth, in most instances, would need extensive occlusal grinding to achieve occlusal harmony. In most instances, this would destroy the posterior denture teeth.

Relining procedures using a simple-addition impression technique

TOOTH-BORNE REMOVABLE PARTIAL DENTURES. This type of RPD needs relining infrequently and usually only for hygienic or esthetic reasons. If the RPD framework fits properly in its terminal position (that is, if all metal rests are completely positioned in their respective rest seats and clasps are in proper relation on the abutment teeth), the entire relining procedure is relatively simple. When it is carried out accurately, the dentist can anticipate little or no change in occlusion on the relined RPD.

The procedure for relining tooth-borne RPDs is presented in step-by-step fashion in the following paragraphs.

Undercuts on the tissue surface of the RPD base must be completely removed by the use of acrylic burs mounted in a low-speed handpiece. This will avoid fracture of the final dental stone cast during both the separation of the impression and the processing procedures.

In addition to undercut removal, an even layer of approximately 1 mm of acrylic resin denture base material should be removed from the tissue surface of the prosthesis with a large acrylic cutting bur mounted in a slow-speed handpiece. This relief will allow sufficient space for the impression material.

If any denture border extension is necessary, this should be accomplished with a suitable material, such as stick modeling compound, before the impressioning procedures are performed.

A final impression is then made with either a zinc oxide–eugenol impression material or one of the elastomeric impression materials, such as thiokol rubber base, silicone, polyether, or the vinyl polysiloxanes. In a tooth-borne RPD, either a closed- or an open-mouth impression technique is used to make the final impression. In either technique, the dentist must be sure that the RPD framework is completely seated in its terminal position while the impression material is setting. After the impression material has completely set, the prosthesis and impression are removed from the mouth.

The tissue-fitting surface is inspected and accepted, and all excess material is removed. If the impression is not accurate, the impression procedures are repeated.

The final impression is replaced in the mouth in its terminal position, and a full-arch irreversible impression in a rim lock or perforated stock tray is made. This impression relates the prostheses to the remaining teeth. The impression is removed after complete gelation and inspected for accurate relationship of the prosthesis to the remaining teeth.

The impression, with the RPD incorporated into it, is poured with dental stone as soon as possible to create a working cast.

The dental stone cast, with the impression of the RPD in place, is separated. The impression material is removed from the tissue-fitting surface and dental stone cast.

The tissue-fitting surface of the prosthesis is processed with new acrylic resin denture base material. It is then finished and polished and returned to the dentist for inspection.

The RPD is inserted and adjusted, according to standard clinical practices (see Chapter 9).

DISTAL-EXTENSION REMOVABLE PARTIAL DENTURES. The distal-extension RPD is more difficult to reline or rebase than the tooth-borne type. The greater the severity of RRR, the greater the dentist's difficulty with all phases of the refitting procedures. In most instances of severe RRR, the occlusion of the prosthesis is so altered after relining that either new denture teeth must be used or, at least, the old ones must be repositioned.

When a maxillary complete denture opposes a mandibular RPD under whose distal-extension denture base severe RRR has taken place, the signs and symptoms of the "combination syndrome" may occur (Kelly, 1972; Saunders and associates, 1979). In this instance, there may be a profound alteration of the occlusal plane on both prostheses. Not only do the denture teeth on the RPD need to be replaced, but it also may be necessary to replace the maxillary complete denture. If this is necessary, it may be prudent and expedient for the dentist to remake the maxillary complete and the mandibular RPD rather than to attempt to either reline or rebase one or both prostheses.

SLIGHT RESIDUAL RIDGE REDUCTION. The procedure for relining distal-extension RPDs when only slight RRR (1 or 2 mm as measured in the first molar area) has occurred is presented in step-by-step fashion in the following paragraphs.

All undercuts on the tissue-fitting surface of the distal-extension denture base of the RPD must be removed by the use of acrylic burs mounted in a low-speed handpiece. Areas that most frequently require removal of undercuts are the mylohyoid ridge and retromylohyoid

fossa. Failure to remove these undercuts in the denture base could lead to fracture of the dental stone cast when the prosthesis is separated from the stone cast to remove the impression material.

The low-speed handpiece and mounted acrylic burs are used to remove an additional 1 mm of acrylic resin denture base material from the entire tissue-fitting surface of the prosthesis.

If any borders of the RPD are improperly extended (such as over the retromolar pads, mylohyoid ridge, or buccal shelf), they should be corrected at this time by use of modeling stick compound.

The final impression may be recorded in any of the elastomeric impression materials (as above) or a zinc oxide–eugenol impression material. The severity of tissue undercuts is one of the determining factors in the dentist's choice of using an inelastic (metallic oxides) over an elastic impression material. In this instance, however, an open-mouth impression technique *must* be employed when the impression is made. The dentist must make certain that the rests, clasps, and indirect retainers are in their terminal position on the abutment teeth and maintained in this position until the impression material sets. Finger pressure on the lingual bar major connector, directly over the occlusal rests and indirect retainers, should be employed and maintained until the impression material sets (Figs. 10-5 through 10-7). At no time during the impression procedures should pressure, finger or occlusal, be applied to the distal-extension denture base.

The RPD with the impression of the tissue-fitting surface should be removed from the mouth and inspected for accuracy. If the impression of the tissues is accurate and no impression material has extruded between the abutment teeth and the metal components of the prosthesis, it can be boxed and poured with dental stone. If the impression is inaccurate so that it exhibits pressure areas or is not fully seated when the impression is made (as determined by impression material under the rests), the impression procedures should be repeated until an accurate impression is made.

The impression should be boxed and poured with dental stone. Before the master cast is separated from the RPD, the entire RPD and

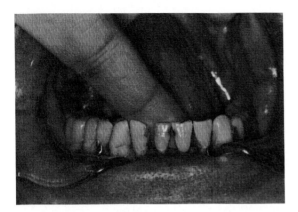

Fig. 10-5. Finger pressure must be maintained on lingual bar (as shown) and directly over rests during relining impression procedures to make certain rests are completely seated.

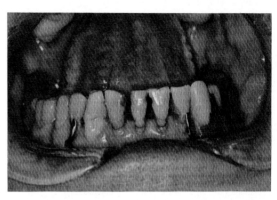

Fig. 10-6. Impression material (thiokol rubber base) is completely polymerized, using an open-mouth technique.

impression is flasked in a denture flask.

After the flasking procedure, the two halves of the denture flasks are opened and the impression material is removed from the tissue surface of the RPD and stone master cast. The tissue surface of the denture bases is cleaned and prepared to receive new heat-cured acrylic denture base material. Standard packing and curing cycles are used to complete the relining of the distal-extension removable partial denture.

In patients with a slight amount of residual ridge reduction, the occlusion of the prosthesis is usually disturbed only minimally, and judicious occlusal adjustment is all that is necessary to bring the RPD back to normal function (Figs. 10-8 and 10-9). The same *clinical* procedure is followed even if the RPD is rebased rather than relined.

MARKED RESIDUAL RIDGE REDUCTION. Reestablishing function for an RPD when there have been significant amounts of RRR (more than 2 mm as measured in the first molar area) is probably the most difficult refitting procedure for the dentist to accomplish accurately. In this instance, it would be more expedient and the patient would be better served if the prosthesis were rebased rather than relined, since the articulation and occlusion of the RPD are usually drastically disturbed. In a majority of these instances, new denture teeth must be used on the RPD to reestablish an adequate occlusion. In patients who exhibit severe RRR, the RPD framework rotates about its fulcrum

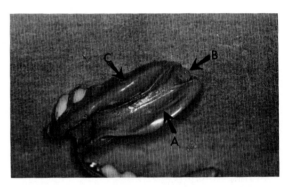

Fig. 10-7. Simple-addition impression showing extension beyond mylohyoid ridge, including retromolar pad, and carried to external oblique ridge on buccal surface. *A,* Mylohyoid ridge; *B,* retromolar pad; *C,* external oblique ridge.

to such a degree that the inferior portion of the major connector compresses the lingual alveolar tissues. This tissue compression usually has caused an ulceration or, if chronic in nature, the formation of hypertrophied tissue (see Figs. 10-3 and 10-10). In many instances, this may be the patient's only complaint and the reason professional care is sought. When occlusal loads are exerted in the first molar region, the prosthesis rotates, causing the occlusal rests to leave the rest seats and the lingual bar to compress the lingual alveolar tissues. When the patient is asked to make light occlusal contact, the dentist will usually find that the RPD is entirely out of occlusal contact (Fig. 10-11).

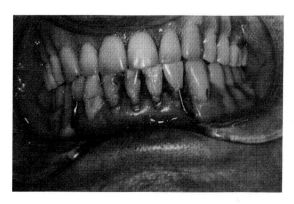

Fig. 10-8. Judicious grinding is performed on occlusion until occlusal load is carried by both RPD and abutment teeth.

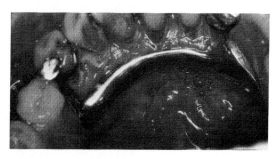

Fig. 10-9. Note that rests are fully seated in completed relining procedure.

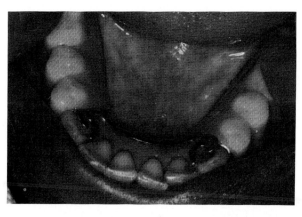

Fig. 10-10. Note that rests are out of rest seats and lingual bar is in contact with tissue when pressure is exerted in first molar area.

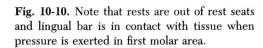

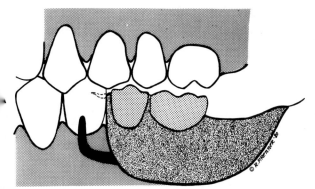

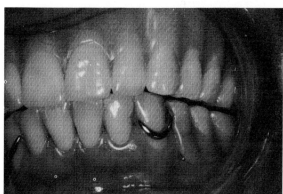

B

Fig. 10-11. In marked RRR, if the patient is asked to close mandible lightly there is no occlusion on RPD. **A,** Diagram. **B,** Photograph.

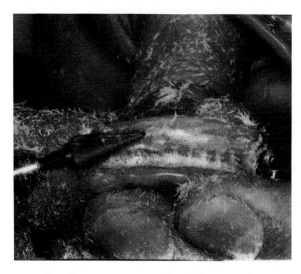

Fig. 10-12. All undercuts are removed with large acrylic cutting bur.

Fig. 10-13. Note that this RPD is underextended in area of mylohyoid ridge and does not extend posteriorly to cover retromolar pad.

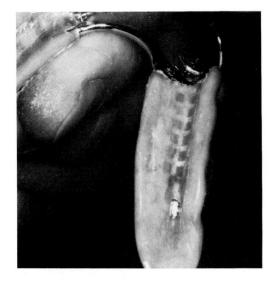

The procedure for relining distal-extension RPDs when marked RRR has occurred is presented in step-by-step fashion in the following paragraphs.

All undercuts are removed from the tissue-fitting surface of the distal-extension denture bases by the use of acrylic burs mounted in a low-speed handpiece (Fig. 10-12). In addition, the entire tissue surface of the RPD is moderately (1 to 2 mm) relieved.

Modeling stick compound must be used wherever necessary to make up any deficiencies in the distal-extension denture base, such as denture border extension (Fig. 10-13). When modeling stick compound or other similar material is used for this purpose, the dentist must always relate the RPD to the abutment teeth in its terminal position. To ensure that the prosthesis is seated in its terminal position while the denture borders are being corrected, the dentist should press down on the occlusal rests, indirect retainers, and lingual bar while

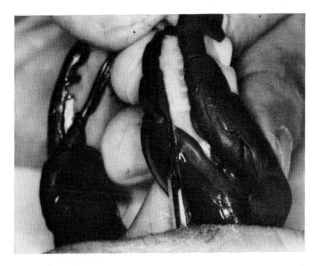

Fig. 10-14. Modeling compound is used to extend borders properly and is relieved over alveolar tissue area.

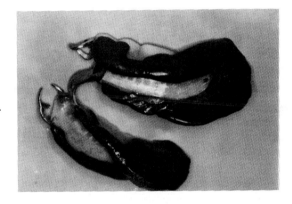

Fig. 10-15. Compound is relieved over alveolar tissue areas before impression is made.

the modeling compound is hardening. Indirect retainers are important components in an RPD in that they allow the dentist to accurately seat the framework in its proper relation to the oral tissues during a relining or rebasing procedure.

After incremental additions of modeling stick compound, the RPD should be removed, chilled, and inspected for accuracy. Additional compound is added until the RPD base is stable and properly extended and the framework is completely seated in its terminal position (Fig. 10-14).

Any modeling stick compound should be re-lieved by about 1 mm at this time in any areas over the alveolar tissue in which it is in tissue contact, by use of a vulcanite scraper or similar instrument (Fig. 10-15). This will allow the impression material to record the denture-bearing tissues in a passive, or mucostatic, state. The compound in contact with the mucosal-tissue area (border tissues) is not relieved when the impression is made.

The final impression is then made with a metallic oxide (zinc oxide and eugenol) or elas-tomeric impression material. The impression is made by use of an open-mouth impression

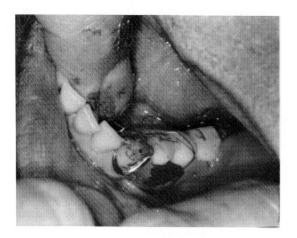

Fig. 10-16. Final wash impression is made with open-mouth technique, making certain finger pressure is applied on lingual bar and over rest areas until impression material polymerizes completely.

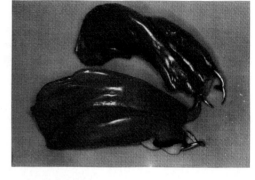

Fig. 10-17. Final wash impression. Note extension beyond mylohyoid ridge and impression material covering retromolar pad.

technique while finger pressure is maintained on the lingual bar and occlusal rest areas until the impression material is set (Figs. 10-16 and 10-17).

When fully set, the impression should be removed from the mouth and examined for accuracy. The distal-extension denture base areas should be examined for pressure areas, voids, or distortion of the tissues. The dentist should examine the inferior surface of the occlusal rests for impression material that may have extruded under the rests and altered the fit of the framework. If any inaccuracies are found, the impression procedures should be repeated until a satisfactory impression is obtained.

When the completed impression is reseated intraorally and the patient is asked to close the mandible, a marked change in the articulation and occlusion will be observed. The patient will, in most cases, occlude only the second molars (Fig. 10-18). If the RPD were reprocessed using this occlusal relationship, the selective grinding procedures necessary to restore proper occlusal articulation would probably completely mutilate the posterior denture teeth. The proper procedure is for the dentist to remove all the denture teeth, whether acrylic resin or dental porcelain, on the RPD. Acrylic resin denture teeth must be removed by grinding them out of the denture base. Dental porcelain denture teeth can be efficiently removed by softening the acrylic resin

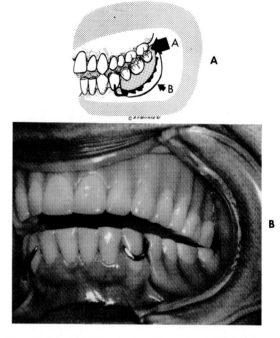

Fig. 10-18. A, Diagram. **B,** Photograph. If RPD is simply relined in this type of refitting procedure, marked change will be observed in occlusion. *A,* Patient will probably occlude only on second molars; *B,* impression material.

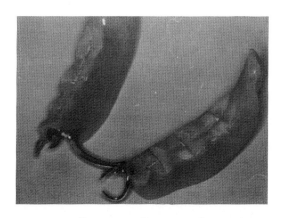

Fig. 10-19. All posterior denture teeth on RPD are ground completely out of occlusion.

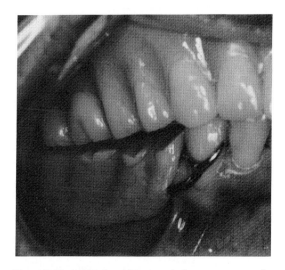

Fig. 10-20. RPD should not occlude in centric occlusion at this stage.

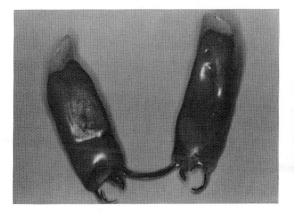

Fig. 10-21. Wax recording medium is added to occlusal surfaces of teeth of RPD.

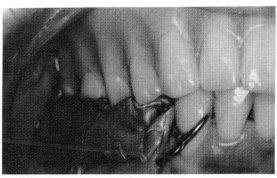

Fig. 10-22. New occlusal registration is made at proper vertical dimension of occlusion.

denture base material lingual to the denture teeth with a hot number 7 spatula or covering it with petroleum jelly and flaming it. The denture teeth can then be pried out of the denture base by a wedging action with a dental instrument (number 7 spatula).

The occlusal portion of the distal-extension denture base should be trimmed until no opposing occlusal contact exists at an appropriate vertical dimension of occlusion (Figs. 10-19 and 10-20). A wax recording material is applied to the occlusal surface of the denture base (Fig. 10-21), and a centric relation record is made at an acceptable vertical dimension of occlusion (Figs. 10-22 and 10-23).

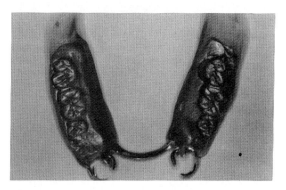

Fig. 10-23. Occlusion recorded in wax. Note uniform contact of teeth.

An overall alginate impression is made in a stock tray over both the RPD and centric relation record and the remaining teeth (Fig. 10-24). This overall impression is boxed and poured with dental stone, the dentist being careful not to disturb the wax centric relation recording (Fig. 10-25).

An alginate impression of the adjusted opposing maxillary dental arch is made and poured with dental stone. The maxillary cast is mounted on a dental articulator by means of a face-bow transfer procedure. The mandibular dental stone cast, with the RPD and impression in place, is articulated by means of the wax centric relation record (Fig. 10-26).

The acrylic resin is removed from the entire occlusal surface of the distal-extension denture base, and new denture teeth are waxed into proper articulation and the occlusion is adjusted.

The polished surface contours are completed by use of set-up wax. The mandibular dental stone cast and RPD are removed from the articulator mounting for the remainder of the laboratory procedures.

The RPD is flasked. After flask separation,

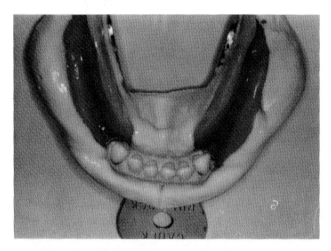

Fig. 10-24. Irreversible hydrocolloid impression is made over RPD and remaining teeth.

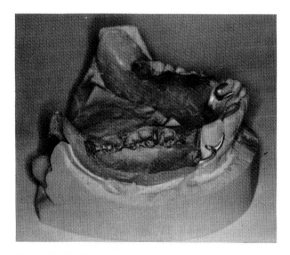

Fig. 10-25. Impression is poured in dental stone, and master cast is recovered.

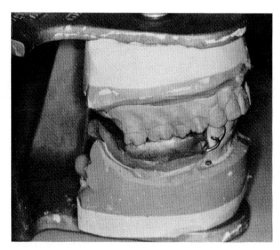

Fig. 10-26. Mandibular cast is luted to articulator by means of occlusal registration.

the impression material and stick compound are removed from the distal-extension denture bases and dental stone master cast. The tissue surface of the distal-extension denture base is prepared to receive new base material, and the prosthesis is packed with new heat-cured acrylic resin. A standard slow-curing acrylic resin cycle is used to cure the acrylic resin.

The processed RPD is deflasked but not removed from the master cast. The prosthesis is rearticulated by the keyed articulator mounting, and a laboratory remounting is performed to correct processing changes.

After the laboratory remounting procedure is completed the RPD is removed from the master cast, finished, and polished. When the prosthesis is viewed from the tissue surface, the metal tissue stop, normally in tissue contact, is not visible but is covered with new acrylic resin denture base material (Fig. 10-27).

Final occlusal corrections are made on the RPD by use of a patient remounting procedure (Fig. 10-28). Insertion of the relined RPD should follow standard insertion procedures as outlined in Chapter 9.

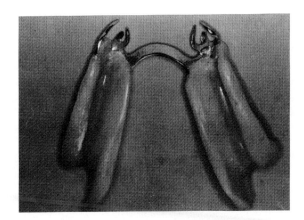

Fig. 10-27. No metal stops, as would normally be seen in new RPD, show through on tissue surface.

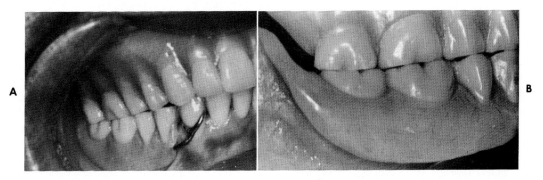

Fig. 10-28. A and **B,** Equilibration of occlusion is completed. Occlusion is borne by RPD and abutment teeth.

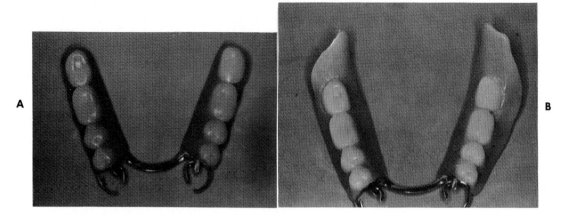

Fig. 10-29. A, RPD before rebasing. **B,** RPD after rebasing. Note difference in border extension of RPD.

When all of the steps have been accomplished, the sequence of relining or rebasing an RPD is similar to treating the patient with an entirely new RPD (Figs. 10-29). Successful treatment depends, in large measure, on the adequacy of fit of the RPD framework.

Relining procedure using the altered cast technique

Another technique, in addition to the two previously described, that is an effective method for relining or rebasing a distal-extension RPD is the altered cast technique, as described in Chapter 6. Mouth temperature wax can be used for denture base development as well as for development of the polished surface contours of the prosthesis in lieu of a metallic oxide or elastomeric impression material. As with any relining or rebasing technique, the adequacy of fit of the RPD framework is the critical factor to the success of the technique.

Use of resilient relining materials

Although the majority of relining and rebasing procedures are carried out by use of hard, heat-cured acrylic resin denture base materials, there are several resilient denture liners commercially available as denture base materials. There are several reported indications for the use of resilient denture liners with complete dentures and distal-extension base RPDs. These include the presence of the following clinical conditions: (1) bilateral, prominent mylohyoid undercuts; (2) multiple, small, opposing bony undercuts; (3) chronic patient

discomfort in the absence of abused oral tissues; (4) knife-edge mandibular residual ridges that cannot be surgically corrected; and (5) marked medical debilitation (Bell, 1970). However, there are a number of disadvantages to using resilient denture liners on RPDs in any of the above clinical conditions. Some of the general disadvantages of these liners are that (1) they are subject to staining and discoloration; (2) they are subject to chemical attack (particularly by alcohol); (3) their surface detail may be altered because of careless handling; (4) they are subject to impregnation with calculus or colonies of *C. albicans;* (5) if not properly prepared and processed, they separate from heat-cured acrylic resin; and (6) the resilient nature of most liners is short lived. One or all of these disadvantages may require the dentist to change the resilient liner frequently (every 6 months to 1 year) when it is used as a relining material for a distal-extension RPD. However, when the dentist chooses to use a resilient relining material instead of a heat-cured acrylic resin, the same clinical and laboratory procedures are used. The soft relining material is substituted for the heat-cured acrylic resin. When an autopolymerizing plastic resin relining material is used, the procedures followed are the same as those used in making a simple-addition relining impression. In this case, the autopolymerizing plastic liner substitutes for the impression material. When any resilient liner is used, the manufacturer's recommended procedures for the preparation of the RPD and the curing of the resin should be

TABLE 10-1
Indications for various procedures to restore function to an RPD

Procedure	Mucosal adaptation	Design and fit of framework	Interocclusal considerations	Condition of denture base material	Condition of remaining denture teeth	Esthetics of RPD
Relining	Unacceptable	Acceptable	Minor change	Acceptable	Acceptable	Acceptable
Rebasing	Unacceptable	Acceptable	Minor change	Unacceptable	Acceptable	Acceptable
Reconstruction (using existing framework)	Unacceptable	Acceptable	Unacceptable	Unacceptable	Unacceptable	Unacceptable
Remaking (creating new framework)	Unacceptable	Unacceptable	Unacceptable	Unacceptable	Unacceptable	Unacceptable
Repair	Acceptable	Varies	Acceptable	Acceptable	Varies	Varies

followed explicitly. At best, however, this type of relining material is of limited clinical value, and close and constant clinical attention is needed during its use (Bell, 1970) (Table 10-1).

Reconstruction of the prosthesis using the existing removable partial denture framework

Many dentists prefer to refit the prosthesis by making an entirely new impression as if a new RPD were being constructed. The RPD framework is fit on the master cast made from this final impression. A new centric relation record is made, and the subsequent procedures are similar to those used in treating a patient with a new RPD. The main advantage, although there are also substantial savings in time and dental laboratory fees, is the use of the existing RPD framework. The double-impression technique, as described by Hindels (1952), is the procedure of choice for making impressions of the tissues supporting the RPD when this reconstruction technique is used.

Simple and complex repairs

The dentist's decision whether to repair or remake an existing RPD is somtimes very difficult. The dentist must evaluate many diagnostic factors before a sound clinical decision can be made. Some of these are (1) the patient's financial status; (2) the patient's biologic age; (3) the frequency of appointments; (4) the patient's medical status; and (5) the degree of difficulty of the impression procedures. Some or all of these factors may influence the decision

whether to repair or remake the prosthesis. Frequently it is more expedient to remake an RPD than to devote the time and effort necessary to repair a framework that is just barely clinically acceptable and may well have to be replaced in the near future. More often than not a prosthesis that has been worn for a considerable amount of time and that is in need of repair has other problems. It is the obligation of the dentist to inform the patient about the relative advantages of either repairing or remaking the prosthesis.

Occasionally, breakage and distortion will occur even on the best designed and executed RPD. The dentist's recognition of the cause of the breakage will help to determine the method of repair and may even help avoid possible future accidents (see Chapters 5 and 6).

An RPD may break for one of several reasons: (1) careless handling or abuse by the patient; (2) loss of adaptation of the prosthesis to teeth and associated tissues, which in turn may cause excessive stress and strain on the components of the framework or denture base; (3) poor execution of the dental laboratory phases of RPD construction; (4) improper mouth preparation or impression procedures performed by the dentist; (5) loss of abutment teeth; and (6) excess abrasion of the teeth, sometimes caused by bruxism or clenching habits.

Once the dentist has established the cause of breakage and the decision to repair, rebase, reline, reconstruct, or remake the RPD has been made, the specific procedure can be done.

Simple repairs

Simple repairs or additions to an RPD can usually be accomplished with or without impressions. Many times, simple repairs can be executed by the dentist in the operatory or in the private office laboratory.

DENTURE BASE REPAIR. Various types of RPD base breakage may occur, ranging from the complete loss of a denture base flange segment to the fracture or loss of a portion of the denture base proper. In the former example, complete loss of a segment of the denture base flange, repair of the prosthesis will require the dentist to use a rebasing or relining impression procedure. Such a procedure is presented in step-by-step fashion in the following paragraphs.

A relining impression in metallic oxide or an elastomeric impression material is obtained, using the RPD as a tray. When an entire portion of the denture base is missing (Fig. 10-30), this area on the RPD must be corrected with autopolymerizing acrylic resin, stick compound, (Fig. 10-31), or both so that the impression material can be accurately carried to place.

The completed impression is boxed and poured with dental stone to secure a master cast (Fig. 10-32).

The new denture flange segment is repaired with either autopolymerizing or heat-cured acrylic resin (Figs. 10-33 and 10-34). If heat-cured acrylic resin is used, the denture flange segment is waxed-up to anatomic contour before the flasking procedures (Fig. 10-35) are performed.

When the fractured segment of the RPD denture flange is still available (Fig. 10-36, *A*), the RPD can be repaired temporarily by ap-

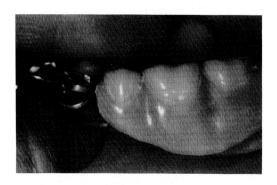

Fig. 10-30. RPD with buccal flange broken off in area of premolar.

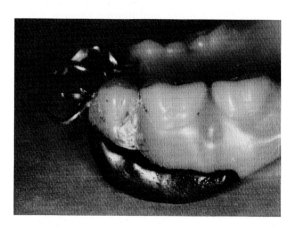

Fig. 10-31. Area border molded with green stick modeling compound recording depth of mucolabial fold.

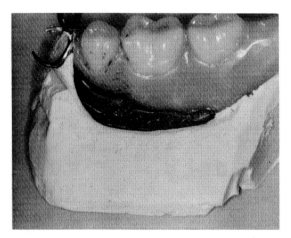

Fig. 10-32. Sectional cast poured in area to be repaired.

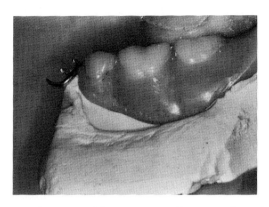

Fig. 10-33. Modeling compound removed with warm water. Area cleaned and prepared with appropriate separating medium.

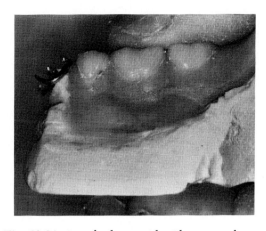

Fig. 10-34. Area built up with either autopolymerizing or heat-cured acrylic resin.

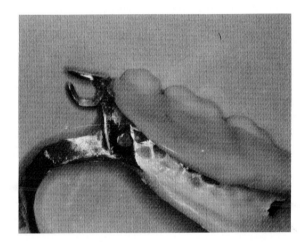

Fig. 10-35. Finished, adjusted, and polished RPD.

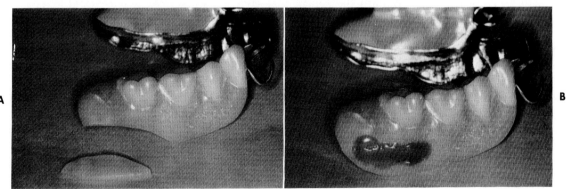

Fig. 10-36. A, Fractured segment of posterior buccal flange still in good condition. **B,** Area opposed and positioned with sticky wax.

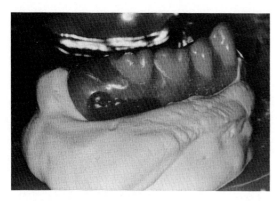

Fig. 10-37. Sectioned stone master cast poured with both segments still in contact.

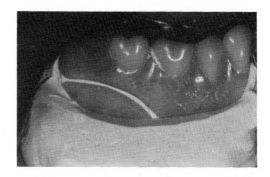

Fig. 10-38. Trough cut for 2 to 3 mm in area of fracture line, with both segments still secured on stone cast.

proximating the fractured segments and joining them together by means of cyanoacrylate cement. The prosthesis then can be repaired as in the first step of this procedure.

The more conventional method of repairing a denture base fracture is to approximate the fractured surfaces and join them with sticky wax (Fig. 10-36, *B*).

The tissue surface of the RPD is poured with dental stone (Fig. 10-37). When the master cast is sufficiently hard, the RPD is removed and the junction of the segments is enlarged to approximately 2 to 3 mm in width (Fig. 10-38).

A separating medium is applied to the working cast, and the RPD segments are replaced on the stone cast.

Autopolymerizing acrylic resin is added in a "salt and pepper" fashion (sprinkled on) to the space between the approximating segments. The acrylic resin monomer and polymer should be applied alternately until the repair site is slightly overfilled (Fig. 10-39).

For creation of a denser repair with less internal porosity, the RPD and dental stone cast should be placed in a temperature-controlled pressure bath at 30 psi at about 120° F for 30 minutes (Fig. 10-40, *A*). The repair should be placed under warm water during this procedure.

The repair site is trimmed and finished with acrylic burs mounted in a low-speed handpiece. Polishing is carried out in a conventional manner, using the various grades of pumice and finally acrylic resin polish (Fig. 10-40, *B*).

REPAIR OF FRACTURED DENTURE TEETH. There are two basic types of denture teeth commonly used in RPD treatment: dental porcelain and acrylic resin. Each has its own inherent problems when fractured and is treated slightly differently during the repair procedure.

DENTAL PORCELAIN DENTURE TEETH. The procedure for repair of dental porcelain denture teeth is presented in step-by-step fashion in the following paragraphs.

Dental porcelain denture teeth are joined to the denture base by the mechanical bonding of the denture tooth to the denture base by means of a diatoric hole or, for an anterior denture tooth, a metal pin. If the denture tooth has loosened from the denture base and the diatoric hole is still intact, the tooth can be mechanically joined to the denture base with new acrylic resin (Fig. 10-41).

When the denture tooth is worn or fractured beyond repair, a new denture tooth must be selected (shade and mold) and used for the repair.

The denture tooth replacement procedure requires removing the worn or fractured segments of the dental porcelain denture tooth by means of judicious application of pin-point heat from a Hanau torch at the junction of the acrylic resin and denture tooth. A thin layer of petroleum jelly should be placed on the denture tooth while the acrylic resin is being softened (Fig. 10-42).

The porcelain denture tooth is removed from the softened acrylic resin by wedging the tooth from the denture base with the rounded end of a number 7 wax spatula.

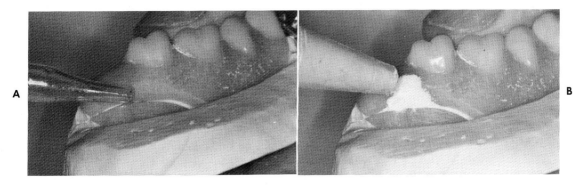

Fig. 10-39. A, Alternate incremental amounts of liquid autopolymerizing acrylic resin monomer are added. B, Excess autopolymerizing polymer is added.

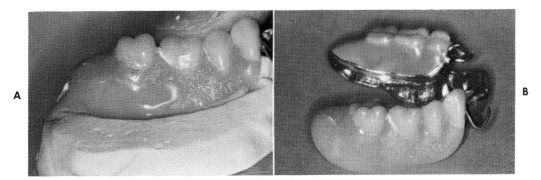

Fig. 10-40. A, Area of fracture is overbuilt and RPD is placed in pressure cooker and processed. B, Finished RPD is adjusted and polished.

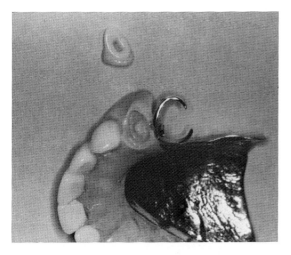

Fig. 10-41. Porcelain tooth lost because of poor mechanical bond between acrylic resin and diatoric hole on porcelain tooth.

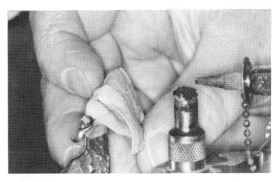

Fig. 10-42. Porcelain denture tooth is removed because of fracture or excessive wear. Tooth is lightly coated with petroleum jelly to distribute heat evenly, and surrounding area is covered with asbestoslike material so as not to harm adjacent denture teeth and acrylic resin, especially in labial gingival area.

The area of acrylic resin surrounding the fracture site is mechanically cleaned, and an area lingual to the replacement denture tooth is prepared to receive an adequate amount of autopolymerizing acrylic resin (Fig. 10-43).

The new denture tooth is positioned into the repair site by luting it to adjacent denture teeth with sticky wax or using a laboratory plaster indexing procedure (Fig. 10-44, A).

New autopolymerizing acrylic resin is then applied to the repair site using an alternate application of acrylic resin polymer and monomer ("salt and pepper," sprinkle-on technique) until it is slightly overfilled (Figs. 10-44, B, through 10-46).

The repair site is pressure and heat cured (30 psi for 30 minutes under water of about 120° F), trimmed, and polished (Figs. 10-47 and 10-48).

If the porcelain denture tooth is basically intact but there is a worn or sharp section that does not compromise the occlusion, this area can be smoothed and polished with a proprietary porcelain finishing kit* and returned to the patient.

ACRYLIC RESIN DENTURE TEETH. The procedure for repair of acrylic resin denture teeth is presented in step-by-step fashion in the following paragraphs.

Fracture or dislogement of an acrylic resin

---

*Porcelain Adjustment Kit, Shofu Dental Corp., Menlo Park, Calif.

denture tooth is treated in a slightly different manner from that of a dental porcelain tooth. If an acrylic resin denture tooth is dislodged from a new RPD, the cause may lie with the formation of an incomplete chemical bond between the acrylic resin denture tooth and the acrylic resin denture base. This incomplete chemical bond may be caused by wax residue or oils left between the two acrylic resins when the RPD was processed.

In these instances, the denture tooth is removed and the area is mechanically cleaned. A

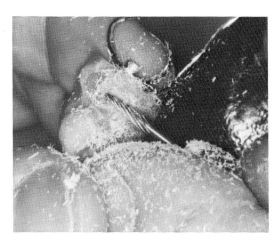

Fig. 10-43. Lingual area is opened and widened for addition of new acrylic resin (autopolymerizing or heat cured).

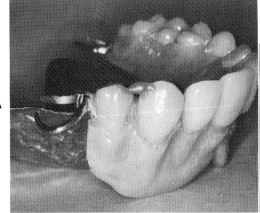
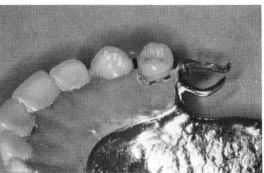

Fig. 10-44. A, Replacement denture tooth is positioned by means of sticky wax on incisal aspect. **B,** Lingual gingival area is enlarged for addition of new autopolymerizing acrylic resin.

boxlike area is removed from the acrylic resin denture base lingual to the dislodged denture tooth (to preserve the esthetics of the facial area). The denture tooth is replaced, secured to the adjacent teeth with sticky wax, and reprocessed with autopolymerizing acrylic resin.

When the acrylic resin denture tooth is abraded or fractured, the defective segments must be removed carefully. The denture tooth must be cut out of the denture base and the surrounding acrylic resin denture base mate-

rial enlarged by use of acrylic resin cutting burs mounted in a low-speed handpiece.

A new denture tooth is selected, adjusted to fit the repair site, and checked to ensure that there is adequate room for the autopolymerizing acrylic resin.

The denture tooth is luted in position, and new autopolymerizing acrylic resin is applied, processed, and finished as above.

Occasionally the anterior denture teeth are positioned against the residual ridge to eliminate a denture flange. In these instances,

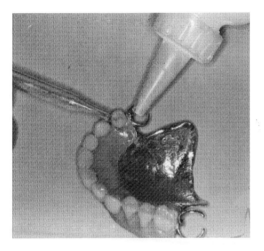

Fig. 10-45. Alternate additions of monomer and polymer are placed into area cut out on lingual gingival aspect of RPD.

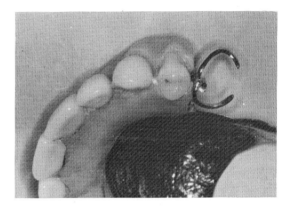

Fig. 10-46. Repair area is overbuilt.

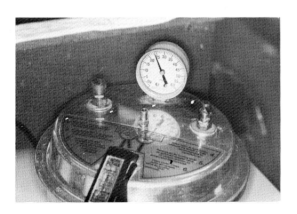

Fig. 10-47. RPD is processed at 30 psi at about 120° F for 30 minutes.

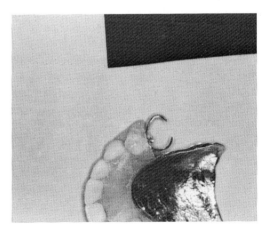

Fig. 10-48. RPD is removed, trimmed, polished, and checked for occlusal discrepancies with articulating paper.

when an anterior denture tooth is fractured, an impression must be made with the RPD in place and the repair must be carried out to completion on a dental stone cast.

An alternate, temporary method to repair a fractured or lost denture tooth on an RPD is to add tooth-colored acrylic resin to the prepared defect site. The mass can be reshaped to simulate the denture tooth after polymerization of the acrylic resin is completed.

When denture teeth are repaired on an RPD, the occlusion of the RPD in centric and eccentric positions must be carefully checked and adjusted if necessary. Traumatic or premature occlusal contacts on denture teeth are a common cause of their fracture.

Complex repairs

There are many complex repairs or modifications that can be made on a defective RPD. These include (1) repair or replacement of a clasp assembly or any part thereof; (2) repair of a major or minor connector; and (3) repair of the RPD after the loss of an abutment tooth. All complex repairs require the use of proper impression procedures by the dentist. It is mandatory that the dentist properly realign the RPD in the patient's mouth before any complex repair procedures are accomplished. This presupposes that the relationship of the residual ridge to the denture base is acceptable and does not require modification.

REPAIR OF A BROKEN CLASP ASSEMBLY. The most frequent type of component breakage on an RPD is the fracture of one or more parts of the clasp assembly (that is, fracture of one or more clasp arms, the occlusal rest, or the area between the minor connector and the major connector). The cause of the fracture should be determined and corrected, if possible, before the repair procedure is carried out (see Chapter 5). If the design of the RPD was inadequate and stress on the RPD framework or parts of it was too great, then a new design and RPD are indicated (see Chapter 3). More commonly the fracture of the framework is caused by patient or dentist mishandling of the chromium-cobalt alloy (such as dropping the prosthesis, bending it on a dental lathe, or adjusting the clasp arm beyond the elastic limit of the metal).

A broken clasp arm is the RPD component that is most subject to fracture, and it can be repaired by either of two techniques: (1) by

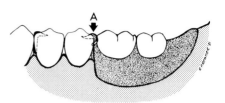

Fig. 10-49. Broken retentive arm is removed, and remnants are polished *(A)*. Overall impression is made intraorally with elastic impression material, and dental stone cast is made from impression. Buccal view.

embedding an 18-gauge wrought wire into the denture base of the RPD as a substitute clasp arm or (2) by constructing a new clasp assembly and soldering or welding it to the existing RPD framework.

The procedure for repair of a broken clasp arm using an 18-gauge platinum-gold-palladium (PGP) wrought wire is presented in step-by-step fashion in the following paragraphs.

The clasp arm of an RPD that usually is fractured or deformed is the retentive arm. An 18-gauge PGP wrought wire can be used as an effective substitute to replace this buccal retentive arm on the RPD (Frank and Nicholls, 1981).

The fractured RPD is placed in the patient's mouth and correctly seated in its terminal position while an irreversible hydrocolloid impression of both the RPD and the natural teeth is made in a stock tray.

This impression is boxed and poured immediately with dental stone to form a working cast on which the repair will be completed (Fig. 10-49).

The fractured portion of the clasp arm is removed from the RPD framework. An area is created in the acrylic resin denture base to mechanically retain the wrought wire (Fig. 10-50).

The 18-gauge PGP wrought wire is contoured to fit the contours of the dental stone replica of the abutment tooth, using orthodontic pliers. A retention loop is fashioned in the distal end of the wire so that it can be mechanically bound into the acrylic resin denture base (Fig. 10-50).

The completed 18-gauge PGP wrought wire is secured in place with sticky wax on the dental stone abutment tooth (Fig. 10-51).

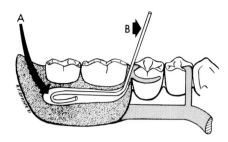

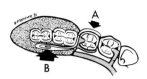

Fig. 10-50. Trough in acrylic resin is made into lingual surface of RPD *(A)*. Either gold or stainless steel wrought wire *(B)* is shaped into loop for retention and carried below occlusal rest area to buccal aspect. Lingual view.

Fig. 10-51. Wrought wire is completely contoured and sticky waxed into position *(A)*. Acrylic resin polymer and monomer are added to fill trough *(B)* to excess. Occlusal view.

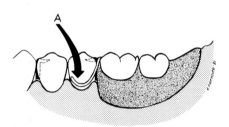

Fig. 10-52. Buccal view of completed wrought wire *(A)* repaired retentive arm.

Autopolymerizing acrylic resin can be added in "salt and pepper" fashion to complete the mechanical retention of the wire in the denture base.

The RPD, 18-gauge PGP wrought wire, and autopolymerizing acrylic resin are cured in a temperature- and pressure-controlled curing unit in warm water (about 120° F) for 30 minutes at 30 psi.

The new buccal retentive arm and acrylic resin are finished and polished (Fig. 10-52). The RPD is checked intraorally for proper contact of the 18-gauge PGP wrought wire arm into the retentive undercut. Adjustments are made when necessary on the wrought wire to increase or decrease the frictional retention of the arm.

When the lingual reciprocal arm is fractured, the buccal retentive arm may cause excessive stress on the abutment tooth in a lingual direction when it is inserted and withdrawn unless proper reciprocation is returned. In this situation, a lingual arm can be incorporated in a fashion similar to that of the 18-gauge PGP wire, but a more rigid metal should be used.

When a bar clasp retentive arm fractures, it may simply be repaired as a circumferential wrought wire clasp. The procedures described above can be used if the undercut is in an acceptable position. If it is necessary to replace a bar-type retentive arm, a new buccal arm must be waxed, cast, and then soldered or welded to the RPD framework at a position near the retentive latticework.

REPAIR OF A BROKEN OCCLUSAL REST. The most common cause for the fracture of an occlusal rest on a clasp is insufficient preparation of the marginal ridge area of the abutment tooth, resulting in inadequate clearance for the metal at the junction of occlusal rest and minor connector.

The procedure for repair of a broken occlusal rest is presented in step-by-step fashion in the following paragraphs.

Before the repair procedures are initiated, proper occlusal clearance should be made between the opposing dentition and the marginal ridge area of the occlusal rest. The proper interarch clearance should be at least 1.5 mm.

Depending on the condition of the existing clasp, one of two procedures can be used to replace the occlusal rest. An alginate impression is made with the prosthesis in place, and the impression is boxed and poured in soldering investment to make a dental cast.

When just the occlusal rest is to be repaired, a platinum foil matrix is placed over the impression of the newly prepared rest seat on the soldering investment cast. An appropriate wire or dental gold solder is used to reconstruct the occlusal rest and solder it to the minor connector. This procedure may require removing the acrylic resin from the adjacent denture teeth and denture base before the soldering procedure.

When the clasp or any part of it is defective a new clasp assembly should be waxed-up and cast. It is soldered or welded to the existing framework at the appropriate junction between the major and the minor connector. This second procedure is more commonly employed, since the clasp is probably distorted after the loss of the occlusal rest.

REPAIR OF A BROKEN MAJOR CONNECTOR. The most common area for distortion or fracture of the major connector is the junction between the major connector and the retentive latticework. The cause is usually a consequence of internal and external finishing lines that are placed too deep or in apposition to one another on the RPD framework, thus weakening the junction. When this area of the framework is too thin, rigorous or even normal treatment may cause the metal to bend or break. Repair procedures would at best be carried out by a reconstruction technique (that is, making a new master cast, pouring matrixes, removing the defective elements, waxing, casting, and soldering or welding the new portion of the framework in position). The RPD is completed as in the other repair techniques described. In clinical practice, however, it is better to remake the RPD than to repair fractured major connectors.

REPAIR OF THE REMOVABLE PARTIAL DENTURE AFTER LOSS OF AN ABUTMENT TOOTH AND MODIFICATION OF A NEW ABUTMENT TOOTH. Occasionally, an abutment tooth must be extracted for any of a number of reasons (Fig. 10-53), and it may be necessary to incorporate the adjacent tooth in the design of the prosthesis. When an abutment tooth has been lost, the patient's oral hygiene and the condition of the remaining dentition should be evaluated carefully by the dentist and consideration should be given to a new RPD design. If, however, repair is indicated, a simple repair using an 18-gauge PGP wrought wire may be made as a temporary measure to retain the prosthesis. If a new abutment tooth is to be used, proper mouth preparations must be made to incorporate design elements of the clasp such as a guiding plane, occlusal or cingulum rests, and retentive and stabilizing arms (Fig. 10-54). After appropriate mouth prepara-

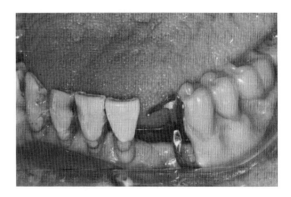

Fig. 10-53. Patient has lost abutment tooth.

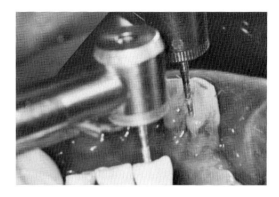

Fig. 10-54. Cingulum area on adjacent tooth is prepared for rest for construction of new clasp assembly.

tion, an impression of the entire dental arch with the RPD framework in place should be made in irreversible hydrocolloid (Fig. 10-55), and this impression should be boxed and poured in dental stone to produce a working cast (Fig. 10-56). The old clasp assembly is removed and a new clasp assembly is waxed, cast, and fitted to the existing RPD framework (Fig. 10-57). A new denture tooth is processed with acrylic resin into the space of the previously extracted abutment tooth.

Frequently a tooth that is not essential to the successful function of the RPD is lost, and its replacement can be carried out in one of two ways. To provide the necessary mechanical retention for the replacement denture tooth, a retentive element must be added to the RPD framework. This is accomplished by making an elastic impression of the dental arch with the

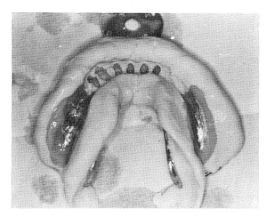

Fig. 10-55. Irreversible hydrocolloid impression has picked up RPD and ridge area where previous abutment tooth was extracted.

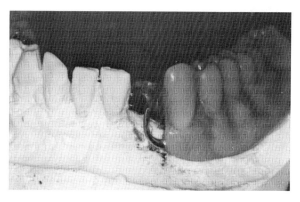

Fig. 10-56. Master cast shows loss of abutment tooth with RPD in place.

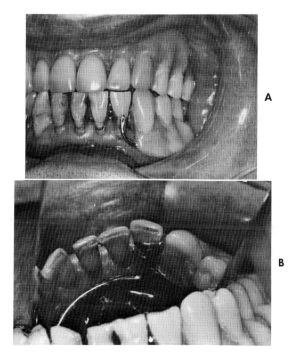

Fig. 10-57. A, Labial view of new clasp assembly with I bar on new abutment tooth. **B,** Lingual view of new clasp assembly with modified cingulum rest on new abutment tooth.

RPD in place intraorally and pouring the impression in dental stone. On this working cast, a retentive element is soldered or brazed to the existing major connector. The replacement denture tooth is processed with acrylic resin to this retentive device. If there is sufficient denture base material adjacent to the denture tooth to be added, it may be processed to the adjacent acrylic resin without the need for additional metal mechanical retention.

Restoration of an abutment tooth under a clasp assembly

Retaining the clasp assembly of an RPD while changing a defective abutment restoration is a very common clinical procedure. The clasp and the remaining portion of the RPD should be evaluated to decide whether it would be more feasible to remake rather than repair the existing prosthesis.

The defective abutment restoration is corrected with a cast restoration, an inlay, or a silver amalgam restoration. If a silver amalgam restoration is used, it is placed in the usual fashion, allowing for proper bulk and strength under occlusal loading. The patient, however, is instructed to leave the RPD out of the mouth until he or she returns to the dentist for its adjustment at least 24 hours later. When the patient returns, the relation of the silver amalgam restoration to the clasp is adjusted by various means (such as pressure indicating paste or other marking devices).

If the restoration is to be a gold inlay, the indirect method for its fabrication is usually preferred. The gross form of the restoration is waxed-up on the working die, and the clasp assembly of the RPD is warmed slightly and gently placed into position. This will help form

the rest seat and other contours being restored. The RPD is removed, the margins of the wax-up are adjusted, and the inlay is cast. Once the inlay is cemented, adjustments can be made as needed for proper fit of the clasp assembly to the restoration, as is done with a silver amalgam restoration technique. Indirect techniques as outlined for cast gold inlay restorations may also be used with full cast crown restorations.

For full cast restorations, various techniques may be used, but the indirect technique seems to be the most feasible and practical (Fig. 10-58). Two indirect techniques are discussed below.

In the first technique, the abutment tooth under consideration is prepared completely and an elastic impression is made of the prepared tooth with the RPD in place (Fig. 10-59). Proper gingival retraction can be accomplished by using either retraction cord or electrosurgery (Fig. 10-60). The prosthesis is removed with the impression material (such as reversible hydrocolloid, thiokol rubber base, or any elastomeric impression material) (Fig. 10-61). The impression is boxed and poured in die stone (Fig. 10-62), and the full cast restoration is waxed according to the characteristics of the tooth to be restored and the existing clasp assembly (Fig. 10-63). The restoration is cast, fitted on the stone cast, and adjusted (Fig. 10-64). The cast restoration is placed in the mouth, and the RPD is seated (Fig. 10-

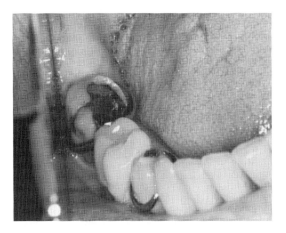

Fig. 10-58. Tooth to be restored with full coverage.

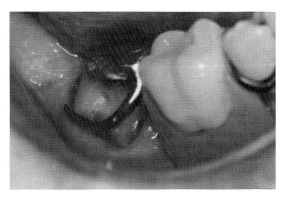

Fig. 10-59. Prepared tooth with RPD clasp assembly is in place to check for adequate clearance for clasp arms and occlusal rest.

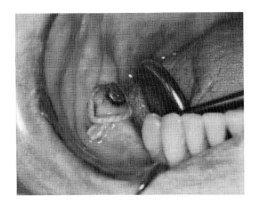

Fig. 10-60. Retraction cord is placed before impression is made.

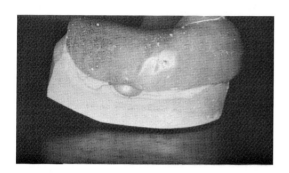

Fig. 10-61. Overall acrylic resin custom tray is made to fit over prepared tooth and RPD.

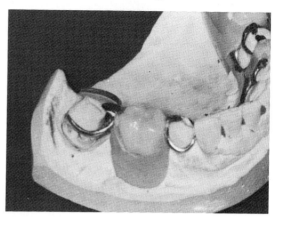

Fig. 10-62. Final master cast with framework in position to check for adequate clearance of clasp assembly over preparation.

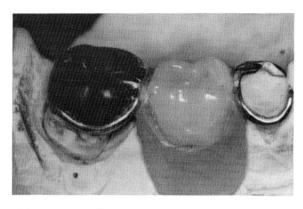

Fig. 10-63. Full coverage restoration waxed-up on stone cast.

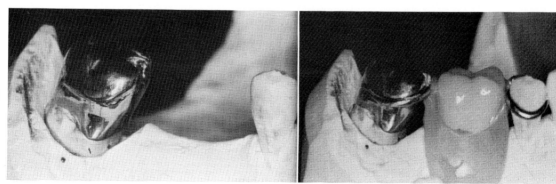

Fig. 10-64. A, Cast crown in place on model. B, Cast crown in place with RPD fitted over it.

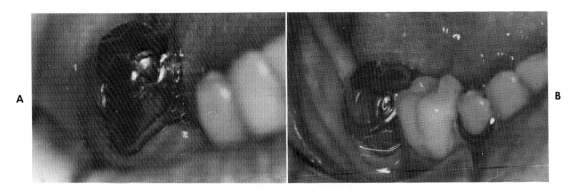

Fig. 10-65. **A,** Cast crown fitted in patient's mouth to check marginal fit and opposing occlusion. **B,** Cast crown in place to check fit of framework after cementation.

65). Slight discrepancies may be treated as outlined previously in the procedure for a silver amalgam restoration.

The second technique involves preparing the abutment tooth, making an accurate copper tube impression of it, and constructing an electroformed die. A transfer coping of either Duralay* or, preferably, a metal alloy, is made and fitted to the tooth, and the RPD is placed in the patient's mouth. The transfer coping and the clasp assembly are fused by means of Duralay, an impression is made over both the coping and the framework, and the impression is poured with the die in place. The same procedures as outlined in the preceding paragraph are then followed.

*Reliance Dental Manufacturing Co., Worth, Ill.

Bibliography

Abel, L.F.: Masticatory function of partial denture patients among navy personnel, J. Prosthet. Dent. 3:382, 1953.

Academy of Denture Prosthetics: Glossary of prosthodontic terms, ed. 4, J. Prosthet. Dent. 38:66, 1977.

Ackerman, A.J.: The prosthetic management of oral and facial defects following cancer surgery, J. Prosthet. Dent. 5:413, 1955.

Adisman, I.K.: The internal clip attachment in fixed-removable partial denture prosthesis, N.Y. J. Dent. 32:125, 1962.

Ainamo, J.: Precision removable partial dentures with pontic abutments, J. Prosthet. Dent. 23:289, 1970.

Alexander, P.C.: Analysis of the cuspid protective occlusion. J. Prosthet. Dent. 13:309, 1963.

Altman, M.D., Yost, K.G., and Pitts, G.: A spectrofluorometric protein assay of plaque on dentures and of denture cleaning efficiency, J. Prosthet. Dent. 42:502, 1979.

American Dental Association: Prosthodontic care: number and types of denture wearers—1975, Chicago, 1976, Bureau of Economic Research and Statistics, American Dental Association.

Amsterdam, M., and Fox, L.: Provisional splinting: principles and technics, Dent. Clin. North Am., p. 73, March 1959.

Anthony, D.H., and Gibbons, P.J.: The nature and behavior of denture cleaners, J. Prosthet. Dent. 8:769, 1958.

Antos, E., Renner, R., Foerth, D.: The swing-lock partial denture: an alternate approach to conventional removable partial denture service, J. Prosthet. Dent. 40:257, 1978.

App, G.R.: Periodontal treatment for the removable partial prosthesis patient: another half century? Dent. Clin. North Am. 17:601, 1973.

Applegate, O.C.: Use of paralleling surveyor in modern partial denture construction, J. Am. Dent. Assoc. 27:1317, 1940.

Applegate, O.C.: The partial denture base, J. Prosthet. Dent. 5:636, 1955.

Applegate, O.C.: Conditions which may influence the choice of partial or complete denture service, J. Prosthet. Dent. 7:182, 1957.

Applegate, O.C.: The interdependence of periodontics and removable partial denture prosthesis, J. Prosthet. Dent. 8:269, 1958a.

Applegate, O.C.: The removable partial denture in the general practice of tomorrow, J. Prosthet, Dent. 8:609, 1958b.

Applegate, O.C.: Factors to be considered in choosing an alloy, Dent. Clin. North Am., p. 583, Nov. 1960a.

Applegate, O.C.: An evaluation of the support for the removable partial denture, J. Prosthet. Dent. 10:112, 1960b.

Applegate, O.C.: The rationale of partial denture choice, J. Prosthet. Dent. 10:891, 1960c.

Applegate, O.C.: Evaluating oral structures for removable partial dentures, J. Prosthet. Dent. 11:882, 1961.

Applegate, O.C.: Essentials of removable partial denture prosthesis, ed. 3, Philadelphia, 1965, W.B. Saunders Co.

Asgar, K., and Peyton, F.A.: Casting dental alloys to embedded wires, J. Prosthet. Dent. 15:312, 1965.

Asgar, K., and others: A new alloy for partial dentures, J. Prosthet. Dent. 23:36, 1970.

Askinas, S.W.: Facings in removable partial dentures, J. Prosthet. Dent. 33:633, 1975.

Atkinson, H.F.: Partial denture problem: surveyors and surveying, Aust. Dent J. 59:28, 1955.

Atkinson, R.A., and Elliot, Jr., R.W.: Removable partial dentures designed for laboratory fabrication by recent dental school graduates: a survey, J. Prosthet. Dent. 22:429, 1969.

Atwood, D.A.: A cephalometric study of the clinical restoration of the mandible. Part II, The variability in the rate of bone loss following the removal of occlusal contacts, J. Prosthet. Dent. 7:544, 1957.

Atwood, D.A.: Practice of prosthodontics: past, present, and future, J. Prosthet. Dent. 21:393, 1970.

Atwood, D.A.: Reduction of residual ridges: a major oral disease entity, J. Prosthet. Dent. 26:266, 1971.

Atwood, D.A.: Reduction of residual ridges in the partially edentulous patient, Dent. Clin. North Am. 17:747, 1973.

Atwood, D.A.: Bone loss of edentulous alveolar ridges. From the proceedings of the James A. English symposium on oral perspectives on bone biology, J. Periodontol. 50:11 (special issue), 1979.

Augsburger, R.H.: The Gilmore attachment, J. Prosthet. Dent. 16:1090, 1966.

Augsburger, R.H.: Evaluating removable partial dentures by mathematical equations, J. Prosthet. Dent. 22:528, 1969.

Austin, K.P., and Lidge, E.F.: Partial dentures: a practical textbook. St. Louis, 1957, The C.V. Mosby Co.

Avant, W.E.: Indirect retention in partial denture design, J. Prosthet. Dent. 16:1103, 1966.

Avant, W.E.: A universal classification for removable partial denture situations, J. Prosthet. Dent. 24:25, 1970.

Avant, W.E.: Factors that influence retention of removable partial dentures, J. Prosthet. Dent. 25:265, 1971a.

Avant, W.E.: Fulcrum and retention lines in planning removable partial dentures, J. Prosthet. Dent. 25:162, 1971b.

Axinn, S.: Preparation of retentive areas of clasps in enamel, J. Prosthet. Dent. 34:405, 1975.

Aydinlik, E., and Akay, H.U.: Effect of a resilient layer in a removable partial denture base on stress distribution to the mandible, J. Prosthet. Dent. **44**:17, 1980.

Backenstose, W.H., and Wells, J.G.: Side effects of immersion-type cleansers on the metal components of dentures, J. Prosthet. Dent. **37**:615, 1977.

Bailey, L.R.: Acrylic resin tray for rubber base impression materials, J. Prosthet. Dent. **5**:658, 1955.

Bailey, L.R.: Rubber base impression techniques, Dent. Clin. North Am., p. 156, March 1957.

Bailyn, M.: Tissue support in partial denture construction, Dent. Cosmos **70**:988, 1928.

Barker, B.C.W.: Dissection of regions of interest to the dentist from a medical approach, Aust. Dent. J. **16**:163, 1971.

Baron H.J.: Psychological aspects of treating denture patients, Morris Plains, N.J., 1974, Warner-Lambert Co., pp. 6-7.

Barone, J.V.: Nutrition of edentulous patients, J. Prosthet. Dent. **15**:804, 1965.

Barrett, D.A., and Pilling, L.O.: The restoration of carious clasp-bearing teeth, J. Prosthet. Dent. **15**:309, 1965.

Bartels, J.C.: Diagnosis and treatment planning, J. Prosthet. Dent. **7**:657, 1957.

Bartlett, A.A.: Duplication of precision attachment partial dentures, J. Prosthet. Dent. **16**:1111, 1966.

Bass, C.C.: An effective method of personal oral hygiene, part II., J. Louisiana St. Med. Soc. **106**:100, 1954.

Bates, J.F.: Studies related to fracture of partial dentures, Br. Dent. J. **120**:79, 1966.

Bates, J.F., Stafford, G.D., and Harrison, A.: Masticatory function: a review of the literature, J. Oral Rehabil. **2**:281, 1975.

Bauman, R.: Inflammatory papillary hyperplasia and home care instructions to denture patients, J. Prosthet. Dent. **37**:608, 1977.

Bauman, R.: Minimizing post-insertion problems: a procedure for removable partial denture placement, J. Prosthet. Dent. **42**:381, 1979.

Beck, H.O.: A clinical evaluation of the Arcon concept of articulation, J. Prosthet. Dent. **9**:409, 1959.

Beck, H.O.: Alloys for removable partial dentures, Dent. Clin. North Am., p. 591, Nov. 1960.

Beck, H.O.: Choosing the articulator, J. Am. Dent. Assoc. **64**:468, 1962.

Beck, H.O.: Denture cleaners and retaining devices, J. Am. Pharm. Assoc. **13**:246, 1972a.

Beck, H.O.: Occlusion as related to complete removable prosthodontics, J. Prosthet. Dent. **27**:246, 1972b.

Beck, H.O., and Morrison, W.E.: Investigation of an Arcon articulator, J. Prosthet. Dent. **6**:359, 1956.

Becker, C.M., Campbell, H.C., and Williams, D.L.: The Thompson dowel-rest system modified for chrome-cobalt removable partial denture frameworks, J. Prosthet. Dent. **39**:384, 1978.

Beckett, L.S.: The influence of saddle classification on the design of partial removable restoration, J. Prosthet. Dent. **3**:506, 1953.

Beckett, L.S.: Accurate occlusal relations in partial denture construction, J. Prosthet. Dent. **4**:487, 1954.

Beckett, L.S.: Partial denture: the rebasing of tissue borne saddles—theory and practice, Aust. Dent. J. **16**:340, 1971.

Beder, D.E.: An evaluation of conventional circumferential clasps, J. Prosthet. Dent. **3**:88, 1953.

Bell, D.H.: Clinical evaluation of a resilient denture liner, J. Prosthet. Dent. **23**:394, 1970.

Bennett, C.C.: Transitional restorations for function and esthetics, J. Prosthet. Dent. **15**:867, 1965.

Bennett, N.G.: A contribution to the study of the movements of the mandible, J. Prosthet. Dent. **8**: 41, 1958.

Benson, D., and Spolsky, V.: A clinical evaluation of removable partial dentures with I-bar retainers: part I, J. Prosthet. Dent. **41**:246, 1979.

Beresin, V.E., and Schiesser, F.J.: The neutral zone in complete and partial dentures, ed. 2, St. Louis, 1978, The C.V. Mosby Co.

Berg, T., Jr., and Caputo, A.A.: Anterior rests for maxillary removable partial dentures, J. Prosthet. Dent. **39**:139, 1978.

Bergman, B., Hogoson, A., and Olsen, C.: Peridontal and prosthetic conditions in patients treated with removable partial dentures and artificial crowns: a longitudinal two year study, Acta Odontol. Scand. **29**:621, 1971.

Berke, J.D., and Moleres, I.: A removable appliance for the correction of maxillomandibular disproportion, J. Prosthet. Dent. **17**:172, 1967.

Berman, M.H.: Accurate interocclusal records, J. Prosthet. Dent. **10**:620, 1960.

Berry, D.C., and Mahood, M.: Oral stereognosis and oral ability in relation to prosthetic treatment, Br. Dent. J. **120**:179, 1966.

Beube, F.E.: Periodontology, New York, 1953, The Macmillan Co.

Beumer, J., III, Curtis, T.A., and Firtell, D.N.: Maxillofacial rehabilitation: prosthodontic and surgical considerations, St. Louis, 1979, The C.V. Mosby Co.

Beyron, H.L.: Characteristics of functionally optimal occlusion and principles of occlusal rehabilitation, J. Am. Dent. Assoc. **48**:648, 1954.

Beyron, H.L.: Occlusion: point of significance in planning restorative procedures, J. Prosthet. Dent. **30**:641, 1973.

Bickley, R.W.: Combined splint–stress breaker removable partial denture, J. Prosthet. Dent. **21**:509, 1969.

Blakeslee, R.W., Renner, R.P., and Shiu, A.: Dental technology: theory and practice, St. Louis, 1980, The C.V. Mosby Co.

Blanchard, C.H.: Filling undercuts on refractory casts with investment, J. Prosthet. Dent. **3**:417, 1953.

Blatterfein, L.: Study of partial denture clasping, J. Am. Dent. Assoc. **43**:169, 1951.

Blatterfein, L.: Design and positional arrangement of clasps for partial dentures, N.Y. J. Dent. **22**:305, 1952a.

Blatterfein, L.: Role of the removable partial denture in the restoration of lost vertical dimension, N.Y. Univ. J. Dent. **10**:274-276, 1952b.

Blatterfein, L.: A systematic method of designing upper partial denture bases, J. Am. Dent. Assoc. **46**:510, 1953.

Blatterfein, L.: The planning and contouring of acrylic resin veneer crowns for partial denture clasping, J. Prosthet. Dent. **6**:386, 1956.

Blatterfein, L.: Rebasing procedures for removable partial dentures, J. Prosthet. Dent. **8**:441, 1958.

Blatterfein, L.: The use of the semiprecision rest in removable partial dentures, J. Prosthet. Dent. **22**:307, 1969.

Blatterfein, L., and others: Minimum acceptable procedures for satisfactory removable partial denture service, J. Prosthet. Dent. 27:84, 1972.

Bliss, C.H.: Psychologic factors involved in presenting denture service, J. Prosthet. Dent. 1:49, 1951.

Bohannan, H.M.: A critical analysis of the mucostatic principle, J. Prosthet. Dent. 4:232, 1954.

Bolender, C.L., and Becker, C.M.: Swinglock removable partial dentures: where and when, J. Prosthet. Dent. 45:4, 1981.

Bolender, C.L., Swenson, R.D., and Yamane, G.: Evaluation of treatment of inflammatory papillary hyperplasia of the palate, J. Prosthet. Dent. 15:1013, 1965.

Bolender, C.L., Swoope, C.C., and Smith, D.E.: The Cornell Medical Index as a prognostic aid for complete denture patients, J. Prosthet. Dent. 22:20, 1979.

Bolouri, A., Hilger, T.C., and Gowrylok, M.D.: Modified flasking technique for removable partial dentures, J. Prosthet. Dent. 34:221, 1975.

Boucher, C.O.: Complete denture impressions based upon the anatomy of the mouth, J. Am. Dent. Assoc. 31:1174, 1944.

Boucher, C.O.: Occlusion in prosthodontics, J. Prosthet. Dent. 3:633, 1953.

Boucher, L.J.: Anatomy of the temporomandibular joint as it pertains to centric relation, J. Prosthet. Dent. 12:464, 1962.

Boucher, L.J.: Decompression stents, J. Prosthet. Dent. 14:1163, 1964.

Boucher, L.J.: Injected silastic in ridge extension procedures, J. Prosthet. Dent. 14:460, 1964.

Boucher, L.J., and Jacoby, J.: Posterior border movements of the human mandible, J. Prosthet. Dent. 11:836, 1961.

Boucher, L.J., and others: Guidelines for advanced prosthodontic education, J. Prosthet. Dent. 23:104, 1970.

Breisach, L.: Esthetic attachments for removable partial dentures, J. Prosthet. Dent. 17:261, 1967.

Breitbart, A.R.: Converting a tooth-supported denture to a distal extension removable partial denture, J. Prosthet. Dent. 18:233, 1967.

Brewer, A.A., and Fenton, A.H.: The overdenture, Dent. Clin. North Am. 17:723, 1973.

Brewer, A.A., and Morrow, R.M.: Overdentures, ed. 2, St. Louis, 1980, The C.V.Mosby Co.

Brill, N.: Factors in the mechanism of full denture retention: a discussion of selected papers, Dent. Prac. Dent. Rec. 18:9, Sept. 1967.

Brill, N., Ashubeler, S., and Tryde, G.: Influence of occlusal patterns on movements of the mandible, J. Prosthet. Dent. 12:255, 1962.

Brill, N., Tryde, G., and Cantor, R.: The dynamic nature of the lower denture space, J. Prosthet. Dent. 15:401, 1965.

Brill, N., Tryde, G., and Schubeler, S.: The role of exteroceptors in denture retention, J. Prosthet. Dent. 9:761, 1959.

Brill, N., and others: Ecologic changes in the oral cavity caused by removable partial dentures, J. Prosthet. Dent. 38:138, 1977.

Brockhurst, P.J.: Comparison of the performance of materials for spring members in dental appliances, using the theory of simple bending, Aust. Dent. J. 15:119, 1970.

Brodbelt, R.H.W.: A simple paralleling template for precision attachments, J. Prosthet. Dent. 27:285, 1972.

Brotman, D.N.: Contemporary concepts of articulation, J. Prosthet. Dent. 10:221, 1960.

Brown, E.T.: The dentist, the laboratory technician, and the prescription law, J. Prosthet. Dent. 15:1132, 1965.

Brudevold, F.: Basic study of the chewing forces of a denture wearer, J. Am. Dent. Assoc. 43:45, 1951.

Brudvik, J.S., and Wormley, J.H.: Construction techniques for wrought wire rentive clasp arms are related to clasp flexibility, J. Prosthet. Dent. 30:769, 1973.

Budtz-Jorgensen, E.: The significance of candida albicans in denture stomatitits, Scand. J. Dent. Res. 82:151, 1974.

Budtz-Jorgensen, E.: Clinical aspects of candida infections in denture wearers, J. Am. Dent. Assoc. 96:474, 1978a.

Budtz-Jorgensen, E.: A 3-month's study of enzymes as denture cleaners, J. Oral Rehabil. 5:35, 1978b.

Budtz-Jorgensen, E.: Materials and methods used for cleaning dentures, J. Prosthet. Dent. 42:619, 1979.

Budtz-Jorgensen, E.: Oral mucosal lesions associated with the wearing of removable dentures, J. Prosthet. Dent. 10:65, 1981.

Budtz-Jorgensen, E., and Kelstrup, J.: Enzymes as denture cleansers, Scand. J. Dent. Res. 85:209, 1977.

Cacciatore, A.: Periodontia related to prosthetics, Dent. Clin. North Am., Nov. 1962.

Caldarone, C.V.: Attachments for partial dentures without clasps, J. Prosthet. Dent. 7:206, 1957.

Campbell, L.D.: Subjective reactions to major connector designs for removable partial dentures, J. Prosthet. Dent. 37:507, 1977.

Carlsson, G.E., Hedegard, B., and Koivumma, K.K.: Studies in partial denture prosthesis: IV, A longitudinal study of mandibular partial dentures with double extension saddles, Acta Odontol. Scand. 23:443-472, 1965.

Carlsson, G.E., Hedegard, B., Koivumma, K.K.: Late results of treatment with partial dentures. J. Oral Rehabil. 3:267, 1976.

Carlsson, G.E., Ingervall, B., and Kocak, G.: Effect of increasing vertical dimension on the masticatory system in subjects with natural teeth, J. Prosthet. Dent. 41:284, 1979.

Carlsson, G.E., and Oberg, T.: Remodeling of the temperomandibular joints, Oral Sci. Rev. 7:58, 1975.

Carlsson, G.E., and Persson, G.: Morphologic changes of the mandible after extraction and wearing of dentures, Odont. Rev. (Malmo) 18:27, 1967.

Cavalaris, C.J.: Pathologic considerations associated with partial dentures, Dent. Clin. North Am. 17:585, 1973.

Cecconi, B.T.: Lingual bar design, J. Prosthet. Dent. 29:635, 1973.

Cecconi, B.T.: Effect of rest designs on transmission of forces to abutment teeth, J. Prosthet. Dent. 32:141, 1974.

Cecconi, B.: Removable partial denture research and its clinical significance, J. Prosthet. Dent. 39:203, 1978.

Cecconi, B.T., Asgar, K., and Dootz, E.: The effect of partial denture clasp design on abutment tooth movement, J. Prosthet. Dent. 25:44, 1971a.

Cecconi, B.T., Asgar, K., and Dootz, E.: Removable partial denture abutment tooth movement as affected by inclination of residual ridges and types of loading, J. Prosthet. Dent. **25:**375, 1971b.

Cecconi, B.T., Asgar, K., and Dootz, E.: Fit of the removable partial denture base and its effect on abutment tooth movement, J. Prosthet. Dent. **25:**515, 1971c.

Cecconi, B.T., Asgar, K., and Dootz, E.: Clasp assembly modifications and their effect on abutment tooth movement, J. Prosthet. Dent. **27:**160, 1972.

Cecconi, B.T., Kaiser, G., and Rahe, A.: Stress-breakers and the removable partial denture, J. Prosthet. Dent. **34:**145, 1975.

Celenza, F.V., and Litvak, H.: Occlusal management in conformative dentistry, J. Prosthet. Dent. **36:**164, 1976.

Cerveris, A.R.: Vibracentric equilibration of centric occlusion, J. Am. Dent. Assoc. **63:**476, 1961.

Chandler, H.T., Brudvik, J.S., and Fisher, W.T.: Surveyed crowns, J. Prosthet. Dent. **30:**775, 1973.

Chase, W.W.: Adaptation of rubber-base impression materials to removable denture prosthetics, J. Prosthet. Dent. **10:**1043, 1960.

Chestner, S.G.: A methodical approach to the analysis of study cases, J. Prosthet. Dent. **4:**622, 1954.

Chick, A.O.: Correct location of clasps and rests on dentures without stress-breakers, Br. Dent. J. **95:**303, 1953.

Christensen, F.G.: Mandibular free end denture, J. Prosthet. Dent. **12:**111, 1962.

Christensen, P.B.: Accurate casts and positional relation records, J. Prosthet. Dent. **8:**475, 1958.

Cinotti, W.R., Grieder, A., and Springob, H.K.: Applied psychology in dentistry, ed. 2, St. Louis, The C.V. Mosby Co., 1972.

Civjan, S., Huget, E.F., and de Simon, L.B.: Surface characteristics of alginate impressions, J. Prosthet. Dent. **28:**373, 1972.

Clark, R.J., and Phillips, R.W.: Flow studies of certain dental impression materials, J. Prosthet. Dent. **7:**259, 1957.

Clayton, J.A., and Jaslo, C.: A measurement of clasp forces on teeth, J. Prosthet. Dent. **25:**21, 1971.

Clayton, J.A., and others: Pantographic tracings of mandibular movements and occlusion, J. Prosthet. Dent. **25:**389, 1971.

Coelho, D.H.: Criteria for the use of fixed prosthesis, Dent. Clin. North Am., p. 299, March 1957.

Cohn, L.A.: The physiologic basis for tooth fixation in precision-attached partial dentures, J. Prosthet. Dent. **6:**220, 1956.

Cohn, L.A.: Occluso-rehabilitation: principles of diagnosis and treatment planning, Dent. Clin. North Am., p. 259, March 1962.

Collett, H.A.: Balancing the occlusion of partial dentures, J. Am. Dent. Assoc. **42:**162, 1951.

Collett, H.A.: Biologic approach to clasp partial dentures, Dent. Dig. **61:**309, 1955a.

Collett, H.A.: Psychodynamic study of abnormal reactions to dentures, J. Am. Dent. Assoc. **51:**541, 1955b.

Collett, H.A.: Complete denture impressions, J. Prosthet. Dent. **15:**603, 1965.

Collett, H.A.: Casting chrome-cobalt alloys in small laboratories, J. Prosthet. Dent. **21:**216, 1969.

Colman, A.J.: Occlusal requirements for removable partial dentures, J. Prosthet. Dent. **17:**155, 1967.

Connor, J.N., Schoenfeld, C.M., and Taylor, R.L.: An evaluation of an enzyme denture cleanser, J. Prosthet. Dent. **37:**147, 1977.

Contino, R.M., and Stallard, H.: Instruments essential for obtaining data needed in making a functional diagnosis of the human mouth, J. Prosthet. Dent. **7:**66, 1957.

Cooper, H.K.: Integration of service in the treatment of cleft lip and cleft palate, J. Am. Dent. Assoc. **47:**27, 1953.

Cooper, T.M., and others: Effect of venting on cast gold full crowns, J. Prosthet. Dent. **26:**621, 1971.

Costa, E.: A simplified system for identifying partially edentulous arches, J. Prosthet. Dent. **32:**639, 1974.

Cowgen, G.T.: Retention, resistance and esthetics of the anterior three-quarter crown, J. Am. Dent. Assoc. **62:**167, 1961.

Coy, R.E., and Arnold, P.D.: Survey and design of diagnostic casts for removable partial dentures, J. Prosthet. Dent. **32:**103, 1974.

Craddock, F.W. Prosthetic dentistry: a clinical outline, ed. 2, St. Louis, 1951, The C.V. Mosby Co.

Craddock, F.W.: Retromolar region of the mandible, J. Am. Dent. Assoc. **47:**453, 1953.

Crosthwaite, H.J.: Fitting removable partial denture frameworks. In Lefkowitz, W., editor: Proceedings of the Second International Prosthodontic Congress, St. Louis, 1979, The C.V. Mosby Co., pp. 94-95.

Crum, R.J., and Loisell, R.J.: Oral perception and proprioception. J. Prosthet. Dent. **28:**215, 1972.

Culpepper, W.D.: A comparative study of shade-matching procedures, J. Prosthet. Dent. **24:**166, 1970.

Cummer, W.E.: Possible combinations of teeth present and missing in partial restorations, Oral Health **10:**421, 1920.

Cummer, W.E.: Partial denture service. In Anthony, L.P., ed.: American textbook of prosthetic dentistry, Philadelphia, 1942, Lea & Febiger.

Cunningham, D.M.: Comparison of base metal alloys and Type IV gold alloys for removable partial denture frameworks, Dent. Clin. North Am. **17:**719, 1973.

Dairy Council of California: Big ideas in nutrition: a self-instructional booklet, Sacramento, 1975, the Council.

Dale, J.W.: A full and partial denture survey, Aust. Dent. J. **15:**225, 1970.

D'Amico, A.: Functional occlusion of the natural teeth of man, J. Prosthet. Dent. **11:**899, 1961.

Dawson, P.E.: Evaluation, diagnosis, and treatment of occlusal problems, St. Louis, 1974, The C.V. Mosby Co.

Demer, W.J.: An analysis of mesial rest–I-bar clasp designs, J. Prosthet. Dent. **36:**243, 1976.

Derry, A., and Bertram, U.: A clinical survey of removable partial dentures after 2 years usage, Acta Odontol. Scand. **28:**581, 1970.

Desjardins, R.P.: Prosthodontic management of the cleft palate patient, J. Prosthet. Dent. **33:**655, 1975.

DeVan, M.M.: The nature of the partial denture foundation: suggestions for its preservation, J. Prosthet. Dent. **2:**210, 1952a.

DeVan, M.M.: Basic principles in impression making, J. Prosthet. Dent. **2:**26, 1952b.

DeVan, M.M.: Preserving natural teeth through the use of clasps, J. Prosthet. Dent. **5:**208, 1955.

DeVan, M.M.: The prosthetic problem: its formulation and suggestions for its solution, J. Prosthet. Dent. **6**:291, 1956.

DeVan, M.M.: The additive partial denture: its principles and design (partial dentures), Northwest Dent. **35**:303, 312, 1956; Dent. Abstr. **2**:468, 1957.

DeVan, M.M.: The appearance phase of denture construction, Dent. Clin. North Am., p. 255, March 1957.

Dietz, W.H.: Modified abutments for removable and fixed prosthodontics, J. Prosthet. Dent. **11**:1112, 1961.

Dinger, E.J., and Peyton, F.A.: Distortion of gold partial denture castings, J. Prosthet. Dent. **1**:443, 1951.

Dirksen, L.C., and Campagna, S.J.: Mat surface and rugae reproduction for upper partial denture castings, J. Prosthet. Dent. **4**:67, 1954.

Dolder, E.J.: The bar joint mandibular denture, J. Prosthet. Dent. **11**:689, 1961.

Dootz, E.R., Craig, R.G., and Peyton, F.A.: Influence of investments and duplicating procedures on the accuracy of partial denture castings, J. Prosthet. Dent. **15**:679, 1965.

Dootz, E.R., Craig, R.G., and Peyton, F.A.: Aqueous acrylamide gel duplicating material, J. Prosthet. Dent. **17**:570, 1967a.

Dootz, E.R., Craig, R.G., and Peyton, F.A.: Simplification of the chrome-cobalt partial denture casting procedure, J. Prosthet. Dent. **17**:464, 1967b.

Draper, D.H.: Forward trends in occlusion, J. Prosthet. Dent. **13**:724, 1963.

Dreizen, S.: Nutritional changes in the oral cavity, J. Prosthet. Dent. **16**:1144, 1966.

Dubin, N.A.: Advances in functional occlusal rehabilitation, J. Prosthet. Dent. **6**:252, 1956.

Dunn, B.W.: Treatment planning for removable partial dentures, J. Prosthet. Dent. **11**:247, 1961.

Dunny, J.A., and King, G.E.: Minor connector designs for anterior acrylic resin bases: a preliminary study, J. Prosthet. Dent. **34**:496, 1975.

Dutton, D.A.: Standard abbreviations (and definitions) for use in dental laboratory work authorizations, J. Prosthet. Dent. **27**:94, 1972.

Dykema, R.W., Cunningham, D.M., and Johnston, J.F.: Modern practice in removable partial prosthodontics, Philadelphia, 1969, W.B. Saunders Co.

Elbert, C.A., and Ryge, G.: The effect of heat treatment on hardness of a chrome-cobalt alloy, J. Prosthet. Dent. **15**:873, 1965.

Ellinger, C.W., and others: Synopsis of complete dentures, Philadelphia, 1975, Lea & Febiger.

Elliott, R.W., Jr.: The effects of heat on gold partial denture castings, J. Prosthet. Dent. **13**:688-698, 1963.

Emig, G.E.: The physiology of the muscles of mastication, J. Prosthet. Dent. **1**:700, 1951.

Emmert, J.H.: A method for registering occlusion in semi-edentulous mouths, J. Prosthet. Dent. **8**:94, 1958.

Enright, C.M.: Dentist-dental laboratory harmony, J. Prosthet. Dent. **11**:393, 1961.

Epstein, S.: Prosthodontic consideration of the aged patient, J. Am. Soc. Geriatr. Dent. **5**:3, 1970.

Ewing, J.E.: The construction of accurate full crown restorations for an existing clasp by using a direct metal pattern technique, J. Prosthet. Dent. **15**:889,1965.

Farrell, J.: Partial denture designing, London, 1970, Henry Kimpton Medical Publisher & Bookseller.

Farrell, J.: Wrought wire retainers: a method of increasing their flexibility, Br. Dent. J. **131**:327, 1971.

Federation of Prosthodontic Organizations: Guidelines for evaluation of completed prosthodontic treatment for removable partial dentures, J. Prosthet. Dent. **27**:326, 1972.

Fedi, P.F.: Cardinal differences in occlusion of natural teeth and that of artificial teeth, J. Am. Dent. Assoc. **62**:482, 1962.

Fenner, W., and Muhlemann, H.R.: Tooth mobility changes during treatment with partial denture prosthesis, J. Prosthet. Dent. **6**:520, 1956.

Fields, H., and Campfield, R.W.: Removable partial prosthesis partially supported by an endosseous blade implant, J. Prosthet. Dent. **31**:273, 1974.

Firtell, D.N.: Effect of clasp design upon retention of removable partial dentures, J. Prosthet. Dent. **20**:43, 1968.

Firtell, D.N., Herzberg, T.W., and Walsh, J.F.: Root retention and removable partial denture design, Prosthet. Dent. **42**:131, 1979.

Fish, E.W.: An analysis of the stabilizing factors in full denture construction, Br. Dent. J. **52**:1, 1931.

Fish, E.W.: Principles of full denture prosthesis, London, 1933, John Bale Sons and Danielsson, Ltd.

Fisher, R.L., and Jaslow, C.: The efficiency of an indirect retainer, J. Prosthet. Dent. **33**:24, 1975.

Foster, T.D.: The use of the face-bow in making permanent study casts, J. Prosthet. Dent. **9**:717, 1959.

Fountain, H.W.: Seating the condyles for centric relation records, J. Prosthet. Dent. **11**:1050, 1961.

Fountain, H.W.: The temporomandibular joints: a fulcrum, J. Prosthet. Dent. **25**:78, 1971.

Frank, R.P.: Fabrication of temporary and treatment partial dentures, J. Prosthet. Dent. **30**:215, 1973.

Frank, R.P., and Nicholls, J.I.: An investigation of the effectiveness of indirect retainers, J. Prosthet. Dent. **38**:494, 1977.

Frank, R.P., Nicholls, J.I.: A study of the flexibility of wrought wire clasps, J. Prosthet. Dent. **45**:259, 1981.

Frantz, W.R.: Variations in a removable maxillary partial denture design by dentists, J. Prosthet. Dent. **34**:625, 1975.

Frechette, A.R.: Partial denture planning with special reference to stress distribution, J. Prosthet. Dent. **1**:710, 1951.

Frechette, A.R.: Partial denture planning with special reference to stress distribution, J. Ont. Dent. Assoc. **30**:318, 1953.

Frechette, A.R.: The influence of partial denture design on distribution of force to abutment teeth, J. Prosthet. Dent. **6**:195, 1956.

Friedman, J.: The ABC classification of partial denture segments, J. Prosthet. Dent. **3**:517, 1953.

Friedman, S.: Effective use of diagnostic data, J. Prosthet. Dent. **9**:729, 1959.

Frost, J.S.: Continuous coverage lower removable partial denture, J. Prosthet. Dent. **11**:894, 1961.

Frush, J.P., and Fisher, R.D.: Introduction to dentogenic restorations, J. Prosthet. Dent. **5**:586, 1955.

Frush, J.P., and Fisher, R.D.: How dentogenic restorations interpret the sex factor, J. Prosthet. Dent. **6**:160, 1956a.

Frush, J.P., and Fisher, R.D.: How dentogenics interprets the personality factor, J. Prosthet. Dent. **6**:441, 1956b.

Fusayama, T., and Nakazato, M.: The design of stock trays and the retention of irreversible hydrocolloid impressions, J. Prosthet. Dent. **21**:136, 1969.

Gabel, A.B.: A new theory of the mechanisms of total support, Dent. Cosmos **76**:677, 1934.

Garver, D.G., Fenster, R.K., and Cannole, P.W.: Vital root retention in humans: an interim report, J. Prosthet. Dent. **41**:255, 1979.

Garver, D.G., and others: Vital root retention in humans: a preliminary report, J. Prosthet. Dent. **40**:23, 1978.

Gaston, G.W.: Rest area preparations for removable partial dentures, J. Prosthet. Dent. **10**:124, 1960.

Gibbons, P., and Bloomer, H.: A supportive-type prosthetic speech aid, J. Prosthet. Dent. **8**:362, 1958.

Gibbs, C.H., and others: Functional movement of the mandible, J. Prosthet. Dent. **26**:604, 1971.

Gill, J.R.: Treatment planning for mouth rehabilitation, J. Prosthet. Dent. **2**:230, 1952.

Gilmore, W.H., Schnell, R.J., and Phillips, R.W.: Factors influencing the accuracy of silicone impression materials, J. Prosthet. Dent. **9**:304, 1959.

Gilson, T.D.: Theory of centric correction in natural teeth, J. Prosthet. Dent. **8**:468, 1958.

Gilson, T.D., Asgar, K., and Peyton, F.A.: The quality of union formed in casting gold to embedded attachment metals, J. Prosthet. Dent. **15**:464, 1965.

Gindea, A.E.: A retentive device for removable dentures, J. Prosthet. Dent. **27**:501, 1972.

Giradot, R.L.: History and development of partial denture design, J. Am. Dent. Assoc. **28**:1399, 1941.

Giradot, R.L.: The physiologic aspects of partial denture restorations, J. Prosthet. Dent. **3**:689, 1953.

Glann, G.W., and Appleby, R.C.: Mouth preparations for removable partial dentures, J. Prosthet. Dent. **10**:698, 1960.

Glickman, I.: The periodontal structures and removable partial denture prosthesis, J. Am. Dent. Assoc. **37**:311, 1948.

Glossary of prosthodontic terms, ed. 4, J. Prosthet. Dent. **38**:66, 1977.

Godfrey, R.J.: Classification of removable partial dentures, J. Am. Coll. Dent. **18**:5, 1951.

Goldman, H.M., and Cohen, D.W.: Periodontal therapy, ed. 6, St. Louis, 1980, The C.V. Mosby Co.

Gomes, B.C., Renner, R.P., and Baer, P.N.: Periodontal considerations in removable partial dentures, J. Am. Dent. Assoc. **101**:496, 1980.

Goodkind, R.J.: The effects of removable partial dentures on abutment tooth mobility: a clinical study, J. Prosthet. Dent. **30**:139, 1973.

Goodman, J.J., and Goodman, H.W.: Balance of force in precision free-end restorations, J. Prosthet. Dent. **13**:302, 1963.

Grant, D.A., Stern, I.B., and Everett, F.G.: Orban's periodontics: a concept—theory and practice, St. Louis, 1972, The C.V. Mosby Co.

Grasso, J.E.: A new removable partial denture clasp assembly, J. Prosthet. Dent. **43**:618, 1980.

Greene, J.H.: The hinge-lock abutment attachment, J. Am. Dent. Assoc. **47**:175, 1953.

Grosser, D.: The dynamics of internal precision attachments, J. Prosthet. Dent. **3**:393, 1953.

Grun, L., and Engelhardt, J.P.: Die Effektivitat von Ultraschall bei der Prothesendisinfektion, Dtsch. Zahnaerztl. Z. **31**:627, 1976.

Grunewald, A.H., Paffenbarger, G.C., and Dickson, G.: The effect of molding processes on some properties of denture resins, J. Am. Dent. Assoc. **44**:269, 1952.

Grunewald, A.H., Paffenbarger, G.C., and Dickson, G.: Dentist, dental laboratory, and the patient, J. Prosthet. Dent. **8**:55, 1958.

Grunewald, A.H., Paffenbarger, G.C., and Dickson, G.: The role of the dental technician in a prosthetic service, Dent. Clin. North Am., p. 359, July 1960.

Gysi, A.: Research in denture construction, J. Am. Dent. Assoc. **16**:199, 1929.

Haines, R.W., and Barnett, S.G.: The structure of the mouth in the mandibular molar region, J. Prosthet. Dent. **9**:962, 1959.

Hall, W.A.: Variations in registering interarch transfers in removable partial denture construction, J. Prosthet. Dent. **30**:548, 1973.

Hanau, R.L.: Articulation defined, analyzed, and formulated, J. Am. Dent. Assoc. **13**:1694, 1926.

Handlers, M., Lenchner, N.H., and Weissman, B.: A retaining device for partial dentures, J. Prosthet. Dent. **7**:483, 1957.

Hanson, J.G., and others: Surveying, J. Am. Dent. Assoc. **91**:826, 1975.

Hardcourt, H.J., and others: The properties of nickel-chromium casting alloys containing boron and silicon, Br. Dent. J. **129**:419, 1970.

Harris, F.N.: The precision dowel rest attachment, J. Prosthet. Dent. **5**:43, 1955.

Harris, W.T., Jr.: Water temperature and accuracy of alginate impressions, J. Prosthet. Dent. **21**:613, 1969.

Harrison, W.M., and Stansbury, B.E.: The effect of joint surface contours on the transverse strength of repaired acrylic resin, J. Prosthet. Dent. **23**:464, 1970.

Harvey, W.L.: A transitional prosthetic appliance, J. Prosthet. Dent. **14**:60, 1970.

Heartwell, C.M.: Psychological considerations in complete denture prosthodontics, J. Prosthet. Dent. **24**:5, 1970.

Heartwell, C.M., Jr., and Rahn, A.O.: Syllabus of complete dentures, ed. 3, Philadelphia, 1980, Lea & Febiger.

Heartwell, C.M., and others: Comparison of impressions made in perforated and nonperforated rimlocks trays, J. Prosthet. Dent. **27**:494, 1972.

Heintz, W.D.: Principles, planning and practice for prevention, Dent. Clin. North Am. **17**:705, 1973.

Hekneby, M.: The spring-slide joint for lower free end removable partial dentures, J. Prosthet. Dent. **11**:256, 1961.

Helkimo, M., Ingervall, B., and Carlsson, G.E.: Variation of retruded and muscular position of mandible under different recording conditions, Acta Odontol. Scand. **29**:423, 1971.

Hembree, M.E., and Hembree, J.H.: Relative abrasiveness of dentrifices, Dent. Hyg. **51**:253, 1977.

Henderson, D.: Writing work authorizations for removable partial dentures, J. Prosthet. Dent. **16**:696, 1966.

Henderson, D.: Occlusion in removable partial prosthodontics, J. Prosthet. Dent. **27**:151, 1972.

Henderson, D.: Major connectors for mandibular removable partial dentures, J. Prosthet. Dent. **30**:532, 1973.

Henderson, D., and Seward, T.E.: Design and force distribution with removable partial dentures: a progress report, J. Prosthet. Dent. **17**:350, 1967.

Henderson, D., and Steffel, V.L.: McCracken's removable partial prosthodontics, ed. 6, St. Louis, 1981, The C.V. Mosby Co.

Herlands, R.E.: Removable partial denture terminology, J. Prosthet. Dent. **8**:964, 1958.

Hickey, J.C.: Responsibility of the dentist in removable partial dentures, J. Ky. Dent. Assoc. **17**:70, 1965.

Hickey, J.C., and Zarb, G.A.: Boucher's prosthodontic treatment for edentulous patients, ed. 8, St. Louis, 1980, The C.V. Mosby Co.

Hindels, G.W.: Load distribution in extension saddle partial dentures, J. Prosthet. Dent. **2**:92, 1952.

Hindels, G.W.: Stress analysis in distal extension partial dentures, J. Prosthet. Dent. **7**:197, 1957.

Hindels, G.W.: Occlusion in removable partial denture prosthesis, Dent. Clin. North Am., p. 137, March 1962.

Hirschtritt, E.: Removable partial dentures with stress-broken extension bases, J. Prosthet. Dent. **7**:318, 1957.

Hobdell, M.H., and others: The prevalence of full and partial dentures in British populations, Br. Dent. J. **128**:437, 1970.

Holmes, J.B.: Influence of impression procedures and occlusal loading on partial denture movement, J. Prosthet. Dent. **15**:474, 1965.

Holmes, J.B.: The altered cast impression procedure for the distal extension removable partial denture, Dent. Clin. North Am. **14**:569, 1970.

House, M.M.: The relationship of oral examination to dental diagnosis, J. Prosthet. Dent. **8**:208, 1958.

Hundson, W.C.: Clinical uses of rubber impression materials and electroforming of casts and dies in pure silver, J. Prosthet. Dent. **8**:107, 1958.

Hughes, G.A.: Facial types and tooth arrangement, J. Prosthet. Dent. **1**:82, 1951.

Hughes, G.A., and Regli, C.P.: What is centric relation? J. Prosthet. Dent. **11**:16, 1961.

Hutchins, D.W., and Parker, W.A.: A clinical evaluation of the ability of denture cleaning solutions to remove dental plaque from prosthetic devices, N.Y. State Dent. J. **39**:363, 1973.

Immekus, J.E., and Aramy, M.: Adverse effects of resilient denture liners in overlay dentures, J. Prosthet. Dent. **32**:178, 1974.

Immekus, J.E., and Aramy, M.A.: A fixed-removable partial denture for cleft palate patients, J. Prosthet. Dent. **34**:286, 1975.

Ingervall, B., Helkimo, M., and Carlsson, G.E.: Recording of the retruded position of the mandible with application of varying external pressure to the lower jaw in man, Arch. Oral. Biol. **16**:1165, 1971.

Isaacson, D.: A biologic concept of occlusion, J. Prevent. Dent. **3**:12, 1976.

Isaacson, G.O.: Telescope crown retainers for removable partial dentures, J. Prosthet. Dent. **22**:436, 1969.

James, A.G.: Stress breakers which automatically return the saddle to rest position following displacement: mandibular distal extension partial dentures, J. Prosthet. Dent. **4**:73, 1954.

James, A.G.: Self-locking posterior attachment for removable tooth-supported partial dentures, J. Prosthet. Dent. **5**:200, 1955.

Jankelson, B.: Physiology of human dental occlusion, J. Am. Dent. Assoc. **50**:664, 1955.

Jankelson, B.: Considerations of occlusion on fixed partial dentures, Dent. Clin. North Am., p. 187, March 1959.

Jeffreys, F.E., and Platner, R.L.: Occlusion in removable partial dentures, J. Prosthet. Dent. **10**:912, 1960.

Jerbi, Frank, C.: Trimming the cast in the construction of immediate dentures, J. Prosthet. Dent. **16**:1047, 1966.

Johnson, E.A., Jr.: Combination of fixed and removable partial dentures, J. Prosthet. Dent. **14**:1099, 1964.

Johnson, H.B.: Technique for packing and staining complete or partial denture bases, J. Prosthet. Dent. **6**:154, 1956.

Johnson, J.F.: The application and construction of the pinledge retainer, J. Prosthet. Dent. **3**:559, 1953.

Johnston, J.F.: Preparation of mouths for fixed and removable partial dentures, J. Prosthet. Dent. **11**:456, 1961.

Johnston, J.F., Cunningham, D.M., and Bogan, R.G.: The dentist, the patient, and ridge preservation, J. Prosthet. Dent. **10**:288, 1960.

Johnston, J.F., Phillips, R.W., and Dykema, R.W.: Modern practice in crown and bridge prosthodontics, Philadelphia, 1971, W.B. Saunders Co.

Jones, D.W.: Thermal analysis and stability of refractory investments, J. Prosthet. Dent. **18**:234, 1967.

Jones, P.: Complete dentures and the associated soft tissues, J. Prosthet. Dent. **36**:136, 1976.

Jones, P.M.: The monoplane occlusion for complete dentures, J. Am. Dent. Assoc. **85**:94, 1972.

Jones, R.R.: The lower partial denture, J. Prosthet. Dent. **2**:219, 1952.

Jordan, L.G.: Designing removable partial dentures with external attachments (clasps), J. Prosthet. Dent. **2**:716, 1952a.

Jordan, L.G.: Mounting master and refractory casts in the articulator in partial denture construction, J. Prosthet. Dent. **2**:108, 1952b.

Jordan, L.G.: Treatment of advanced periodontal disease by prosthodontic procedures, J. Prosthet. Dent. **10**:908, 1960.

Jordan, L.G.: Arrangement of anatomic-type artificial teeth into balanced occlusion, J. Prosthet. Dent. **39**:484, 1978.

Kabcenell, J.L.: Stress breaking for partial dentures, J. Am. Dent. Assoc. **63**:593-602, 1961.

Kabcenell, J.L.: Effective clasping of removable partial dentures, J. Prosthet. Dent. **12**:104, 1962.

Kaires, A.K.: Effect of partial denture design on bilateral force distribution, J. Prosthet. Dent. **6**:373, 1956a.

Kaires, A.K.: Partial denture design and its relation to force distribution and masticatory performance, J. Prosthet. Dent. **6**:672, 1956b.

Karies, A.K.: A study of partial denture design and masticatory pressures in a mandibular bilateral distal extension case, J. Prosthet. Dent. **8**:340, 1958.

Kane, B.E.: Buoyant stress equalizer, J. Prosthet. Dent. **14**:698, 1964.

Kane, B.E.: Improved buoyant stress equalizer, J. Prosthet. Dent. **17**:365, 1967.

Kantor, M.E., Silverman, S.I., and Garfinkle, L.: Centric-relation recording techniques: a comparative investigation, J. Prosthet. Dent. **28**:593, 1972.

Kapur, K.K.: The comparison of different methods of recording centric relation, Tufts Univ. Dent. Abstr. **2**:508, 1957.

Katulski, E.M., and Appleyard, W.N.: Biological concepts of the use of the mechanical cast surveyor, J. Prosthet. Dent. **9**:629, 1959.

Kelly, E.: Fatigue failure in denture base polymers, J. Prosthet. Dent. **21**:257, 1969.

Kelly, E.: Changes caused by a mandibular removable partial denture opposing a maxillary complete denture, J. Prosthet. Dent. **27**:140, 1972.

Kelly, E.K.: The physiologic approach to partial denture design, J. Prosthet. Dent. **3**:699, 1953.

Kelly, E.K.: Partial denture design applicable to the maxillofacial patient, J. Prosthet. Dent. **15**:168, 1965.

Kennedy, E.: Partial denture construction, Brooklyn, N.Y., 1928, Dental Items of Interest Publishing Co.

Kessler, B.: An analysis of the tongue factor and its functioning areas in dental prosthesis, J. Prosthet. Dent. **5**:629, 1955.

Killebrew, R.H.: Crown construction for broken down partial denture abutments, J. Prosthet. Dent. **11**:93, 1961.

Kimball, H.D.: The role of periodontia in prosthetic dentistry, J. Prosthet. Dent. **1**:286, 1951.

Klein, I.E., and others: Minimum clinical procedures for satisfactory complete denture, removable partial denture, and fixed partial denture services, J. Prosthet. Dent. **22**:4, 1969.

Knodle, J.M.: Experimental overlay and pin partial denture, J. Prosthet. Dent. **17**:472, 1967.

Knowles, L.E.: The biomechanics of removable partial denture and its relationship to fixed prosthesis, J. Prosthet. Dent. **8**:426, 1958.

Knowles, L.E.: A dowel attachment removable partial denture, J. Prosthet. Dent. **13**:679, 1963.

Koper, A.: An intracoronal semiprecision retainer for removable partial dentures: the Thompson dowel, J. Prosthet. Dent. **30**:759, 1973.

Kornfeld, M.: The problem of function in restorative dentistry, J. Prosthet. Dent. **5**:670, 1955.

Kotowicz, W.E., and others: The combination clasp and the distal extension removable partial denture, Dent. Clin. North Am. **17**:651, 1973.

Kramer, H.M.: Impression technique for removable partial dentures, J. Prosthet. Dent. **11**:84, 1961.

Kratochvil, F.J.: Influence of occlusal rest position and clasp design on movement of abutment teeth, J. Prosthet. Dent. **13**:114, 1963.

Kratochvil, F.J.: Maintaining supporting structures with a removable partial prosthesis, J. Prosthet. Dent. **25**:167, 1971.

Kratochvil, F.J., and Caputo, A.A.: Photoelastic analysis of pressure on teeth and bone supporting removable partial dentures, J. Prosthet. Dent. **32**:52, 1974.

Krikos, A.A.: Artificial undercuts for teeth which have un-favorable shapes for clasping, J. Prosthet. Dent. **22**:301, 1969.

Krikos, A.A.: Preparing guide planes for removable partial dentures, J. Prosthet. Dent. **34**:152, 1975.

Krogh-Poulsen, W.: Partial denture design in relation to occlusal trauma in periodontal breakdown, Int. Dent. J. **4**:847, 1954; also Acad. Rev. **3**:18, 1955.

Krol, A.J.: Clasp design for extension-base removable partial dentures, J. Prosthet. Dent. **29**:408, 1973a.

Krol, A.J.: RPI clasp retainer and its modifications, Dent. Clin. North Am. **17**:631, 1973b.

Kurth, L.E.: Mandibular movement and articulator occlusion, J. Am. Dent. Assoc. **39**:37, 1949.

Kurth, L.E.: Centric relation and mandibular movement, J. Am. Dent. Assoc. **50**:309, 1955.

Lambson, G.O.: Papillary hyperplasia of the palate, J. Prosthet. Dent. **16**:636, 1966.

Lammie, G.A., and Osborne, J.: The bilateral free-end saddle lower denture, J. Prosthet. Dent. **4**:640, 1954.

Landa, J.S.: The troublesome transition from a partial lower to a complete lower denture, J. Prosthet. Dent. **4**:42, 1954.

Landa, J.S.: The prosthodontist views the rehabilitation of the cleft-palate patient, J. Prosthet. Dent. **6**:421, 1956.

Laney, W.R., and Desjardins, R.P.: Comparison of base metal alloys and Type IV gold alloys for removable partial denture framework, Dent. Clin. North Am. **17**:611, 1973.

Lanier, B.R., and others: Making chromium-cobalt removable partial dentures: a modified technique, J. Prosthet. Dent. **25**:197, 1971.

Lauritzen, A.G., and Bodner, G.H.: Variations in location of arbitrary and true hinge axis points, J. Prosthet. Dent. **11**:224, 1961.

Lavelle, W.E., and Zach, G.E.: The tissue bar and Ceka anchor as aids in cleft palate rehabilitation, J. Prosthet. Dent. **30**:321, 1973.

LaVere, A.M.: Denture education for edentulous patients, J. Prosthet. Dent. **16**:1013, 1966.

LaVere, A.M., and Krol, A.J.: Selection of a major connector for the extension base removable partial denture, J. Prosthet. Dent. **30**:102, 1973.

Lazarus, A.H.: Partial denture design, J. Prosthet. Dent. **1**:710, 1951.

Lee, John, H.: Sectional partial metal dentures incorporating an internal locking bolt, J. Prosthet. Dent. **13**:1067, 1963.

Leff, A.: Precision attachment dentures, J. Prosthet. Dent. **2**:84, 1952.

Lefkowitz, W., editor: Proceedings of the Second International Prosthodontic Congress, St. Louis, 1979, The C.V. Mosby Co.

Lenchner, N.H., Handlers, M., Weissman, B. A modification of special retaining device for partial dentures, J. Prosthet. Dent. **8**:973, 1958.

Leupold, R.J.: A comparative study of impression procedures for distal extension removable partial dentures, J. Prosthet. Dent. **16**:708, 1966.

Leupold, R.J., and Kratochvil, F.J.: An altered-cast procedure to improve support for removable partial dentures, J. Prosthet. Dent. **15**:672, 1965.

Levin, B.: Personal communication, 1979.

Levitch, H.C.: Physiologic stress-equalizer, J. Prosthet. Dent. 3:232, 1953.

Lloyd, R.S., Pruzansky, and Subtelny, J.D.: Prosthetic rehabilitation of a cleft palate patient subsequent to multiple surgical and prosthetic failures, J. Prosthet. Dent. 7:216, 1957.

Long, J.H., Jr.: Location of the terminal hinge axis by intraoral means, J. Prosthet. Dent. 23:11, 1970.

Longwell, W.H.: The cleaning of artificial dentures, Br. Dent. J. 99:337, 1955.

Lord, J.L., and Teel, S.: The overdentures: patient selection, use of copings, and follow-up evaluation, J. Prosthet. Dent. 32:41, 1974.

Lott, F., and Levin, B.: Flange technic: an anatomic and physiologic approach to increased retention, function, comfort and appearance of dentures, J. Prosthet. Dent. 16:394, 1966.

Lowe, R.O., and others: Swallowing and resting forces related to lingual flange thickness in removable partial dentures, J. Prosthet. Dent. 23:279, 1970.

Lucia, V.O.: The gnathological concept of articulation, Dent. Clin. North Am., p. 183, March 1962.

Lundeen, H.C.: Centric relation records: the effect of muscle action, J. Prosthet. Dent. 31:244, 1974.

Lundquist, D.O., and Fiebiger, G.E.: Registrations for relating the mandibular cast to the maxillary cast based on Kennedy's classification system, J. Prosthet. Dent. 35:371, 1976.

MacCallum, M., and others: Which cleaner?, Dent. Practit. and Dent. Rec. 19:83, 1968.

MacGregor, A.R., and Farah, J.W.: Stress analysis of mandibular partial dentures with bounded and free-end saddles. J. Dent. 8:27, 1980.

MacGregor, A.R., Miller, T.P.G., and Farah, J.W.: Stress analysis of partial dentures, J. Dent. 6:2 125, 1978.

MacKinnon, K.P.: Indirect retention in partial denture construction, Dent. J. Aust. 27:221, 1955.

Mahalick, J.A., Knap, F.J., and Weiter, E.S.: Occlusal wear in prosthodontics, J. Am. Dent. Assoc. 82:154, 1971.

Mahler, D.B., and Ady, A.B.: The influence of various factors on the effective setting expansion of casting investments, J. Prosthet. Dent. 13:365, 1963.

Maison, W.G.: Instructions to denture patients, J. Prosthet. Dent. 8:825, 1959.

Mann, A.W.: The lower distal extension partial denture using the Hart-Dunn attachment, J. Prosthet. Dent. 8:282, 1958.

Mann, A.W., and Pankey, L.D.: Oral rehabilitation utilizing the Pankey-Mann instrument and a functional bite technique, Dent. Clin. North Am., p. 215, March 1959.

Mann, A.W., and Pankey, L.D.: Oral rehabilitation. I. Use of the P-M instrument in treatment planning and restoring the lower posterior teeth, J. Prosthet. Dent. 10:135, 1960a.

Mann, A.W., and Pankey, L.D.: Oral rehabilitation. II. Reconstruction generated path technique, J. Prosthet. Dent. 10:151, 1960b.

Mann, A.W., and Pankey, L.D.: The P.M. philosophy of occlusal rehabilitation, Dent. Clin. North Am., p. 621, Nov. 1963.

Markov, N.: Cytologic study of the effect of toothbrush physiotherapy on the mucosa of the edentulous ridge, J. Prosthet. Dent. 18:122, 1967.

Marris, F.N.: The precision dowel rest attachment. J. Prosthet. Dent. 5:43, 1955.

Martone, A.L.: The effects of oral prostheses on the production of speech sounds, Ohio State Univ. Dent. Abstr. 2:508, 1957.

Martone, A.L.: The challenge of the partially edentulous mouth, J. Prosthet. Dent. 8:942, 1958.

Martone, A.L., and others: Anatomy of the mouth and related structures, J. Prosthet. Dent.; Part I, 11:1009, 1961; Part II, 12:4, 1962; Part III, 12:206, 1962; Part IV, 12:409, 1962; Part V, 12:629, 1962; Part VI, 12:817, 1962; Part VII, 13:4, 1963; Part VIII, 13:204, 1963.

Massler, M., Geriatric nutrition I: osteoporosis, J. Prosthet. Dent. 42:252, 1979a.

Massler, M., Geriatric nutrition II: dehydration in the elderly, J. Prosthet. Dent. 42:489, 1979b.

Mauk, E.H.: Classification of mutilated dental arches requiring treatment by removable partial dentures, J. Am. Dent. Assoc. 29:2121, 1942.

McCall, J.O.: The periodontal element in prosthodontics, J. Prosthet. Dent. 16:585, 1966.

McCollum, B.B.: The mandibular hinge axis and a method of locating it, J. Prosthet. Dent. 10:428, 1960.

McCracken, W.L.: A comparison of tooth-borne and tooth-tissue—borne removable partial dentures, J. Prosthet. Dent. 3:375, 1953.

McCracken, W.L.: Mouth preparations for partial dentures, J. Prosthet. Dent. 6:39, 1956.

McCracken, W.L.: Functional occlusion in removable partial denture construction, J. Prosthet. Dent. 8:955, 1958a.

McCracken, W.L.: Impression materials in prosthetic dentistry, Dent. Clin. North Am., p. 671, Nov. 1958b.

McCracken, W.L.: Partial denture construction, St. Louis, 1960, The C.V. Mosby Co.

McCracken, W.L.: Differential diagnosis: fixed or removable partial dentures, J. Am. Dent. Assoc. 63:767, 1961.

McCracken, W.L.: Occlusion in partial denture prosthesis, Dent. Clin. North Am., p. 109, March 1962a.

McCracken, W.L.: Survey of partial denture designs by commercial dental laboratories, J. Prosthet. Dent. 12:1089, 1962b.

McCracken, W.L.: A philosophy of partial denture treatment, J. Prosthet. Dent. 13:889, 1963.

McGill, W.J.: Acquiring space for partial dentures, J. Prosthet. Dent. 17:163, 1967.

McKenzie, J.S.: Mutual problems of the periodontist and prosthodontist, J. Prosthet. Dent. 5:37, 1955.

McLean, D.W.: The partial denture as a vehicle for function, J. Am. Dent. Assoc. 23:1272, 1936.

McLeod, N.S.: Improved design for the Thompson dowel semiprecision intracoronal retainer, J. Prosthet. Dent. 40:513, 1978.

McMillen, L.B.: Border movements of the human mandible, J. Prosthet. Dent. 27:524, 1972.

Means, C.R., and Flenniken, I.E.: Gagging: a problem in prosthetic dentistry, J. Prosthet. Dent. 23:614, 1970.

Mehta, J.D., and Joglekar, A.P.: Vertical jaw relations as a factor in partial dentures, J. Prosthet. Dent. 21:618, 1969.

Mensor, M.C.: Classification and selection of attachments, J. Prosthet. Dent. **29**:494, 1973.

Merkeley, H.J.: The labial and buccal accessory muscles of mastication, J. Prosthet. Dent. **4**:327, 1954.

Merkeley, H.J.: Cleft palate prosthesis, J. Prosthet. Dent. **9**:506, 1959a.

Merkeley, H.J.: Mandibular rearmament, I. Anatomic considerations, J. Prosthet. Dent. **9**:559, 1959b.

Messerman, T.: A concept of jaw function with a related clinical application, J. Prosthet. Dent. **13**:130, 1963.

Meyer, F.S.: The generated path technique in reconstruction dentistry, I and II, J. Prosthet. Dent. **9**:354, 432, 1959.

Meyers, H.M., and Krol, A.J.: Effectiveness of sonic-action denture cleaning program, J. Prosthet. Dent. **32**:613, 1974.

Miller, D.A.: Complete dentures supported by natural teeth, J. Prosthet. Dent. **8**:924, 1958.

Miller, E.L.: Systems for classifying partially dentulous arches, J. Prosthet. Dent. **24**:25, 1970.

Miller, E.L.: Planning partial denture construction, Dent. Clin. North Am. **17**:571, 1973.

Miller, E.L.: Critical factors in selecting removable prostheses, J. Prosthet. Dent. **34**:486, 1975.

Miller, E.L., and Grasso, J.E.: Removable partial prosthodontics, ed. 2, Baltimore, 1981, The Williams & Wilkins Co.

Miller, P.A.: Complete dentures supported by natural teeth, J. Prosthet. Dent. **8**:924, 1958.

Miller, S.: Textbook of periodontia, New York, 1950, The Blakiston Co.

Mills, M.: Mouth preparation for the removable partial denture, J. Am. Dent. Assoc. **60**:154, 1960.

Millstein, P.L., Clark, R.E., and Myerson, R.L.: Differential accuracy of silicone-body interocclusal records and associated weight loss due to volatiles, J. Prosthet. Dent. **33**:649, 1975.

Millstein, P.L., and others: Determination of the accuracy of wax interocclusal registrations, J. Prosthet. Dent. **24**:189, 1971.

Miner, J.F.: The nature of a denture base: a key factor in denture sore mouth, J. Prosthet. Dent. **29**:250, 1973.

Mitchell, J.V., and Damele, J.J.: Influence of tray design upon elastic impression materials, J. Prosthet. Dent. **23**:51, 1970.

Moore, A.W.: Ideal versus adequate dental occlusion, J. Am. Dent. Assoc. **55**:51, 1957.

Moore, D.S.: Some fundamentals of partial denture design to conserve the supporting structures, J. Ont. Dent. Assoc. **32**:238, 1955.

Morden, J.F.C., Lammie, G.A., and Osborne, J: Effect of various denture cleaning solutions on chrome-cobalt alloys, Dent. Practit. and Dent. Rec. **6**:504, 1956.

Morris, H.F., and Asgar, K.: Physical properties and microstructure of four new commercial partial denture alloys, J. Prosthet. Dent. **33**:36, 1975.

Morrison, M.L.: Internal precision attachments retainers for partial dentures, J. Am. Dent. Assoc. **64**:209, 1962.

Morrow, R.M.: Tooth-supported complete dentures: an approach to preventive prosthodontics, J. Prosthet. Dent. **21**:513, 1969.

Morrow, R.M., and others: Compatibility of alginate impression materials and dental stones, J. Prosthet. Dent. **25**:556, 1971.

Morse, P.K., and Boucher, L.J.: What a prosthodontist does, J. Prosthet. Dent. **21**:402, 1969.

Morstad, A.T., and Petersen, A.D.: Postinsertion denture problems, J. Prosthet. Dent. **19**:126, 1968.

Moses, C.H.: The significance of some natural laws in the practice of preventive and restorative dentistry, J. Prosthet. Dent. **3**:304, 1953.

Mosteller, J.H.: Use of prednisolone in the elimination of postoperative thermal sensitivity, J. Prosthet. Dent. **12**:1176, 1962.

Moulton, G.H.: The importance of centric occlusion in diagnosis and treatment planning, J. Prosthet. Dent. **10**:921, 1960.

Muenchinger, F.: Evaluation of an electronic denture cleaner, J. Prosthet. Dent. **33**:610, 1975.

Muhler, J.C.: The development and evaluation of an improved denture cleaning and polishing paste, J. Ind. Dent. Assoc. **48**:17, 1969.

Murrell, G.A.: Phonetics, function, and anterior occlusion, J. Prosthet. Dent. **33**:23, 1974.

Myers, G.E., Wepfer, G.G., and Peyton, F.A.: The thiokol rubber base impression materials, J. Prosthet. Dent. **8**:330, 1958.

Myerson, R.L.: The use of porcelain and plastic teeth in opposing complete dentures, J. Prosthet. Dent. **7**:625, 1957.

Nairn, R.I.: The problem of free-end denture bases, J. Prosthet. Dent. **16**:522, 1966.

Nassif, J., and Blumenfeld, W.L.: Joint consultation services by the periodontist and prosthodontist, J. Prosthet. Dent. **29**:55,1973.

Naylor, J.: What the patient should know about complete dentures, J. Prosthet. Dent. **9**:832, 1959.

Naylor, J.G.: Role of the external pterygoid muscles in tempormandibular articulation, J. Prosthet. Dent. **10**:1037, 1960.

Neill, D.J.: The problem of the lower free-end removable partial denture, J. Prosthet. Dent. **8**:623, 1958.

Neill, D.J.: A study of materials and methods employed in cleaning dentures, Br. Dent. J. **124**:107, 1968.

Neufeld, J.O.: Changes in the trabecular pattern of the mandible following the loss of teeth, J. Prosthet. Dent. **8**:685, 1958.

Neurohr, F.: Partial dentures: a system of functional restoration, Philadelphia, 1939, Lea & Febiger.

Nevin, R.B.: Periodontal aspects of partial denture prosthesis, J. Prosthet. Dent. **5**:215, 1955.

Nickolson, R.J., Stark, M.M., and Scott, H.E.: Calculus and stain removal from acrylic resin dentures, J. Prosthet. Dent. **20**:326, 1968.

Nuttall, E.B.: Establishing posterior functional occlusion for fixed partial dentures, J. Am. Dent. Assoc. **66**:341, 1963.

Oddo, V.J., Jr.: The movable-arm clasp for complete passivity in partial denture construction, J. Am. Dent. Assoc. **74**:1009, 1967.

O'Leary, T.J., and others: Tooth mobility in cuspid-protected and group-function occlusion, J. Prosthet. Dent. **27**:21, 1972.

Olinger, N.A.: Cleft palate prosthesis rehabilitation, J. Prosthet. Dent. **2**:117, 1952.

Orban, B.S.: Biologic principles in correction of occlusal disharmonies, J. Prosthet. Dent. **6**:637, 1956.

Osborne, J., and Lammie, G.A.: The bilateral free-end saddle lower denture, J. Prosthet. Dent. **4**:640, 1954.

Osborne, J., and Lammie, G.A.: Partial dentures, ed. 4, Oxford, 1974, Blackwell Scientific Publications.

Overby, G.E.: Esthetic splinting of mobile periodontally involved teeth by vertical pinning, J. Prosthet. Dent. **11**:112, 1961.

Overton, R.G., and Bramblett, R.M.: Prosthodontic services: A study of need and availability in the United States, J. Prosthet. Dent. **27**:329, 1972.

Parker, H.M.: Impact reduction in complete and partial dentures: a pilot study, J. Prosthet. Dent. **16**:227, 1966.

Parmeijer, J.H.N., and others: Intraoral occlusal telemetry: Part IV, Tooth contact during swallowing, J. Prosthet. Dent. **24**:396, 1970.

Patur, B.: The role of occlusion and the periodontium in restorative procedures, J. Prosthet. Dent. **21**:371, 1969.

Payne, A.G.L.: Factors influencing the position of artificial upper anterior teeth, J. Prosthet. Dent. **26**:26, 1971.

Payne, S.H.: Diagnostic factors which influence the choice of posterior occlusion, Dent. Clin. North Am., p. 203, March 1957.

Pendleton, E.C.: Anatomy of the face and mouth from the standpoint of the denture prosthetist, J. Am. Dent. Assoc. **33**:219, 1946.

Pendleton, E.C.: Changes in the denture supporting tissues, J. Am. Dent. Assoc. **42**:1, 1951.

Perel, M.L.: Periodontal consideration of crown contours, J. Prosthet. Dent. **26**:627, 1971.

Perry, C.: Philosophy of partial denture design, J. Prosthet. Dent. **6**:775, 1956.

Perry, C.: Nutrition for senescent denture patients, J. Prosthet. Dent. **11**:73, 1961.

Perry, C.K.: Transfer base for removable partial dentures, J. Prosthet. Dent. **31**:582, 1974.

Peyton, F.A., and Anthony, D.H.: Evaluation of dentures processed by different techniques, J. Prosthet. Dent. **13**:269, 1963.

Peyton, F.A., and Craig, R.G.: Restorative dental materials, ed. 5, St. Louis, 1975, The C.V. Mosby Co.

Pfeiffer, K.A.: Clinical problems in the use of alginate hydrocolloid, Dent. Abstr. **2**:82, 1957.

Phillips, R.N.: A problem of retention in a lower partial denture, J. Prosthet. Dent. **6**:213, 1956.

Phillips, R.W.: Factors influencing the accuracy of reversible hydrocolloid impressions, J. Am. Dent. Assoc. **43**:1, 1951.

Phillips, R.W.: Factors affecting the surface of stone dies poured in hydrocolloid impressions, J. Prosthet. Dent. **2**:390, 1952.

Phillips, R.W.: The physical properties of hydrocolloids and alginates and factors influencing their work qualities and accuracy, Fortn. Rev. Chic. Dent. Soc. **26**:9, 1953.

Phillips, R.W.: Elastic impression materials: a second progress report of a recent conference, J. South. Calif. Dent. Assoc. **26**:150, 1958.

Phillips, R.W.: Physical properties and manipulation of rubber impression materials, J. Am. Dent. Assoc. **59**:454, 1959.

Phillips, R.W.: Skinner's science of dental materials, ed. 7, Philadelphia, 1973, W.B. Saunders Co.

Phillips, R.W., and Leonard, L.J.: A study of enamel abrasion as related to partial denture clasps, J. Prosthet. Dent. **6**:657, 1956.

Phillips, R.W., and Price, R.R.: Some factors which influence the surface of stone dies poured in alginate impressions, J. Prosthet. Dent. **5**:72, 1955.

Pipko, D.J.: Combinations in fixed-removable prostheses, J. Prosthet. Dent. **26**:481, 1971.

Pipko, D.J., and El-Sadek, M.: An in vitro investigation of abrasion and staining of dental resins, J. Dent. Res. **51**:689, 1972.

Plainfield, S.: Communication distortion. The language of patients and practitioners of dentistry, J. Prosthet. Dent. **22**:11, 1969.

Plotnick, I.J.: Internal attachment for fixed removable partial dentures, J. Prosthet. Dent. **8**:85, 1958.

Plotnick, I.J.: Stress regulator for complete and partial dentures, J. Prosthet. Dent. **17**:166, 1967.

Plotnick, I.J., Beresin, V.E., and Simkins, A.B.: The effects of variations in the opposing dentition on changes in the partially edentulous mandible, J. Prosthet. Dent.; Part I, **33**:278, 1975; Part II, **33**:403, 1975; Part III, **33**:529, 1975.

Pokorny, D.K., and Blake, F.P.: Principles of occlusion, Anaheim, Calif., 1980, Denar Corp.

Posselt, U.: Studies in the mobility of the human mandible, Acta Odontol. Scand. [Suppl.] **10**:3, 1952.

Posselt, U.: Movement areas of the mandible, J. Prosthet. Dent. **7**:375, 1957a.

Posselt, U.: Terminal hinge movement of the mandible, J. Prosthet. Dent. **7**:787, 1957b.

Posselt, U., and Franzen, G.: Registration of condyle path inclination by intraoral wax records: variation in three instruments. J. Prosthet. Dent. **10**:441, 1960.

Potter, R.B., Appleby, R.C., and Adams, C.D.: Removable partial denture design: a review and a challenge, J. Prosthet. Dent. **17**:63, 1967.

Pound, E.: The problem of the lower anterior bridge, J. Prosthet. Dent. **5**:543, 1955.

Pound, E.: Applying harmony in selecting and arranging teeth, Dent. Clin. North Am., p. 241, March 1962.

Pound, E.: Cross-arch splinting vs. premature extractions, J. Prosthet. Dent. **16**:1058, 1966.

Preiskel, H.: Precision attachments for free-end saddle prostheses, Br. Dent. J. **127**:462, 1969.

Preiskel, H.: Screw retained telescopic prostheses, Br. Dent. J. **130**:107, 1971.

Prieskel, H.W.: Impression techniques for attachment-retained distal extension removable partial dentures, J. Prosthet. Dent. **25**:620, 1971.

Preiskel, H.W.: Precision attachments in dentistry, ed. 3, St. Louis, 1979, The C.V. Mosby Co.

Prince, I.B.: Conservation of the supportive mechanism, J. Prosthet. Dent. **15**:327, 1965.

Quinlivan, J.T.: Fabrication of a simple ball-socket attachment, J. Prosthet. Dent. **32**:222, 1974.

Quinn, I.: Status of the dental laboratory work authorization, J. Am. Dent. Assoc. **79**:1189, 1969.

Rahn, A.O., and Boucher, L.J.: Maxillofacial prosthetics, Philadelphia, 1970, W.B. Saunders Co.

Ramfjord, S.P.: Dysfunctional temperomandibular joint and muscle pain, J. Prosthet. Dent. **11**:353, 1961.

Ramfjord, S.P., and Ash, M.M., Jr.: Occlusion, ed. 2, Philadelphia, 1971, W.B. Saunders Co.

Ramsey, W.O.: The relation of emotional factors to prosthodontic service, J. Prosthet. Dent. 23:4, 1970.

Rantanen, T., Surila, H.S., and Lehvila, P.: Effect of instruction and motivation on dental knowledge and behavior among wearers of partial dentures, Acta Odont. Scand. 38:1, 1980.

Rapuano, J.A.: Single tray dual-impression technique for distal extenion partial dentures, J. Prosthet. Dent. 24:41, 1970.

Raybin, N.H.: The polished surface of complete dentures, J. Prosthet. Dent. 13:236, 1963.

Reitz, P.V.: Technique for mounting removable partial dentures on an articulator, J. Prosthet. Dent. 22:490, 1969.

Renner, R.P., and others: The role of *C. albicans* in denture stomatitis, Oral Surg. 47:323, 1979.

Renner, R.P. Complete dentures: a guide for patient treatment, New York, 1981, Masson Publishing USA, Inc.

Reynolds, J.M.: Crown construction for abutments of existing removable partial dentures, J. Am. Dent. Assoc. 69:423, 1964.

Reynolds, J.M.: Occlusal wear facets, J. Prosthet. Dent. 24:367, 1970.

Rieder, C.E.: Occlusal considerations in preventive care, J. Prosthet. Dent. 28:462, 1972.

Roberts, B.W.: The recall system: a necessary part of a partial denture service, Br. Dent. J.149:46, 1980.

Robinson, M.J.: Centric position, J. Prosthet. Dent. 1:384, 1951.

Roche, A.F.: Functional anatomy of the muscles of mastication, J. Prosthet. Dent. 13:548, 1963.

Roraff, A.R.: Instant photographs for developing esthetics, J. Prosthet. Dent. 26:21, 1971.

Rosenstiel, E.: Rubber base elastic impression materials, Dent. Abstr. 1:55. 1956.

Rothman, R.: Phonetic considerations in denture prosthesis, J. Prosthet. Dent. 11:214, 1961.

Rudd, K.D., and Dunn, B.W.: Accurate removable partial dentures, J. Prosthet. Dent. 18:559, 1967.

Rudd, K.D., Morrow, R.M. and Bange, A.A.: Accurate casts, J. Prosthet. Dent. 21:545, 1969.

Rudd, K.D., Morrow, R.M., and Strunk, R.R.: Accurate alginate impressions, J. Prosthet. Dent. 22:294, 1969.

Rudd, K.D., and O'Leary, T.J.: Stabilizing periodontally weakened teeth by using guide plane removable partial dentures: a preliminary report, J. Prosthet. Dent. 16:721, 1966.

Rudd, K.D., and others: Comparison of effects of tap water and slurry water on gypsum casts, J. Prosthet. Dent. 24:563, 1970.

Rushford, C.B.: A technique for precision removable partial denture construction, J. Prosthet. Dent. 31:377, 1974.

Russotto, S.B.: The role of *Candida albicans* in the pathogenesis of angular cheilosis, J. Prosthet. Dent. 44:243, 1980.

Rybeck, S.A., Jr.: Simplicity in a distal extension partial denture, J. Prosthet. Dent. 4:87, 1954.

Ryge, G., Kozak, S.F., and Fairhurst, C.W.: Porosities in dental gold castings, J. Am. Dent. Assoc. 54:746, 1957.

Saizar, P.: Centric relation and condylar movement, J. Prosthet. Dent. 26:581, 1971.

Saunders, T.R., Gillis, R.E., Jr., and Desjardins, R.P.: The maxillary complete denture opposing the mandibular bilateral distal extension partial denture: treatment considerations, J. Prosthet. Dent. 41:124, 1979.

Sauser, C.W.: Pretreatment evaluation of partially edentulous arches, J. Prosthet. Dent. 11:886, 1961.

Savage, R.D., and MacGregor, A.R.: Behavior therapy in prosthodontics, J. Prosthet. Dent. 24:126, 1970.

Scaife, R.R., Jr., and Holt, J.E.: Natural occurrence of cuspid guidance, J. Prosthet. Dent. 22:225, 1969.

Schabel, R.W.: Dentist-patient communication: a major factor in treatment prognosis, J. Prosthet. Dent. 21:3, 1969.

Schabel, R.W.: The psychology of aging, J. Prosthet. Dent. 27:569, 1972.

Schireson, S.: Grinding teeth for masticatory efficiency and gingival health, J. Prosthet. Dent. 13:337, 1963.

Schmidt, A.H.: Planning and designating removable partial dentures, J. Prosthet. Dent. 3:783, 1953.

Schmidt, A.H.: Repairing chrome-cobalt castings, J. Prosthet. Dent. 5:385, 1955.

Schole, M.L.: Management of the gagging patient, J. Prosthet. Dent. 9:578, 1959.

Schopper, A.F.: Removable appliances for the preservation of the teeth, J. Prosthet. Dent. 4:634, 1954.

Schopper, A.F.: Loss of vertical dimension: causes and effects—diagnosis and various recommended treatments, J. Prosthet. Dent. 9:428, 1959.

Schorr, L., and Clayman, L.H.: Reshaping abutment teeth for reception of partial denture clasps, J. Prosthet. Dent. 4:625, 1954.

Schuyler, A.F.: Planning the removable partial denture to restore function and maintain oral health, N.Y. Dent. J. 13:4, 1947.

Schuyler, C.H.: Fundamental principles in the correction of occlusal disharmony: natural and artificial (grinding), J. Am. Dent. Assoc. 22:1193, 1935.

Schuyler, C.H.: The partial denture and a means of stabilizing abutment teeth, J. Am. Dent. Assoc. 28:1121, 1941.

Schuyler, C.H.: Correction of occlusal disharmony of the natural dentition, N.Y. Dent. J. 13:445, 1947.

Schuyler, C.H.: Factors of occlusion applicable to restorative dentistry, J. Prosthet. Dent. 3:772, 1953.

Schuyler, C.H.: An evaluation of incisal guidance and its influence on restorative dentistry, J. Prosthet. Dent. 9:374, 1959.

Schuyler, C.H.: Factors contributing to traumatic occlusion, J. Prosthet. Dent. 11:708, 1961.

Schuyler, C.H.: Stress distribution as the prime requisite to the success of a partial denture, J. Am. Dent. Assoc. 20:2148, 1963.

Schwalm, C.A., Smith, D.E., and Erickson, J.D.: A clinical study of patients 1 to 2 years after placement of removable partial dentures, J. Prosthet. dent. 38:380, 1977.

Schwartz, W.D., and Barsby, M.J.: Design of partial dentures in dental practice, J. Dent. 6:166, 1978.

Schwartz, W.D., and Barsby, M.J.: A survey of the practice of partial denture prosthetics in the United Kingdom, J. Dent. 8:95, 1980.

Schweitzer, J.M.: Open bite from the prosthetic point of view, Dent. Clin. North Am., p. 269, March 1957.

Schweitzer, J.M.: Masticatory function in man, J. Prosthet. Dent. **11**:625, 1961.

Schweitzer, J.M.: Oral rehabilitation problem cases, 2 vols., St. Louis, 1964, The C.V. Mosby Co.

Scott, D.C.: Suggested designs for metal partial dentures, Dent. Tech. **2**:21, 1954.

Sears, V.H.: Occlusion: the common meeting ground in dentistry, J. Prosthet. Dent. **2**:15, 1952.

Sears, V.H.: Occlusal pivots, J. Prosthet. Dent. **6**:332, 1956.

Sears V.H.: Centric and eccentric occlusions, J. Prosthet. Dent. **10**:1029, 1960.

Sears, V.H.: Mandibular equilibration, J. Am. Dent. Assoc. **65**:45, 1962.

Seiden, A.: Occlusal rests and rest seats, J. Prosthet. Dent **8**:431, 1958.

Sekine, H., and others: Dynamic investigation of the lingual bar (5th report), Bull. Tokyo Dent. Coll. **6**:126, 1965.

Sexson, J.C., and Phillips, R.W.: Studies on the effects of abrasives on acrylic resins, J. Prosthet. Dent. **1**:454, 1951.

Shafagh, I., Yoder, J.L., and Thayer, K.E.: Diurnal variance of centric relation position, J. Prosthet. Dent. **34**:574, 1975.

Shanahan, T.E.J., and Leff, A.: Interocclusal records, J. Prosthet. Dent. **10**:842, 1960.

Shannon, I.L., Terry, J.M., and Nakamoto, R.Y.: Palatal coverage and parotid flow rate, J. Prosth. Dent. **24**:601, 1970.

Sharry, J.J., editor: Complete denture prosthodontics, ed. 3, New York, 1974, McGraw-Hill Book Co.

Sheppard, I.M., and Sheppard, S.M.: Denture occlusion, J. Prosthet. Dent. **20**:307, 1968.

Shohet, H.: Relative magnitudes of stress on abutment teeth with different retainers, J. Prosthet. Dent. **21**:267, 1969.

Shore, N.A.: Educational program for patients with temporomandibular joint dysfunction (ligaments), J. Prosthet. Dent. **23**:691, 1970.

Sicher. H., and DuBrul, E.L.: Oral anatomy, ed. 5, St. Louis, 1970, The C.V. Mosby Co.

Silver, M.: Impressions and silver-plated dies from a rubber impression material, J. Prosthet. Dent **6**:543, 1956.

Silverman, M.M.: Determination of vertical dimension by phonetics, J. Prosthet. Dent. **6**:465, 1956; Dent. Abstr. **2**:221, 1957.

Silverman, S.I.: Denture prosthesis and the functional anatomy of the maxillofacial structures, J. Prosthet. Dent. **6**:305, 1956.

Silverman, S.I.: The psychologic considerations in denture prosthesis, J. Prosth. Dent. **8**:582, 1958.

Simmons, J.J., Swing-lock clinical manual, Dallas, 1968, Idea Development Co.

Simpson, D.H.: Considerations for abutments, J. Prosthet. Dent. **5**:375, 1955.

Singer, F.: Functional impressions and accurate interocclusal records for removable partial dentures, J. Prosthet. Dent. **12**:536, 1962.

Singer, F.: Improvements in precision attached removable partial dentures, J. Prosthet. Dent. **17**:69, 1967.

Skinner, C.N.: A classification of removable partial dentures based upon the principles of anatomy and physiology, J. Prosthet. Dent. **9**:240, 1959.

Skinner, E.W., and Hobbit, N.E.: A study of the accuracy of hydrocolloid impressions, J. Prosthet. Dent. **6**:80, 1956.

Smedley, V.C.: Discussion: partial denture planning with special reference to stress distribution, J. Prosthet. Dent. **1**:725, 1951.

Smith, B.H.: Changes in occlusal face height with removable partial dentures, J. Prosthet. Dent. **34**:278, 1975.

Smith, D.C.: The cleaning of dentures, Dent. Practit. and Dent. Rec. **17**:39, 1966.

Smith, F.W., and Applegate, O.C.: Roentgenographic study of bone changes during exercise stimulation of edentulous areas, J. Prosthet. Dent. **11**:1086, 1961.

Smith, G.P.: Objectives of a fixed partial dentures, J. Prosthet. Dent. **11**:463, 1961.

Smith, G.P.: The responsibility of the dentist toward laboratory procedures in fixed and removable partial denture prosthesis, J. Prosthet. Dent. **13**:295, 1963.

Smith, J.P.: Care of dentures, Dent. Practit. and Dent. Rec. **6**:121, 1955.

Smith, P.K.: The effect on the accuracy of polysulphide impression material after treating preparations with various agents, Aust. Dent. J. **16**:337, 1971.

Smith, R.A., and Rymarz, F.P.: Cast clasp transitional removable partial dentures, J. Prosthet. Dent. **22**:381, 1969.

Smith, R.A.: Secondary palatal impressions for major connector adaptation, J. Prosthet. Dent. **24**:108, 1970.

Smith, R.A.: Clasp repair for removable partial dentures, J. Prosthet. Dent. **29**:231, 1973.

Smutko, G.E. In Winkler, S.W.: Essentials of complete denture prosthodontics, Philadelphia, 1979, W.B. Saunders Co.

Smyd, E.S.: Bio-mechanics of prosthetic dentistry, J. Prosthet. Dent. **4**:368, 1954.

Smyd, E.S.: The role of tongue, torsion, and bending in prosthodontic failures, J. Prosthet. Dent. **11**:95, 1961.

Solle, W.: An improved dental surveyor, J. Am. Dent. Assoc. **60**:727, 1960.

Sostenbo, H.R.: C.E. Luce's recordings of mandibular movement, J. Prosthet. Dent. **11**:1068, 1961.

Staffanou, R.S., and Thayer, K.E.: Reverse pin-porcelain veneer and pontic technique, J. Prosthet. Dent. **12**:1138, 1962.

Stafford, G.D., and MacCulloch, W.T.: Radiopaque denture base materials, Br. Dent. J. **131**:22, 1971.

Stansbury, B.E.: A retentive attachment for overdentures, J. Prosthet. Dent. **35**:228, 1976.

Starcke, E.N., Jr.: A historical review of complete dentures impression materials, J. Am. Dent. Assoc. **91**:1037, 1975.

Starshak, T.J., and Sanders, B.: Preprosthetic oral and maxillofacial surgery, St. Louis, 1980, The C.V. Mosby Co.

Steffel, V.L.: Simplified clasp partial dentures designed for maximum function, J. Am. Dent. Assoc. **32**:1093, 1945.

Steffel, V.L.: Fundamental principles involved in partial denture designs: with special reference to equalization of tooth and tissue support, Aust. J. Dent. **54**:328, 1950; Dent. J. Aust. **23**:68, 1951.

Steffel, V.L.: Relining removable partial dentures for fit and function, J. Prosthet. Dent. **4**:496, 1954.

Steffel, V.L.: Planning removable partial dentures, J. Prosthet. Dent. **12**:524, 1962.

Steffel, V.L.: Current concepts in removable partial denture service, J. Prosthet. Dent. **20**:387, 1968.

Steiger, A.A., and Boitel, R.H.: Precision work for partial dentures, Zurich, 1959, Buchdruckerei Berichthaus.

Steinberg, G.J.: The telescopic type of fixed partial denture abutment, J. Prosthet. Dent. **9**:863, 1959.

Stern, W.J.: Guiding planes in clasp reciprocation and retention, J. Prosthet. Dent. **34**:408, 1975.

Sternlicht, H.C.: Prosthetic treatment planning for the periodontal patient, Dent. Abstr. **2**:81, 1957.

Stipho, H.D.K., Murphy, W.M., and Adams, D.: Effect of oral prosthesis on plaque accumulation, Br. Dent. J. **145**:47, 1978.

Stratemann, M.W., and Shannon, I.L.: Control of decalcification in orthodontic patients by daily self-administered application of a water-free 0.4 percent stannous fluoride gel, Am. J. Orthod. **66**:273, 1974.

Strauss, R., and others: Behavioral factors and denture status, J. Prosthet. Dent. **37**:264, 1977.

Strohaver, R.A., and Trovillion, H.M.: Removable partial overdentures, J. Prosthet. Dent. **35**:624, 1976.

Stuart, C.E.: Accuracy in measuring functional dimensions and relations in oral prosthesis, J. Prosthet. Dent. **9**:220, 1959.

Sunoo, Y.G.: Fatique properties and corrosion resistance of some chromium-cobalt alloys used in partial dentures, J. Korea Res. Soc. Dent. Mater. **4**:4, 1969.

Swartz, M.L., and Phillips, R.W.: Cleaning, polishing and abrasion techniques (in vitro) Ann. N.Y. Acad. Sci. **153**:120, 1968.

Sweeney, W.T., and others: Proposed specification for plastic teeth, J. Prosthet. Dent. **7**:420, 1957.

Sykora, O., and Calikkocaoglu, S.: Maxillary removable partial denture designs by commercial dental laboratories, J. Prosthet. Dent. **22**:633, 1970.

Talkov, L.: Lining up multiple abutments, J. Prosthet. Dent. **1**:727, 1951.

Talkov, L.: Survey of complete periodontal prosthesis, J. Prosthet. Dent. **11**:124, 1961.

Tallgren, A.: Alveolar bone loss in denture wearers as related to facial morphology, Acta Odontol. Scand. **28**:251, 1970.

Tallgren, A.: The continuing reduction of the residual alveolar ridge in complete denture wearers: a longitudinal study covering 25 years, J. Prosthet. Dent. **27**:120, 1972.

Tallgren, A., and others: Roentgen cephalometric analysis of ridge resorption and changes in jaw and occlusal relationships in immediate complete denture wearers, J. Oral Rehabil. **7**:77, 1980.

Tautin, F.S.: Should dentures be worn continuously?, J. Prosthet. Dent. **39**:372, 1978.

Teppo. K.W., and Smith, F.W.: A method of immediate clasp repair, J. Prosthet. Dent. **30**:77, 1975.

Terkla, L.G., and Laney, W.R.: Partial dentures, ed. 3, St. Louis, 1963, The C.V. Mosby Co.

Terrell, W.H.: Split bar technic applicable to both precision attachment and clasp cases, J. South. Calif. Dent. Assoc. **9**:10, 1942.

Teteruck, W.R., and Lundeen, H.C.: The accuracy of an ear face-bow, J. Prosthet. Dent. **16**:1039, 1966.

Theilade, J.: Om rengoring af proteser, Tandlaegebladet **62**:41, 1958.

Theilade, J., and Budtz-Jorgensen, E.: Electron microscopic study of denture plaque, J. Dent. Res. **56**:554, 1977 (Abst).

Tillman, E.J.: Molding and staining acrylic resin anterior teeth, J. Prosthet. Dent. **5**:497, 1955; Dent. Abstr. **1**:111, 1956.

Tillman, E.J.: Removable partial denture upper and complete lower denture, J. Prosthet. Dent. **11**:1098, 1961.

Tomlin, H.R., and Osborne, J.: Cobalt-chromium partial dentures: a clinical survey, Br. Dent. J. **110**:307, 1961.

Trainor, J.E., and Elliott, R.W., Jr.: Removable partial dentures designed by dentists before and after graduate level instruction: a comparative study, J. Prosthet. Dent. **27**:509, 1972.

Trapozzano, V.R., and Winter, G.R.: Periodontal aspects of partial denture design, J. Prosthet. Dent. **2**:101, 1952.

Tryde, G., and Brantenberg, F.: Den sublinguale barre, Tandlaegebladet **69**:873, 1965.

Tsao, D.H.: Designing occlusal rests using mathematical principles, J. Prosthet. Dent. **23**:154, 1970

Tuccillo, J.J., and Nielsen, J.P.: Compatibility of alginate impression materials and dental stones, J. Prosthet. Dent. **25**:556, 1971.

Turck, D.A.: A histologic comparison of the edentulous denture and non-denture bearing tissues, J. Prosth. Dent. **15**:419, 1965.

Turrell, A.J.: Clinical assessment of vertical dimension, J. Prosthet. Dent. **28**:238, 1972.

Tylman, S.D.: Theory and practice of crown and fixed partial prosthodontics (bridge), ed. 6, St. Louis, 1970, The C.V. Mosby Co.

Ulrich, J.: The human temporomandibular joint: kinematics and actions of the masticatory muscles, J. Prosthet. Dent. **9**:399, 1959.

United States Air Force: Dental laboratory technicians manual, Air Force Manual 160-27, Washington, D.C., 1959, U.S. Government Printing Office.

Vasic, S., and others: An aesthetic clasp for acrylic partial dentures, J. Can. Dent. Assoc. **37**:38, 1971.

Vig, R.G.: Splinting bars and maxillary indirect retainers for removable partial dentures, J. Prosthet. Dent. **13**:125, 1963.

Waerhaug, J.: Justification for splinting in periodontal therapy, J. Prosthet. Dent. **22**: 201, 1969.

Wagman, S.S.: Tissue management for full cast veneer crowns, J. Prosthet. Dent. **15**:106, 1965.

Wagner, A.G.: Instructions for the use and care of removable partial dentures, J. Prosthet. Dent. **26**:481, 1971.

Wagner, A.G.: A technique to record jaw relations for distally edentulous dental arches, J. Prosthet. Dent. **29**:405, 1973.

Wagner, A.G., and Forque, E.C.: A study of four methods of recording the path of insertion of removable partial dentures, J. Prosthet. Dent. **35**:267, 1976.

Wagner, A.W., Burkhart, J.W., and Fayle, H.E., Jr.: Contouring abutment teeth with cast gold inlays for removable partial dentures, J. Prosthet. Dent. **201**:330, 1968.

Waldron, C.A.: Oral leukoplakia, carcinoma, and the prosthodontist, J. Prosthet. Dent. **15**:367, 1965.

Wallace, D.H.: The use of gold occlusal surfaces in complete and partial dentures, J. Prosthet. Dent. **14**:327, 1964.

Waller, N.I.: The root rest and the removable partial denture, J. Prosthet. Dent. **33**:16, 1975.

Walter, J.D.: Anchor attachments used as locking devices in two-part removable prostheses, J. Prosthet. Dent. **33**:628, 1975.

Waltz, M.E.: Ceka extracoronal attachments, J. Prosthet. Dent. **29**:167, 1973.

Ward, H.L., and Weinberg, L.A.: An evaluation of periodontal splinting, J. Am. Dent. Assoc. **63**:48, 1961.

Warr, J.A.: Numerical system of clasp design, J. Prosthet. Dent. **11**:1105, 1961.

Weinberg, L.A.: Lateral force in relation to the denture base and clasp design, J. Prosthet. Dent. **6**:785, 1956.

Weinberg, L.A.: An evaluation of the face-bow mounting, J. Prosthet. Dent. **11**:32, 1961.

Weinberg, L.A.: Atlas of removable partial denture prosthodontics, St. Louis, 1969, The C.V. Mosby Co.

Weinberg, L.A.: An evaluation of occlusal factors in TMJ dysfunction-pain syndrome, J. Prosthet. Dent. **41**:198, 1979.

Wheeler, R.C.: Complete crown form and the periodontium, J. Prosthet. Dent. **11**:722, 1961.

Wical, K.E., and others: Studies of residual ridge resorption. Part I. Use of panoramic radiography for evaluation and classification of mandibular resorption, J. Prosthet. Dent. **32**:7, 1974a.

Wical, K.E., and others: Studies of residual ridge resorption. Part II. The relationship of dietary calcium and phosphorus to residual ridge resorption, J. Prosthet. Dent. **32**:13, 1974b.

Wictorin, L.: Effect of toothbrushing on acrylic resin veneering material. II. Abrasive effect of selected dentifrices and toothbrushes, Acta Odontol. Scand. **30**:383, 1972.

Wictorin, L., Hedegard, B., and Lundberg, M.: Cineradiographic studies of bolus position during chewing, J. Prosthet. Dent. **26**:236, 1971.

Williams, A.G.: Technique for provisional splint with attachment, J. Prosthet. Dent. **21**:555, 1969.

Wilson, J.H.: Partial dentures: rebasing the saddle supported by the mucosa and alveolar bone, Dent. J. Aust. **24**:185, 1952.

Wilson, J.H.: Partial dentures: relining the saddle supported by the mucosa and alveolar bone, J. Prosthet. Dent. **3**:807, 1953.

Wilson, J.H.: Some clinical and technical aspects of partial dentures, Dent. J. Aust. **26**:176, 1954.

Wilson J.H.: The use of partial dentures in the restoration of occlusal standards, Aust. Dent. J. **1**:93, 1956.

Winkler, S.: Essentials of complete denture prosthodontics, Philadelphia, 1979, W.B. Saunders Co.

Wolfson, E.: Staining and characterization of acrylic teeth, Dent. Abstr. **1**:41, 1956.

Yalisove, I.L.: Crown and sleeve-coping retainers for removable partial prostheses, J. Prosthet. Dent. **16**:1069, 1966.

Young, H.A.: Factors contributory to success in prosthodontic practice, J. Prosthet. Dent. **5**:354, 1955.

Young, J.M.: Surface characteristics of dental stone: impression orientation, J. Prosthet. Dent. **33**:336 1965.

Young, J.M.: The prosthodontist's role in total treatment of patients, J. Prosthet. Dent. **27**:399, 1972.

Yurkstas, A., Fridley, H.H., and Manly, R.S.: A functional evaluation of fixed and removable bridgeworks, J. Prosthet. Dent. **1**:570, 1951.

Zach, G.A.: Advantages of mesial rests for removable partial dentures, J. Prosthet. Dent. **33**:32, 1975.

Zarb, G.A., and MacKay, H.F.: The partially edentulous patient: the biologic price of prosthodontic intervention, Aust. Dent. J. **25**:63, 1980.

Zarb, G.A., and MacKay, H.F.: Cosmetics and removable partial dentures: the Class IV partially edentulous patient, J. Prosthet. Dent. **46**:360, 1981.

Zarb, G.A., and others: Prosthodontic treatment for partially edentulous patients, St. Louis, 1978, The C.V. Mosby Co.

Zerosi, C.: A new type of removable splint: its indications and function, Dent. Abstr. **1**:451, 1956.

Zinner, I.D.: Semiprecision rest system for distal-extension removable partial dentures, J. Prosthet. Dent. **42**:4, 1979.

Zoeller, G.N.: Block form stability in removable partial dentures, J. Prosthet. Dent. **22**:633, 1969.

Zoeller, G.N., and Kelly, W.J., Jr.: Block form stability in removable partial prosthodontics, J. Prosthet. Dent. **25**:515, 1971.

Index

A

Abscesses, 106
Abutment teeth
  angle of cervical convergence of, 57
  axial loading of, 174
  cast restorations for, 156-159
    intracoronal direct retainers in, 56
    ledges in, crown, 159
    tooth preparation for, 159
  crown preparations on, 120
  effect of bruxing on, 2
  effect of direct retainer on, 36, 55
  effect of minor connector on, 36
  encirclement of, by clasp arms, 23, 59
  evaluation of, on mounted diagnostic casts, 108
  evaluation of, for relining procedures, 288-289
  fitting of framework to, 170, 171
  gingiva of, 93
  height of contour, 57
    survey of, 83, 84
  ideal placement of rests on, 36
  impressions of, 162
  increased plaque on, 252-253
  infrabulge area of, 57
  long axis of, occlusal load directed along, 36
  loss of, repair of prosthesis with, 310-314
  marginal ridge of, in rest preparation, 146
  methods of reducing stress to, 34
  mobility of, decreasing, 34
  overdenture, 133
  position of clasp components by, 59-60
  position of rest on, 60
  position of retentive clasp arm on, 57
  preservation of, 174
  recontouring of, in clasp design, 60, 62, 108
  recontouring of, in establishing path of placement, 83
  restoration of, under clasp assembly, 311-314
  retentive areas of
    location of, 60-62, 64
    measuring depth of, 86
    for use of bar clasps, 72
  selection of, for removable partial denture, 118
    vs fixed partial denture, 6
  stresses on, 5
  survey of, 60-61
  surveyed crown of, 156-159
  torquing forces on, 56
  transferance of forces to
    by bracing clasp arm, 56-57
    by minor connector, 56-57
    by rest, 56
  trauma to, and periodontium, 275
  undercut area of
    for cast circumferential clasp, 24, 65
    for circumferential C clasp, 67

Abutment teeth—cont'd
  undercut area of—cont'd
    for I-bar clasp, 75
    for ring clasp, 65
    for RPI-bar clasp, 75
    in selection of clasp arm metals, 8-9
    in selection of clasp assembly design, 60
    survey of, 83-84
    for T-bar clasp, 26
Acid denture cleaners, 261
Acrylic resin
  autopolymerizing
    in repair of acrylic resin denture teeth, 307
    in repair of broken clasp arm, 309
    in repair of denture base, 304
    in repair of porcelain denture teeth, 306
  for complete palate major connector, 17, 49
    with cast metal, 49
  for construction of record bases, 223
  for custom tray fabrication, 161
  denture bases of, 80
    advantages of, 80
    in combination with cast metal, 31
    processing of, problems from, 269
    retention of
      with mesh type minor connector, 54
      with metal base minor connector, 54
      with open latticework type minor connector, 52
  denture teeth of, 3, 235
    anatomic considerations of, 237
    fractured, 266
      repair of, 306-308
    removal of, from dentures, 296
  dimensional change of, 256
  in fabrication of jig for centric relation positioning, 219
  in fabrication of record bases, 221
  nodules of, on tissue surface of prosthesis, 265
  polymerization of, 248
  porosity in, 266
  in relining procedures, 300
  in replacement of denture teeth, 311
  for retention of denture teeth to framework, 3
  toothbrushing, 259
  for trays in altered cast impression technique, 176, 177, 178, 179, 186, 187, 188, 189
Adhesive for impression trays, 162, 163, 164
Adjustment
  occlusal
    of opposing removable partial dentures, 278
    after processing removable partial denture, 248-249
    after relining prosthesis, 292
    prior to restorative and prosthetic treatment, 130
    in sequence of mouth preparations, 137
    of single removable partial denture, 278
  postinsertion, 279-285